MAR - 5 2018

3 1994 01564 0425

SANTA

P9-EJI-347

Praise for *The Harvard Medical School Guide to Yoga*

"*The Harvard Medical School Guide to Yoga* is a wonderful addition to the yoga library that helps bridge the gap between East and West. The yoga world has to clean up its act in order to find its deserved place in the world of medicine, and this manual is a necessary step. The practices and research are sound."

—RODNEY YEE, internationally renowned yoga instructor

"Every so often a manual emerges from the sea of 'how-to' yoga books and startles by virtue of its eminent accessibility, its breathtaking comprehensiveness, its scientific underpinnings, its remarkable clarity, and its immediate applicability. Dr. Marlynn Wei and Dr. James Groves's *The Harvard Medical School Guide to Yoga* is just such a manual. Inspired and inspirational, this book includes a treasure trove of easy-to-follow illustrations of numerous yoga poses; it will be an invaluable resource for all students of yoga interested not only in toning their body and reducing their stress but also, more generally, in evolving their health to ever-higher levels of mental, physical, and spiritual well-being."

—MARTHA STARK, MD, author of *Relentless Hope: Refusal to Grieve*
and six other award-winning integrative psychiatry books

"Wei and Groves are reaching out to you, inspiring, coaxing, and above all informing about the path you can take for health and wellness of your inseparable body, mind, and soul. The lessons contained herein are encyclopedic in scope, but the message is of a journey that lies ahead for you, within you, accessible and transformative. Whether needed to enhance well-being and facilitate recovery for those who suffer or are ill or to just make this one life at once more peaceful, reflective, calm, and energetic, *The Harvard Medical School Guide to Yoga* can be your itinerary."

—JERROLD F. ROSENBAUM, MD, chief of psychiatry, Massachusetts General
Hospital; Stanley Cobb Professor of Psychiatry, Harvard Medical School

"Marlynn Wei and James Groves have done the public a great service. They are physicians who've learned by acquaintance how yoga can be a powerful aid to health. Consequently they have produced a thorough and very accessible guide replete with tables and summaries and simple drawings, which leaves the reader with an excellent grasp of this particular pathway to wellness."

—GREGORY L. FRICCHIONE, MD, director, Benson Henry Institute for Mind Body Medicine at Harvard Medical School

"It is amazing to me that yoga has become popular enough that professors at Harvard Medical School would publish a book on the subject. Giving people more information and helping them find their way is what I see as being the great purpose of a book on the subject of yoga. Blessings to Marlynn Wei and James E. Groves for helping make this Divine Knowledge available to you, and may all achieve success in yoga."

—SRI DHARMA MITTRA, creator of the *Master Yoga Chart of 908 Postures*

THE HARVARD MEDICAL SCHOOL

GUIDE *to* YOGA

8 Weeks to Strength, Awareness, and Flexibility

BY MARLYNN WEI, MD, JD
AND JAMES E. GROVES, MD

613.7046 GRO
Groves, James E.
The Harvard Medical School
    guide to yoga

$19.99
31994015640425

CENTRAL

Da Capo
LIFE
LONG

Many of the designations used by manufacturers and sellers to distinguish their products are claimed as trademarks. Where those designations appear in this book and Da Capo Press was aware of a trademark claim, the designations have been printed in initial capital letters.

Copyright © 2017 by Harvard University

Illustrations, Figures, and Tables: Marlynn Wei, MD, JD

All rights reserved. No part of this publication may be reproduced, stored in a retrieval system, or transmitted, in any form or by any means, electronic, mechanical, photocopying, recording, or otherwise, without the prior written permission of the publisher. Printed in the United States of America. For information, address Da Capo Press, 53 State Street, 9th floor, Boston, MA 02109.

Designed by Jeff Williams
Set in 11.25 point Fairfield by the Perseus Books Group

Library of Congress Cataloging-in-Publication Data

Names: Groves, James E., author. | Wei, Marlynn, author.
Title: The Harvard Medical School guide to yoga : eight weeks to strength,
    awareness, and flexibility / by Marlynn Wei, MD, JD and James Groves MD.
Description: First Da Capo Press edition. | Boston, MA : Da Capo Lifelong
    Books, a member of the Perseus Books Group, 2017.
Identifiers: LCCN 2016057402 | ISBN 9780738219363 (paperback) | ISBN
    9780738219370 (ebook)
Subjects: LCSH: Hatha yoga—Popular works. | Self-care, Health—Popular
    works. | BISAC: HEALTH & FITNESS / Yoga. | BODY, MIND & SPIRIT /
    Meditation.
Classification: LCC RA781.7 .G77 2017 | DDC 613.7/046—dc23 LC record available at https://
lccn.loc.gov/2016057402

Published by Da Capo Press, an imprint of Perseus Books, LLC, a subsidiary of Hachette Book Group, Inc.
www.dacapopress.com

Note: The information in this book is true and complete to the best of our knowledge. This book is intended only as an informative guide for those wishing to know more about health issues. In no way is this book intended to replace, countermand, or conflict with the advice given to you by your own physician. The ultimate decision concerning care should be made between you and your doctor. We strongly recommend you follow his or her advice. Information in this book is general and is offered with no guarantees on the part of the authors or Da Capo Press. The authors and publisher disclaim all liability in connection with the use of this book.

Da Capo Press books are available at special discounts for bulk purchases in the U.S. by corporations, institutions, and other organizations. For more information, please contact the Special Markets Department at the Perseus Books Group, 2300 Chestnut Street, Suite 200, Philadelphia, PA, 19103, or call (800) 810-4145, ext. 5000, or e-mail special.markets@perseusbooks.com.

LSC-C

10 9 8 7 6 5 4 3 2 1

To our wise and compassionate teachers,

To you, the reader, and

To the teacher who lives within each of us.

Contents

Disclaimer

While the authors of this book have taken great care in presenting the material you will find in this book, the book is not intended as a substitute for professional medical advice. The medical information is provided as an information resource only and is not to be used or relied on for any diagnostic or treatment purposes. This information is not intended to be patient education, does not create any patient-physician relationship, and should not be used as a substitute for professional diagnosis and treatment. If you have any health concerns or conditions that warrant special attention, please seek the advice of a health professional before beginning a yoga practice or attempting any of the practices or poses described in this book. If you experience pain or other side effects when trying the poses presented here, please seek appropriate medical attention.

Cautions on Rapid or Forceful Yoga Breathing

For beginners, rapid and forceful breathing exercises, such as the Breath of Fire (see page 98), should be done only with the guidance and supervision of a certified yoga teacher. Rigorous, forceful breathing should also be avoided during pregnancy. People with medical conditions, such as high blood pressure, such respiratory issues as asthma, seizure disorders, panic or anxiety disorders, or bipolar disorder should check with their doctor first before doing such yoga breathing because it can lead to high blood pressure and hyperventilation, which can then trigger such medical issues as seizures, panic attacks, or asthma episodes.

It's important to remember that yoga breathing exercises should never be painful. If you experience sudden pain or difficulty breathing during or after intense yoga breathing, you should stop immediately and seek medical attention. The risk of yoga breathing is unclear since it is not yet studied on a large scale, so it's important to discuss it with your own doctor before trying these techniques.

Cautions on Hot Yoga

Hot yoga is a version of yoga done in a heated and humidified room. Since over-heating can occur around 104 to 105 degrees Fahrenheit and some forms of hot yoga have been shown to raise the core body temperature to 103 to 104 degrees, we recommend that heated yoga should be done with caution. Hot yoga has a greater risk of musculoskeletal injury because of the increased laxity of ligaments and tendons in heated conditions, so people may unknowingly overstretch their muscles or joints. Pregnant women should be cautious of hot yoga, given the risk of overheating and dehydration to both mother-to-be and baby, and should speak with their doctor first. If you have any medical conditions, speak to your doctor first to determine whether hot yoga is safe for you.

Reference List

Historical Frameworks of Yoga

Basic Principles

Breathing Techniques

Poses

Pose by Category

Yoga Precautions

Muscle Locks and Hand Expressions

Meditations

Putting It All Together

PART I

The Art and Science of Yoga

Why Do Yoga?

Yoga does not just change the way we see things, it transforms
the person who sees.

B. K. S. IYENGAR, *LIGHT ON LIFE*

Welcome to the practice of yoga. You may have come to yoga to feel stronger, get more flexible, or relieve stress. You are part of a growing community interested in yoga, a modern practice rooted in thousands of years of ancient Indian texts and traditions. Yoga encompasses physical postures, breathing techniques, meditation, and ethical principles. Archaeologists have found soapstone seals from over five thousand years ago that have yoga postures engraved on them. Yoga is first mentioned in the Vedic texts of Indian literature from 1700 to 500 BCE. The word itself comes from the Sanskrit root *yuj*, which means to yoke, to join, or to unite. While the practice continues to be taught (for hundreds of generations now) and continues to evolve, the fundamental idea that yoga *unites* our body, mind, and being remains.

Yoga is fast becoming a well-known practice in the American household. A 2016 survey conducted by Yoga Alliance and *Yoga Journal* found that the number of Americans doing yoga has grown by over 50 percent in the last four years to over 36 million as of 2016, up from 20.4 million in 2012. Nine out of ten Americans have heard of yoga, and one in three Americans has already tried yoga at least once. More than a third of Americans say they are very likely to try yoga in the next year. While yoga is currently more popular with women, more and more men are doing yoga, too. More older adults are trying yoga. Yoga is also gaining popularity with children and in schools.

When you do yoga, you will notice many benefits, ranging from stress relief and physical fitness to better flexibility and strength. Yoga builds your capacity to handle mental and physical stress and provides you with the flexibility and confidence to get through what you are experiencing—no matter where you are. People who do yoga are 20 percent more likely to have a positive image of their own physical and mental health, including a stronger sense of mental clarity, physical fitness, flexibility, and strength. The physical and psychological health benefits are real.

Over 90 percent of all current research on yoga has found that yoga has a positive impact on health.[1] Our book is different from many other yoga books in that it provides you with a scientific and researched-based understanding of yoga. We also share our perspective as medical professionals who both practice yoga and use yoga in our clinical practice to treat stress, anxiety, depression, addictions, and post-traumatic stress disorder.

Benefits of Yoga

Yoga has many scientifically proven benefits for the mind and body.

+ **Yoga builds strength and endurance.** Many styles of yoga provide low-impact aerobic exercise and are good for your heart. One study found that 24 rounds of sun salutations 6 times a week significantly improved upper-body strength over 6 months. Another study found that an hour of rigorous yoga twice a week for 8 months increases leg strength.

+ **Yoga improves balance and flexibility.** Your sense of knowing where your body is in space and being able to balance will improve and have the potential to improve your overall athletic or fitness performance. A twice-weekly yoga program helped improved flexibility and balance in college athletes in just 10 weeks.[2]

+ **Yoga builds your awareness of and connection to your body.** The more that you can tune into your body, the more that you are able to listen to it and protect it from injury.

+ **Yoga builds the mind-body connection.** Your body and mind are powerfully connected to each other. Stress and emotions can have a major impact on your body and health. Building your mind-body connection helps you feel more whole and empowered to improve your health.

- **Yoga helps people who are already healthy.** Yoga has been shown to improve the performance, wellness, and fitness of people who are already healthy, including athletes. Many professional athletes in football, basketball, baseball, tennis, and golf do yoga to help with their athletic performance.

- **Yoga encourages you to pursue a healthier lifestyle.** Yoga motivates nearly two thirds of people to exercise more and 40% to eat healthier.[3] Yoga practitioners are more likely to live green and eat sustainable food. Yoga may also inspire you to pursue many other physical or self-care activities.

- **Yoga gives you stronger "body-responsiveness."** Body-responsiveness refers to our relationship with our own body, and, like any other relationship, listening and trust are essential for a strong relationship. A strong relationship with your body means: "I am confident that my body lets me know what is good for me" or "I am able to 'listen' to my body and what it needs."

- **Yoga improves your sleep.** Yoga, including poses, breathing techniques, and meditation, are useful research-backed methods to help improve quality of sleep and treat insomnia. Sixty percent report that yoga helps them get better sleep.[4]

- **Yoga improves your immune system.** At the biochemical level, yoga boosts your immune system so you're better able to fight off illnesses and heal faster.

- **Yoga is beneficial during healthy pregnancies.** Prenatal yoga reduces stress and anxiety and helps women feel connected with their changing body during pregnancy.

- **Yoga is adaptable and useful to help with medical conditions.** The most common health problems that lead people to try yoga are back pain, stress, and arthritis—all conditions that research has shown improve with practicing yoga regularly. Yoga has been shown to be helpful as part of treatment for a variety of medical conditions, including chronic lower back or neck pain, fatigue, obesity, asthma, irritable bowel syndrome, osteoarthritis, rheumatoid arthritis, carpal tunnel syndrome, Parkinson's disease, migraines, diabetes mellitus, kidney disease, multiple sclerosis, and for cancer survivors.

+ **Yoga helps you cope with health problems.** Yoga not only can be integrated into the treatment of many different health issues, but it can ease coping with health problems. Yoga is adaptable and focuses on the individual's needs, so it be tailored to people who are frail or bedbound or not used to being physically active.

+ **Yoga relieves stress.** More than 80% of people who do yoga report that it reduces stress.[5] You'll feel more calm and grounded with yoga. You don't have to escape your inner thoughts and feelings. You aren't encouraged to push your body too far. The original purpose of yoga and its poses is to calm the mind and prepare you for meditation, which is considered an important part of yoga. Stress is the leading cause for visits to the doctor and wreaks havoc on your physical body, so being able to relax is essential for your physical health as well.

+ **Yoga improves your mood.** More than two thirds of people who do yoga notice that it improves their mood.

+ **Yoga creates a more flexible mind.** Yoga's effects are not all just physical. By using a comprehensive yoga approach, including breathing, meditation, self-reflection, and poses, you will improve your ability to stay with the moment with an open, uncritical attitude. This starts building a more flexible mind.

+ **Yoga gives you tools to balance your mind (and body).** Yoga offers both energizing and calming principles (*brahmana* and *langhana* in Sanskrit) and the combination of the two can produce a balancing (*samana*) effect on both body and mind.

+ **Yoga puts you more in your body and less in your head.** With the breathing techniques, postures, and also meditations, contrary to what you might assume, you will be less "stuck" in your head and better able to escape the self-criticism and judgments that might live there.

+ **Yoga builds self-esteem and confidence.** The more you do yoga, the more you will feel empowered and confident about both your body and mind as a whole.

+ **Yoga improves your memory and attention.** Studies show that yoga strengthens the parts of the brain that are responsible for memory and attention. An 8-week yoga program helped older adults improve their memory and decision-making capabilities.[6] Yoga also improves academic performance and classroom behavior in children and teens.

+ **Yoga helps with such problems as depression, anxiety.** Growing research shows that yoga can be integrated successfully into treatment for mental health problems such as depression, anxiety, insomnia, binge eating disorder, and schizophrenia.

+ **Yoga helps people cut back on drinking and smoking.** Yoga reduces cravings and helps people who are interested in using less alcohol, tobacco or other substances.

+ **Yoga builds your relationship with yourself.** Yoga encourages you to be more self-aware and self-reflective, while letting go of any self-criticism.

+ **Yoga helps you connect better with others.** Yoga fosters empathy and compassion. Yoga is rooted in ethical principles of self-compassion and awareness that can both increase your empathy for yourself and others. Yoga expands your awareness and helps you discover the powerful connection between your body and your mind.

+ **Yoga encourages you to give back to your community.** One form of yoga is called *seva*, or selfless service. The philosophy of yoga encourages you to be aware of what's happening around you and to follow a sense of purpose or intention. Nearly 50% of yoga practitioners report that they donate time to the community.

+ **Yoga may lead you to delve into self-reflective and spiritual explorations.** Yoga is more commonly a secular practice in the United States, but you may be inspired to explore the spiritual dimension of yoga.

These are just a sampling of potential reasons to do yoga, and you may discover a whole host of other benefits in your own practice. Your reasons for doing yoga can also change along the way. Even though most come to yoga for stress relief or fitness, two thirds of yoga students and the majority of yoga teachers continue yoga for different reasons over time. Yoga opens the door to many new and exciting parts of your life—you can't predict the impact yoga will have on your life until you try it out for yourself.

Our Stories

Yoga has played an important role in our lives and in those of the people we treat. Our hope is to make yoga as accessible as possible for all levels of experience and flexibility and be inclusive of all sociocultural, racial, and spiritual backgrounds. We teach yoga by paying close attention to your body, building up from basic poses, using props to support the body, and encouraging you to not care about being "perfect."

Everyone comes to yoga with his or her own story. We encourage you to reflect on and welcome your own story. Here are our own personal stories of how we found yoga and what it has done for us.

DR. MARLYNN WEI'S STORY

When I first started doing yoga over a decade ago, I was looking for relief from the physical and mental stress of training to be a doctor and psychiatrist. If you had asked me what yoga was before I started doing yoga, I probably would have said it was just another way to work out.

During my medical training, I witnessed profound suffering: family members when their loved ones died in the intensive care unit, parents who could no longer recognize their children because of end-stage Alzheimer's disease, and patients with terminal illness. There were times when I felt somewhat effective in being able to help people, but there were equally—if not more—times when I felt helpless in the face of the enormity of their pain.

It was through wanting to be better able to sit with suffering that I found yoga. Although I am not a morning person, I went every weekday morning at six a.m. before going to hospital rounds, to clear my head and center myself. The flow of the postures, breathwork, and meditations freed my mind. It felt as if yoga was a deep well with nourishing waters that replenished my mind, body, and soul. Yoga taught me how to expand my own capacity to witness, hold, and *sit with* suffering—and to do so with compassion. A mentor once told me that when a patient asked her, "How can you help me when you haven't experienced my suffering?" she responded, "I haven't had your life experience, but I will sit with you." Yoga helps you listen and sit with yourself and others.

In psychiatry training, I learned how to treat such disorders as anxiety and depression with medication and psychotherapy. When I started my own therapy practice, I had the opportunity to develop my own style and integrate components of yoga, mindfulness, and meditation—elements found in what is termed the new "third wave" of cognitive behavioral psychotherapies (the first wave focused on behavior; and the second wave, on cognitive factors, such as thought processes). I had many clients who had severe anxiety and panic attacks on a weekly and, sometimes, daily basis. I taught yoga breathing skills and meditation methods to help calm both the body and mind.

Over the years I have seen yoga skills help people stop panic attacks from spiraling out of control, reduce stress, and get better sleep, and give them more of a sense of control and endurance to witness chaos. All of this eased their anxiety. I encouraged people to practice these yoga techniques daily for at least fifteen minutes a day—because being able to relax is like a mental muscle that needs to be worked out daily so that when you need it, the ability to cope and calm down will be a lot more accessible. People got better. Many were able to feel back to themselves within a few months and take these lifelong skills with them.

At the same time, I discovered more and more scientific research that backed the healing power of yoga. Although most psychotherapists have been taught to deal primarily with the mind, I have found that by approaching the mind and body as a whole, I can address the whole person and teach people to participate in healing themselves in lasting ways that deepen and, sometimes, even go beyond more traditional methods.

At its heart, I have found that yoga goes beyond the physical and even the psychological. Yoga deepens the connection and understanding we have for ourselves and others and provides us with the opportunity to treat ourselves with kindness and love—and this naturally extends to the people around us.

Finally, I am deeply grateful to be part of a tradition that can be traced throughout many generations of my family—my mother, grandmother, and great-grandmother (who had her feet bound!)—all of whom practiced meditation along with other forms of yoga. These inspirational women led their families with much strength and resilience while facing wartime conflict and significant discrimination. It proves that the power of yoga simply requires you to be present. It is inspiring to know that the power of yoga and meditation has been and continues to be a natural and empowering practice that transcends time and place.

DR. JAMES GROVES'S STORY

When I think of yoga, what comes to mind is, **Yoga is with me**. But why would it come to me this way? My guess is that yoga is like a friend, or a mate, or someone in my family. It's something that is always there, something that I can even take for granted, something that makes no demands on me but is reliable.

And it's with me in different ways at different times. As my life moves along, it becomes both more familiar—and more surprising. That paradox of familiarity and newness keeps it always with me. And it gives me the gift of compassion toward myself on a regular basis.

How I got into yoga is probably unusual. At age fifty I was treating a well-known scientist for combat-related trauma. And fairly soon in the relationship I came to understand how important—life saving, even—yoga had become to him. He kept mentioning his teacher, Tom Stiles, later Makunda, and eventually I asked him whether he would mind if I saw Stiles as my yoga instructor. He didn't, and I contacted Tom for private lessons, weekly for about an hour, just like psychotherapy, something I was quite familiar with.

The lessons were standard Ashtanga yoga with *pranayama*, poses, and meditation. I also had a regular personal practice, about an hour a day. It all went well, I had more serenity, was calmer, felt fitter, lost weight—the usual things. But then about six months into my practice, I was trapped in the back of a runaway taxi in Boston that leaped the median and hurtled toward oncoming traffic. I had just time to see we were about to crash and brace myself. The driver was killed; I had fractures of legs, pelvis, spine, sternum—but no serious head injury or internal damage.

I healed fast physically; my major residual effect of the accident was severe post-traumatic stress disorder with insomnia, nightmares, flashbacks, chronic anxiety, and some depression. I threw myself into yoga even more intensively, but I really didn't get better mentally until I stumbled onto yoga nidra sleep, mentioned in one of the dozens of yoga books I owned and studied. Once I realized that I could function just as well after a night of nidra sleep, I slowly got better over the next year or so, until I was almost back to normal. "Almost," because you never really lose your sense of how close death came, but that changed from a bad thing into something that almost amounted to a gift. A gift of awareness of how precious life is.

My picture of myself is that I'm not a very spiritual person, but rather am a fairly skeptical fan of scientific medicine. But I was lucky that my yoga introduction was through another scientist, another skeptic, so I didn't have the feeling that I was yielding to superstition. Maybe I'm more spiritual than I think, coming from the working class of West Texas, dour German Catholics on one side of my family, rather fundamentalist Southern Baptists on the other—but it was fortunate that I didn't feel I was getting into some kind of cult. I confess that meditation is not my favorite thing: it still makes me somewhat anxious at times, and I find reasons to put it off.

But yoga is so big, so diverse—it has so many options that it's still a great place for me to live in.

We each come to yoga with our different personal stories. We also have an enormous respect and immense gratitude toward the cultural roots and ancient traditions from which yoga has arisen. It would have been well beyond the scope of this book to cover in depth the rich historical, philosophical, and spiritual traditions of yoga, but we hope we can pique your curiosity and encourage you to continue to read more about yoga.

✦

At the end of the day, yoga means to yoke, to unite, to connect. We hope this book will help you connect more deeply with the people in your life—and with yourself.

How to Use This Book

This book has something to offer no matter your level of experience. Beginners will learn the main elements of yoga through our 8-week program of breathing techniques, poses, and meditations. You will become familiar enough with yoga to build your own home yoga practice or feel ready to take a class in a yoga studio.

If you already practice yoga, this book will deepen your practice by explaining the science behind yoga and how to build on your practice by adding breathing skills, muscle locks, mudras, and meditation. Experienced yoga teachers will discover the exciting new research findings on yoga, breathing, and meditation. This book can also serve as a reference guide for yoga teachers who are interested in knowing the science and research behind yoga benefits and to use research-based principles to minimize the risk of injuries.

If you're new to yoga, by the end of this book you will learn nearly one hundred poses, dozens of meditation and breathing techniques, and the science behind it all. So, how do we get started?

If you're someone who would like to know the science of yoga before you get started on the yoga mat, then we suggest reading Chapters 2 and 3 first to get a better understanding of all the modern scientific research. But if you prefer to get started with yoga right away, just skip ahead to Chapters 4 and 5 to get down the basics. Then, read the overview sections for Chapters 6, 7, and 9 to learn the basics of yoga breathing, poses, and meditation. Just remember, you don't have to learn all the breathing exercises, poses, and meditations at once!

Instead, use our 8-week program outlined in Chapter 10 as a way to get a weekly sampling of each component of yoga (breathing, poses, meditation, self-reflection). Each week ties together these components by theme. As you practice week to week, you can then go back and read Chapters 2 and 3. Finally, take a look at Chapter 8 to refine your practice.

Since our program requires you to move back and forth throughout the book, we have provided a reference list for you on pages xiii–xviii.

We also will continue to update our website (www.harvardguidetoyoga.com) with additional resources.

How Can I Figure Out the Right Style of Yoga for Me?

Finding the right style of yoga depends on your personal preferences, goals, what's available where you live, any past and present injuries or medical conditions, and the integration of spirituality. If you're interested in doing yoga, try a variety of styles to find out what works for you. Over 90 percent of yoga research studies, covering over fifty styles of yoga, found that yoga has positive results.[7] So as long as you show up to your mat, you're going to reap the benefits.

The majority of styles in the United States fall under the umbrella term *hatha yoga*, which is a generic term for yoga with physical poses. The majority of yoga in the United States are hatha yoga. But sometimes studios use "hatha yoga" to indicate that the class is slower and has static postures compared to a moving flow, or vinyasa class.

Yoga styles have different pacing of poses, set series or a variety of poses, and environments, such as a heated studio. Some forms of yoga, such as Kundalini yoga or Jivamukti yoga, include yoga breathing, chanting, and meditation. Power and Ashtanga yoga classes are rigorous and sweaty. Restorative yoga and yin yoga are slower, but restorative yoga uses bolsters and blankets so you're fully supported on the ground. In yin yoga, you actively stay in poses for up to ten minutes and letting gravity do the work. Iyengar classes can spend an entire class focusing on the proper alignment of one or two poses, using such props as blocks, straps, and folded blankets. Here is a list of yoga styles to help you navigate your search. There are many more styles of yoga that might not be on the list, and we encourage you to explore.

Table 1.1 Traditions and Styles of Yoga Common in the United States*

Tradition and Styles of Yoga	Founder/Date	Description
AcroYoga	Two schools: Jessie Goldperg and Eugene Poku in 1999 in Montreal; Jason Nemer and Jenny Klein, term trademarked in 2006 in California	Combines acrobatics, yoga, and dance. Typically done as partner yoga with a third person as the "spotter" to ensure safety.
Aerial or AntiGravity Yoga	Aerial performer Christopher Harrison in New York in 2007	Uses special hanging hammocks to support a combination of yoga, Pilates, and dance poses
Ananda Yoga	Swami Kriyananda in the 1960s	Uses silent affirmations during poses. The affirmations are intended to deepen the practice and a typical sequence includes gentle hatha poses.
Anusara Yoga	Established in 1997 by John Friend; the school was reestablished in 2012 under new leadership as the Anusara School of Hatha Yoga	School of hatha yoga. The practice is based in Tantra philosophy, which teaches that all beings are essentially good and emphasizes heart-opening. Focused on an aspirational attitude, awareness of alignment, and action as an expression of freedom.
Ashtanga Yoga or Ashtanga Vinyasa Yoga	Founded in 1948 by K. Pattabhi Jois (1915–2009)	Physically demanding, fast-paced flowing practice. The system is based on six series of asanas, progressing in difficulty.
Baptiste Power Vinyasa Yoga	Founded in 1950s by Baron Baptiste and his father Walton Baptiste; Baptiste is the son of two prominent yoga teachers who opened the first yoga studio in San Francisco in 1955	Practiced in a heated room and has flowing sequences that are physically challenging and last 90 minutes
Bikram Yoga	Founded by Bikram Choudhury in 1971 in the United States	Practiced in rooms heated to 105 degrees Fahrenheit. The sequence is fixed and has 45 minutes of standing poses and 45 minutes of floor postures (26 poses total).
Chair Yoga	General term for gentle yoga done with the support of a chair	Gentle form of yoga practiced using a chair to support the body in seated and standing poses. Useful for people who may have difficulty standing, limited mobility, or are at higher risk for falls.
Forrest Yoga	Founded by Ana Forrest in 1982	Combines physically challenging sequences with emotional exploration
Hatha Yoga	Generic term that is the foundation for the majority of Western yoga styles that use physical postures	Umbrella term that covers practices that focuses on physical posture. This can also be used as a term to emphasize static postures compared to styles with more movement.
Hot Yoga	General term for yoga practiced in heated environment	Different styles of yoga are practiced in heated rooms, including Bikram yoga, Forrest yoga, power yoga, and TriBalance yoga.

*This list is by no means exhaustive as there are dozens of yoga styles and traditions. *(continued)*

Tradition and Styles of Yoga	Founder/Date	Description
Integral Yoga	Founded by Swami Satchidananda in 1966	Gentle practice that uses classical hatha postures and combines chanting, relaxation, meditation, and breathing
Integrative Yoga Therapy	Founded by Joseph Le Page in 1993 in San Francisco	Focuses on yoga in health settings, such as hospitals and rehabilitation centers.
Iyengar Yoga	Founded by B. K. S. Iyengar who moved to Pune, India, to teach yoga in 1937	B. K. S. Iyengar developed a style of yoga that focuses on alignment. The practice uses yoga props to achieve proper alignment in poses and teacher training is extensive for several years.
Jivamukti Yoga	Founded by Sharon Gannon and David Life in 1984	Flowing physical practice that focuses on nonharming (*ahimsa*) principles and spiritual development. The practice is meditative, including chanting, music, and affirmations.
Kripalu Yoga	Founded by Amrit Desai in 1965 and established in Stockbridge, Massachusetts, in 1982	Form of hatha yoga that combines postures, breath control, meditation, and relaxation techniques
Kriya Yoga	Revived by Mahavatar Babaji and Lahiri Mahasaya and Paramahansa Yogananda's book in 1920	Focuses on self-discipline, self-study, and devotion through breathing techniques, mantra, and mudra to work toward spiritual development
Kundalini Yoga	Introduced in the United States by Yogi Bhajan in 1969	Referred to as the Yoga of Awareness, with the primary goal to awaken and liberate healing energy at the base of the spine and drawing it upwards. The practice includes chanting, breathing exercises, poses, mantras, and meditations.
ParaYoga	Founded by Rod Stryker in 1995	Combines Tantric philosophy with yoga and examines how asana affects energy
Power Yoga	The term originates from Bender Birch's 1995 Power Yoga written to introduce Ashtanga yoga to Westerners.	Power yoga is a term referring to rigorous yoga practices in the tradition of Ashtanga yoga.
Prana Flow Yoga	Founded by Shiva Rea in 2005, who has a background in dance and Ayurveda	An energetic flow sequence that incorporates dance and moving meditation.
Prenatal Yoga	General term of yoga for pregnant women	Poses and breathing exercises are tailored to different stages of pregnancy. Prenatal yoga avoids pressure on the abdomen and focuses on stability, support, and strength rather than flexibility and endurance.
Purna Yoga	Founded in 2003 by Aadil and Mirra Palkhivala	Focuses on asana as well as meditation, breath control, applied philosophy, nutrition, and lifestyle

Table 1.1 Traditions and Styles of Yoga Common in the United States (*continued*)

Tradition and Styles of Yoga	Founder/Date	Description
Restorative Yoga	Derived from the Iyengar style of yoga	Gentle and relaxing practice that uses bolsters, blankets, and blocks as props to help support passive poses
Senior Yoga	General term for yoga for seniors	Gentle form of yoga for people over the age of 65
Sivananda Yoga	Sivananda yoga is a spiritual practice based on the teachings of Swami Sivananda and founded by his student Swami Vishnu-devananda in 1957	Focuses on 12 core poses and Sanskrit chanting, breathing, meditation, and relaxation. The five main principles are: proper exercise (*asanas*); proper breathing (*pranayama*); proper relaxation (*savasana*); proper diet (*vegetarian*); and positive thinking (*Vedanta*), and meditation (*dhyana*).
Sudarshan Kriya	Taught through the Art of Living nonprofit educational organization founded in 1981 by Sri Sri Ravi Shankar	Breathing techniques that focus and integrate the mind and body.
Svaroopa Yoga	Founded in 1992 by Swami Nirma-lananda Saraswati (formerly Rama Berch)	Focuses on inner opening and releasing tension of the deeper muscles of the spine. Svaroopa means "the bliss of your own Being."
Tibetan or Trul-khor Yoga	Trul-khor is the Tibetan generic term for movement practices. Two forms are being taught in the West: — Yantra yoga by Chogyal Namkhai Norbu — Trul-Khor yoga by Tenzin Wangyal Rinpoche, who founded Ligmincha Institute in 1992	The practice has been less known in the West. Tibetan yoga is described in the 1939 book by Peter Kelder, *Ancient Secret of the Fountain of Youth*. The form known as Yantra yoga has 108 movements and has a continuous series of movement compared to hatha yoga. Trul-Khor yoga has an emphasis on breath and movement and continuous movement.
Trauma-Sensitive or Trauma-Informed Yoga	Founded by David Emerson and informed by clinical research by Dr. Bessel van der Kolk	Style of yoga geared to help people who have experienced trauma or have post-traumatic stress disorder. Principles include creating a safe space, providing choices, and using invitational language.
TriBalance Yoga	Corey Kelly and Shawnda Falvo opened TriBalance Yoga in 2007 near Chicago.	Form of hot yoga that draws from several styles of yoga, including Ashtanga yoga, Iyengar yoga, Yin yoga, and therapeutic yoga. Sequences can vary by class (there is no set pose sequence) and poses can be held for longer to provide fascia release.
TriYoga	Founded by Kali Ray in Santa Cruz, California	Kundalini-inspired hatha yoga with flowing, dancelike movement

(continued)

Tradition and Styles of Yoga	Founder/Date	Description
Viniyoga	Developed and taught by T. Krishnamacharya and his son T. K. V. Desikachar	A gentle and individualized therapeutic style of hatha yoga that includes poses, breathing, chanting, meditation, prayer, and ritual. The American Viniyoga Institute was founded in 1999 by Gary Kraftsow, who studied with Desikachar.
Vinyasa	General term for several styles of yoga using "flow" of movement with breath	Vinyasa yoga includes many styles of yoga in which there is rhythmic breath synchronized and connected with movement. Breath and asanas are aligned in a smoothly flowing sequence, leading to vinyasa yoga also being known as "flow" yoga.
Yin Yoga	Founded in the 1970s by Taoist Paulie Zink	Slow-paced, steady yoga in which poses are held for 6 to 10 minutes and aim to increase circulation, affect deep connective tissue, and improve flexibility. Although slower and inward focused, yin yoga is still challenging and active in a way that is very different than restorative yoga.
YogaFit	Yoga fitness education school developed by Beth Shaw in 1994	YogaFit is designed to improve fitness and combines fitness moves, such as pushups and sit-ups. The style is modified for a health club setting, eliminating Sanskrit terms and chanting.
Yoga Nidra	Term describing "yogic sleep," a state of deep conscious sleeplike state	Peaceful practice, a relaxed state described during yoga meditations. The practice is becoming popularized as a form of meditation or mind-body practice to increase relaxation and improve sleep.
Yoga Therapy	General term describing the use of yoga to improve health and wellness	Individualized practice of yoga intended to improve overall physical, emotional, mental, and spiritual health. The International Association of Yoga Therapists (IAYT), founded in 1989, provides an online directory of certified yoga therapists (www.iayt.org) and accredited yoga therapy training programs.

How Do I Find a Yoga Teacher?

There are many varieties of yoga and teachers with their unique styles, so finding the right yoga teacher(s) for you is a process. In general, a yoga teacher is there to guide you through safe alignment for your body, expand mind-body awareness, and nurture your ability to listen to your individual needs.

There is no official state licensing authority that credentials yoga professionals in the same way that states oversee licenses for such professionals as doctors or lawyers. Yoga Alliance, a national organization that emerged in the 1990s, has created standards to certify certain yoga schools and yoga teachers. Credentialing includes 200-hour, 300-hour, and 500-hour classifications to become a registered yoga teacher (RYT). Experienced RYT (E-RYT) designates a teacher with significant yoga teaching experience. Yoga Alliance has a directory of certified yoga teachers and registered yoga schools (www.yogaalliance.org/directory).

If you have any medical conditions, you should talk to your doctor first before starting yoga and may want to consider working with a yoga therapist. The term *yoga therapists* refers to teachers who use yoga practices, such as poses, breathing, and meditation, to help people with medical conditions. Yoga therapists typically have additional advanced training for specific medical conditions so that they can integrate yoga safely into conventional medical care. However, yoga therapists are not licensed by a state authority, but receive certification through third-party organizations, such as the International Association of Yoga Therapists, which lists yoga therapists in its online directory (www.iayt.org). A growing number of hospitals and clinics are also starting to offer yoga programs that are available to people with medical conditions.

CHAPTER 2

Historical Frameworks of Yoga

The success of Yoga does not lie in the ability to perform postures but in how it positively changes the way we live our life and our relationships.

T. K. V. DESIKACHAR

Ancient ways of understanding the body and mind are intertwined with the tradition of yoga. While we have a deep respect for the cultural history, traditions, and philosophy of yoga, it is beyond the scope of this book to delve into them deeply, but we hope we can pique your curiosity so you will be inspired to read more about yoga. First, we'd like to introduce you to the eight limbs, or paths, of yoga to show you the basic components of classical yoga.

Eight Paths of Classical Yoga

In the first or second century CE, Maharishi Patanjali, who is sometimes called the father of yoga, wrote about classical yoga in the ancient text *Yoga Sutras*. The word sutras is Sanskrit for "threads," and the yoga sutras are the core principles of classical yoga. Back then, the goal was not fitness or flexibility, but it was to prepare you for meditation. Patanjali's text mentions physical poses in only three of the over two hundred principles, or sutras, of yoga. This might surprise you because most people think about challenging poses when they think about yoga. But this was actually not the case when yoga originated—or even how it is practiced in other parts of the world today.

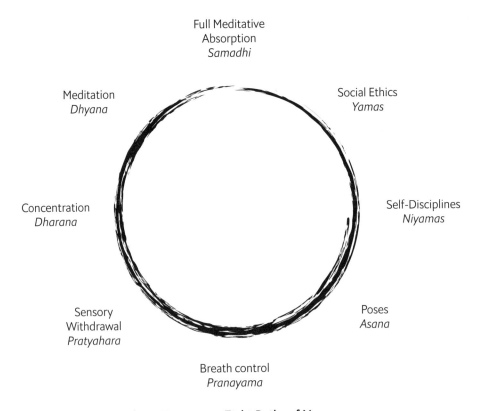

Full Meditative
Absorption
Samadhi

Meditation
Dhyana

Social Ethics
Yamas

Concentration
Dharana

Self-Disciplines
Niyamas

Sensory
Withdrawal
Pratyahara

Poses
Asana

Breath control
Pranayama

Figure 2.1   Eight Paths of Yoga

Classical yoga describes eight paths, or "limbs," of yoga to guide a purposeful life.

Classical yoga is also called *Ashtanga* yoga, Sanskrit for "eight-limbed." These eight "limbs," or paths (see Figure 2.1), include ethical principles, self-discipline guidelines, yoga breathing, poses, and four levels of meditation. Each path prepares you toward full self-realization—or what some might call enlightenment. That being said, our 8-week program in Chapter 10 most likely won't get you to the final stage, but we still think it's important to practice many of the paths, including breathing, poses, and meditation. We believe this not only out of respect for the wisdom of thousands of years of tradition, but also because modern scientific studies of yoga over the past decade have found that each of these components—not just the poses—help you feel better physically and emotionally. We discuss many of these modern scientific findings in the Chapter 3 and will provide a roadmap for you in Chapter 10 toward building a well-rounded yoga practice.

The first two paths of yoga are guidelines on how to be a moral and good person.

First Path: Social Ethics (*Yamas*)

The first path describes social ethical principles (*yamas*), including nonviolence or compassion (*ahimsa*), truthfulness (*satya*), moderation (*brahmacharya*), generosity without jealousy or envy (*aparigraha*), and not stealing because we are worried we can't generate what we need (*asteya*). These ethical principles are intended to build integrity and can be applied to the poses and the entire yoga practice as well. By not forcing your body into a pose that feels painful, you are practicing compassion and nonviolence. By recognizing what your body needs and adding blocks for support, rather than try to do a pose because you feel it needs to look impressive, you are expressing truthfulness. By not comparing yourself to others in the yoga studio, you practice being generous and not coveting what others have.

Second Path: Self-Disciplines (*Niyamas*)

The second path is self-discipline (*niyama*). We learn how to behave toward ourselves, encouraging values of cleanliness (*saucha*), being content (*samtosa*), self-disciplined (*tapas*), self-reflective (*svadhyaya*), and to surrender to the fact that we are not in control (*isvara pranidhana*). Self-discipline is associated with the element of fire and the transformative nature of fire. You can practice this self-discipline and ignite change by dedicating daily time to your yoga practice. Chapters 9 and 10 introduce meditations and self-reflective questions to help you examine your feelings. The concept of surrendering can, just as in the Alcoholics Anonymous program, be interpreted in a spiritual devotion manner, but can also be acknowledged in a secular manner of letting go of the idea that you are able to control everything. Through surrender, you will see, we are better able to flow with uncertainty.

Third Path: Postures (*Asana*)

The third limb (discussed in Chapter 7) is probably the most familiar one—yoga postures. Patanjali also talked about poses in terms of being "seated," which can refer to both the physical position as well as the understanding that we all are "seated" in our own subjective version of reality. By being situated in your body, you realize that your perspective is uniquely your own: How you are in a pose will be different from anyone else's pose.

Fourth Path: Breath Control (*Pranayama*)

The fourth limb (discussed in Chapter 6) is breath control, or *pranayama*, which is an umbrella term for a variety of different yoga breathing techniques ranging from slow and steady varieties to more rapid and forceful exercises. Using your breath is an important part of yoga practice. Breathing exercises can be done in separate seated session or during poses.

Fifth Path: Withdrawal to Internal Mind (*Pratyahara*)

In archery, you must first pull back in order to shoot your bow the farthest. The fifth path is about a similar process, where you step away from the distractions of the outside world, your phone, the television, the e-mails coming into your inbox. You redirect your attention to your own internal and external experiences of your mind. This doesn't mean you have to shut everything out and try to ignore noise or sights, but you are simply taking a step back and getting some space from which to observe the busy world around you.

When you step back, you start to develop an "observing self." You discover that you are a being who has thoughts and feelings. Rather than getting swept up in those thoughts and feelings, you can simply observe them passing through you.

Sixth Path: Concentration (*Dharana*)

The sixth path is a form of meditation (discussed in Chapter 9) called concentration (*dharana*), or what scientists call focused awareness meditation. Whether you are gazing at a candle flame or observing your breath, you practice concentration by focusing your attention onto a point of internal or external sensation or feeling.

Seventh Path: Meditation (*Dhyana*)

The seventh path is meditation or contemplation, *dhyana*, or an unbroken flow of awareness. This is a more challenging form of meditation that is also described as effortless presence, natural presence, or choiceless awareness.

Eighth Path: Full Meditative Absorption (*Samadhi*)

The final path of yoga is a state of very focused, absorbed meditation, or *samadhi*. This is a state of peace and pure awareness without having a specific point of focus. But remember, just because you don't feel this sense of "enlightenment" at the end of the practice doesn't mean that you haven't done yoga or that you should be disappointed in yourself. The idea of full meditative absorption doesn't need to be the ultimate end-goal when you do yoga, but it can serve as a reminder and hope for growth through yoga.

Now that you have a framework for classical yoga, we turn to the three approaches to the human body that are frequently referenced in yoga: the chakra system, Ayurvedic tradition, and the meridian system from Traditional Chinese Medicine.

Historical Approaches to the Human Body

Traditional yogic approaches to the body focus on the importance of energy, or life force. In yoga texts and in Ayurveda, an ancient Indian system of natural healing, the essential life force, or life energy, is called *prana*. The ancient text *Varaha Upanishad* describes the body as a "jewel" filled with essential elements. In Traditional Chinese Medicine, this energy is called qi or chi. Both systems have similar metaphors for describing energy and its flow throughout the body. When your body is healthy, then your energy flows smoothly and fully. When your energy is blocked, deficient, or overactive, then this imbalance is thought to cause physical illness or psychological problems. Yoga and other practices, such as tai chi, qi gong, acupressure, or acupuncture, are intended to release congested energy, strengthen weak energy, or calm excessive energy.

This emphasis on a life force is historically different from the European scientific approach to the body, which had turned to anatomical dissection of cadavers as early as the third century BCE as well as the second century CE. The first public human dissection occurred in Bologna, Italy, in 1315. Understanding the body through dissection became a standard practice in sixteenth-century Europe, but that did not occur until much later in Asia. Anatomical dissection of a cadaver did not reach India until 1836. This first human dissection in Asia was met with controversy and viewed as disruptive to the fabric of the ancient Indian medicine Ayurvedic traditions. One historian describes that after the introduction of anatomical dissection to Indian medicine, "the role of the 'divine' was banished forever," and the body became viewed as an "animated corpse."[1]

Anatomical dissection of the human body was also resisted in China for many years, because practitioners of Chinese medicine did not believe examining a dead body, emptied of its life force, would accurately represent the internal workings of the human body. The first public human dissection in China occurred in 1913. Today, these traditions of the energetic and physical perspective of the body merge in mind-body practices. These approaches to the body coexist, like different languages to help us understand and interpret the body.

The Chakra System

The chakra system (Table 2.1) is a metaphysical understanding of human physiology and personal growth that is closely linked to yoga. Chakras are nonphysical energy fields, analogous to electromagnetic fields, and also map onto our physical body as ascending points along the spine. In the ancient texts, the *Yoga Upanishads* and in the *Yoga Sutras of Patanjali*, chakras were described as centers of consciousness. The word *chakra* initially might raise the red flag of pseudoscience, but the seven major chakras do in fact correspond anatomically to prominent and large clumps of nerve ganglia, or plexuses, along the spine and also with different endocrine glands that have different functions in the body.

The Tantric teachings, a spiritual tradition in India, describes seven basic chakras. These chakras are connected by a network of energy channels throughout the body called *nadis*. The Sanskrit word *nadi* comes from the root *nad*, which means flow, movement, or vibration. Ancient texts mention a network of 72,000 to 350,000 energy channels throughout the human body, called *nadis*. All channels originate from one of two centers in the body, either in the area right below the navel or the heart.

Yoga is supposed to strengthen your body by helping energy flow freely through these channels. Three channels are particularly relevant to yoga. The first is the *sushumna nadi,* which is considered one of the main channels in the body, starting at the base of the spine to the crown of the head. The chakras are aligned along this main channel and energy flows upward toward the crown of the head.

Two other channels, *ida* and *pingala nadis*, wind around the central spine. These channels meet at the sixth chakra, or the third eye chakra, located between your brows. The *ida* channel is associated with the left side; feminine, lunar, cool qualities; and the color white. The *pingala* channel is associated with the right side; masculine, solar, warm qualities; and the color red.

Wellness today is defined as a healthy balance of the mind and body, a state that nurtures well-being. Yoga is meant to balance the energy between the *ida* and *pingala* channels with such exercises as alternate nostril breathing (Chapter 6). Relaxing poses, such as forward folds and seated poses, increase the flow of energy in the *ida* channel. Energizing poses, such as backbends, standing poses, inversions, and twists, increase the flow of energy in the *pingala* channel.

Balance in the energy centers also is important to wellness in the chakra system. Each chakra has a physical location in the body and psychological or emotional themes. The theory is that deficiencies or excesses in certain chakras, or "blocked" or "open" chakras, lead to certain physical or psychological problems.

Chakras open and close (become blocked) based on patterns of our behavior and interactions. Insecurity and fear are symptoms originating in the first chakra.

Table 2.1 The Chakra System

Major Chakra	One	Two	Three	Four	Five	Six	Seven
Sanskrit Name	*Muladhara*	*Swadhisthana*	*Manipura*	*Anahata*	*Vissudha*	*Ajna*	*Sahasrara*
Function	Grounding	Sexuality	Strength	Love	Creativity	Intuition	Understanding
Physical Location	Perineum	Sacrum	Behind navel	Heart	Throat	Brow/forehead	Top of head
Spinal Vertebrae	Lumbar 1–5 Sacral 1–5	Thoracic 9–12 Sacral 1–5	Thoracic 5–9	Thoracic 1–5	Cervical 3–7	Cervical 1–2	Cerebral cortex
Nerve Plexus	Coccygeal	Sacral	Solar plexus	Pulmonary, cardiac	Pharyngeal	Carotid	Brain
Gland	Adrenal	Ovaries, testicles	Pancreas	Thymus	Thyroid	Pineal	Pituitary
Body Areas	Legs, feet, large intestine	Hips, pelvis, genitals, kidney, bladder, lower back	Stomach, liver, gallbladder	Lungs, heart, arms, hands	Throat, ears, neck and shoulders, hands	Eyes, brow	Head, brain
Theme, Motivation	Survival	Desire	Power	Compassion	Communication	Vision	Consciousness
Inner Sense	Security Stability Stillness	Emotion Nurture Pleasure	Energy Anger Self-esteem	Balance Unity Healing	Creation Vibration Resonance	Imagination Seeing Third Eye	Knowing Transcendence Bliss
Matter	Solid	Fluid	Plasma	Gas	Vibration	Color	None
Element	Earth	Water	Fire	Air	Sound	Light	Thought
Problems	Weight, sciatic, constipation	Sexual, urinary issues	Digestion problems, fatigue	Respiratory issues, heart disease	Thyroid, sore throat	Vision issues, headaches	Mood or memory issues
Color	Red	Orange	Yellow	Green	Blue	Indigo	Violet or white
Yoga	Hatha	Tantra	Karma	Bhakti	Mantra	Yantra	Jnana
Seed Mantra	Lam	Vam	Ram	Yam	Ham	Om	None
Action	To be	To feel	To act	To love	To speak	To see	To know
Animal Representation	Elephant, ox, bull	Fish, ocean creatures	Ram	Birds, antelope	Bull, lion	Owl	None

(continued)

Table 2.1   The Chakra System (*continued*)

Major Chakra	One	Two	Three	Four	Five	Six	Seven
Yoga Exercises	Mountain, Knee to Chest, Locust, Standing Forward Bend, Legs up the Wall	Goddess, Happy Baby, Reclining Bound Angle, Lizard, Half Pigeon, Half Moon	Bow, Reverse Plank, Fierce, Breath of Fire	Victorious Breath, Alternate Nostril Breathing, Cobra, Upward Facing Dog, Camel, Fish	Sound of Om, singing, chanting, Lion's Breath, Shoulder Stand, Fish, Camel	Guided imagery, meditation	Meditation and meditation poses
Meditation	Grounding	Water	Energy	Compassion	Breath, Mantra	Color	Simple

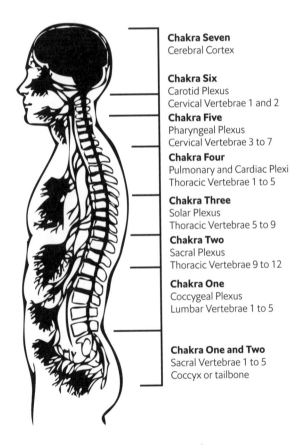

Chakra Seven
Cerebral Cortex

Chakra Six
Carotid Plexus
Cervical Vertebrae 1 and 2

Chakra Five
Pharyngeal Plexus
Cervical Vertebrae 3 to 7

Chakra Four
Pulmonary and Cardiac Plexi
Thoracic Vertebrae 1 to 5

Chakra Three
Solar Plexus
Thoracic Vertebrae 5 to 9

Chakra Two
Sacral Plexus
Thoracic Vertebrae 9 to 12

Chakra One
Coccygeal Plexus
Lumbar Vertebrae 1 to 5

Chakra One and Two
Sacral Vertebrae 1 to 5
Coccyx or tailbone

Figure 2.2   Chakras and Nerve Plexuses

The ancient chakra system corresponds to anatomical nerve plexuses, or clusters of nerves in the body.

For example, someone with difficulty getting emotionally close with people, has a "blocked" fourth or heart chakra. When you feel all tangled up in your thoughts, your seventh chakra, which is associated with cognition, may be overactive.

Thinking about chakras can be conceptually helpful in organizing your yoga sequence and tailoring poses based on a specific type of energy or theme that you want to focus on. For example, if you are having a hectic day and you feel flighty, you may wish to practice yoga poses that are grounding, that focus more on chakra one (located near the tailbone). If you feel heavy and sluggish, chakra three exercises offer more energy and strength. When you feel unheard or that you're having a hard time expressing yourself, choose chakra five exercises, which include mantras. All of the chakras are considered equally important for personal growth. The goal is to pay attention to and balance all of the chakras to promote wellness and wholeness.

Chakra One: Root Chakra, Center of Stability and Support

The first chakra starts at the base of the spine, located at the lower lumbar, sacral, and pelvic region. The theme of the root chakra is to feel grounded and solid. This chakra is characterized by simplicity and stability, like its Sanskrit name, which means "root support." Its element is earth. When this first chakra is blocked or deficient, you may experience insecurity or fear. Many of us spend little time truly connected to the earth. We spend most of our day rushing from one event to the next. We get stuck in our own thoughts and worry. It can be difficult to slow down and keep things simple. Yoga exercises that focus on the first chakra connect your body with the earth and provide stability and stress reduction.

Yoga for Root Chakra: Even ratio breathing (page 90), Easy Pose (page 110), Child's Pose (page 112), Standing Forward Bend (page 129), Pyramid Pose (page 136), Mountain Pose (page 114), Low Lunge Pose (page 143), Extended Triangle Pose (page 148), Yogi Squat (page 186), Seated Head to Knee Forward Bend (page 201), Breath Meditation (page 241)

Chakra Two: Sacral Chakra, Center of Sexuality and Imagination

Chakra two is in the lower abdomen between the navel and the genitals at the sacral plexus and is connected with emotions, empathy, and sexuality. Its element is water and has the theme of letting go and creating flow. The translation of its name is "sweetness," which corresponds to the healing aspect of the second chakra—to nurture, to create harmony, and to soothe. The second chakra is the center of identity, sexuality, emotions, pleasure, sensation, and movement. When the second chakra is deficient, there is a loss of creativity, imagination, sex drive, or empathy. An overactive second chakra leads to excessive focus on sexuality. When the second chakra is balanced, then you are able to be creative and have a balanced sex life. Exercises for opening the second chakra focus on moving and relaxing the hips and lower abdomen.

Yoga for Sacral Chakra: Child's Pose (page 112), Goddess Pose (page 187), Bound Angle Pose (page 188), Reclining Bound Angle Pose (page 189), Lizard Pose (page 190), Reclining Pigeon Pose (page 192), Half Pigeon Pose (page 193)

Chakra Three: Solar Plexus Chakra, Center of Self-Esteem

Chakra three is located at the heart center, or solar plexus at the center of the chest. The translation of its Sanskrit name is "lustrous gem," a bright, radiant center of light. The purpose of the third chakra is to be active and transform, similar to the combustion of fire and the sun, which change matter and generate energy and heat. A balanced and active third chakra provides a strong self-esteem and allows us to overcome inertia or a lack of motivation. It is associated with power, self-esteem and strength. The location of the third chakra also makes it a balancing point between the lower and higher chakras. When the third chakra is overactive, it manifests in a greed for power or control. Yoga exercises that stimulate the third chakra heat the body and fill us with energy.

Yoga for Solar Plexus Chakra: Breath of Fire (page 98), backbends (pages 169–184), twisting poses (pages 150–157)

Chakra Four: Heart Chakra, Center of Love and Self-Acceptance

Chakra four is located at the upper chest at the heart area and represents love and compassion. A healthy fourth chakra means that you are both able to feel love and self-acceptance and share love and compassion. The first opportunity to practice unconditional and nonjudging love is with ourselves. The healing nature of the heart chakra is in its compassion and ability to bring unity. The experience of love in this chakra is different from passion or desire of the second chakra because, here, love is experienced as a state of being not focused on an outside object. The translation for the Sanskrit name of the fourth chakra is "sound that is made without any two things striking," "unhurt," or "unstruck." This reinforces the idea that there is a loving connection and shared energy without any actual physical elements involved at all. The theme of the fourth chakra is acceptance, unity, and expansiveness, like its element air. Breath, as a source of energy, is essential to keeping this chakra balanced. A blocked heart chakra can lead to judging yourself or others harshly or closing yourself off from friendships and relationships.

Yoga for the Heart Chakra: Backbends (pages 169–184), Compassion Meditation (page 245)

Chakra Five: Throat Chakra, Expression and Communication

Chakra five is located in the throat area and is associated with expression, communication, and creativity. The elements of fifth chakra are sound, vibration, and speech. The Sanskrit name means "purification." Imagine how sound can be cleansing—the vibration of music at a concert washing over you, laughing with others, or singing. If you have an overactive fifth chakra, you might find yourself talking more than usual or having trouble keeping a secret. When you find it difficult to express yourself and speak up, this suggests a deficient fifth chakra. Yoga focused on the throat chakra uses your body and voice as the instrument with mantras.

Yoga for Throat Chakra: Baby Cobra Pose (page 173), Cobra Pose (page 172), Supported Fish Pose (page 182), Supported Shoulder Stand (page 206), Legs up the Wall Pose (page 207), Mantra Meditation (page 246)

Chakra Six: Third Eye Chakra, Wisdom and Intuition

Chakra six, also called the "third eye" or "brow chakra," is located in the center of the forehead. Its theme is imagination, wisdom, and intuition, and its element is light. The translation of the sixth chakra is "to perceive and command." The sixth chakra gland is the pineal gland, which is actually stimulated and regulated by light. A blocked third eye may be someone who has a busy mind or indecisiveness. An overactive sixth chakra is when you are distracted with daydreaming and imagination. Yoga exercises for the third eye include meditations, including meditations on color, and guided visualizations.

Yoga for Third Eye Chakra: Child's Pose (page 112), Standing Forward Bend (page 129), Dolphin Pose (page 125), Seated Head to Knee Pose (page 201), Gazing Candle Meditation (page 244), *Om* Meditation (page 249)

Chakra Seven: Crown Chakra, Knowing and Enlightenment

Chakra seven is at the top of the head and represents knowledge and understanding. The seventh chakra is also known as the "crown chakra" or "thousand-petal lotus," from its name, *sahasrara*, which means "thousandfold." The crown chakra is considered the seat of enlightenment in yoga—the ultimate state of consciousness, which transcends the mind and physical body. The goal of a balanced crown chakra is to experience knowing and awareness. Deficiencies in the crown chakra leads to a lack of self-awareness. The goal of meditation is to open the seventh chakra.

Yoga for Crown Chakra: Alternate Nostril Breathing (page 94), Upward Salute (page 120), Eagle Pose (page 165), Tree Pose (page 163)

The practice of yoga aims to balance the chakras. Some forms of yoga have another goal, which is to allow Kundalini energy, or a construct of cosmic energy, to rise in the body. Kundalini energy is symbolized by a coiled serpent sitting dormant at the base of the spine at the first chakra. Yoga seeks to stimulate this energy and allow it to ascend through aligned chakras of the spine and leave up through the top of the head. Shaktii Parwha Kaur Khalsa, in *Kundalini Yoga: The Flow of Eternal Power*, describes the "proof" that kundalini has risen in a person is "in the upgrading of that person's attitude toward life, his relationships with other people and with himself." This tradition informs modern exercises of yoga and mindfulness. For example, when you perform a body scan (see Chapter 9) where you focus on and release tension in parts of the body, you move your attention in an ascending direction—from the soles of your feet to the top of your head—in the same direction of the ascending chakras, or rising Kundalini energy.

Ayurvedic Tradition

Ayurveda is a five-thousand-year-old system of natural healing that focuses on the science of life and longevity. Many of the Ayurvedic and yoga traditions overlap as they both grew from similar ancient texts. Both share the same understanding of the body and mind. Ayurveda has three types of fundamental energies: wind (*vata*), fire (*pitta*), and earth (*kapha*). Our balance—or imbalance—of these three elements determine our nature and physical and mental state. Mind-body types are called *doshas*, which describe your physical body type, sleep patterns, temperament, and how you handle stress. If you are predominantly wind, then you may tend to be thin, energetic, and spontaneous. Fire types are intense, focused, and goal-oriented. Those who possess predominantly the earth element are nurturing, grounded, and methodical. Different yoga poses and exercises stimulate or suppress different energies as with chakras.

Traditional Chinese Medicine Meridians

Traditional Chinese Medicine's understanding of the body also influences yoga. This approach to human physiology originates from Taoism, which was developed by Lao-tzu about 600 CE. The core philosophy is that we are part of nature and in constant flux. The goal is to maintain balance amidst constant change. It is based on energy, or qi. Qi would be similar to *prana* in the yoga tradition. The body is made whole and balanced through an interconnected network of energy pathways called meridians, or *jinglou*—this is the equivalent of the subtle channels in yoga. These pathways create a continuous flow of information and energy and link the connective tissues of the body with different organs and parts of the body. This flow of energy allows you to be whole and healthy. Similar to chakras, *qi* can be blocked or weak, creating physical or psychological issues.

Yin and Yang

The pathways have different properties in terms of yin or yang. Yin and yang are complementary forces that need each other to be in balance. Yin is feminine and dark, associated with such properties as being slow, soft, cold, and wet. Yin is represented by water, earth, moon, and nighttime. Yang is masculine and light, linked with action, speed and, aggressiveness. Yang is associated with the sun, sky, and daytime. Everyone, both women and men, has properties of both yin and yang. Balance of these forces are important to keep the body and mind healthy and in harmony.

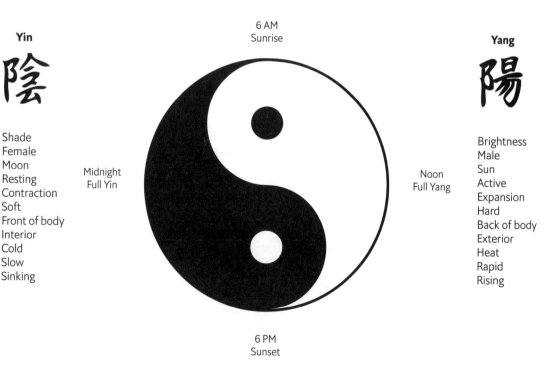

Figure 2.3 Yin and Yang Principles

In Traditional Chinese Medicine and philosophy, the elements of yin and yang energy balance each other. This understanding of the balance of energy is integrated into many styles of yoga.

When you have too much yin or too little yang, your body is cold and slow, such as problems of low thyroid or slow metabolism. When you have too much yang or too little yin, you are hot and overstimulated, like being in a high thyroid state.

Different yoga exercises stimulate different meridians of the body and can activate more yin or yang energy. Such poses as Low Lunge Pose (see page 143) and forward bends stir the dark, slow, evening feminine energy of yin. Sun salutation sequences (see pages 260–268) and twisting poses create hot, bright, morning masculine energy of yang.

The energy lines of the body are also characterized by the five main elements. There are five "elements" of energy: fire, earth, metal, water, and wood. The body is divided into two categories of function: *zang*, or "solid," organs, which collect and store; and *fu*, or "hollow," organs, which transform and transport. Yin organs are solid and actively produce and store energy and body fluids. Yang organs are hollow, constantly transporting, transforming, and moving energy and body fluids.

There are twelve major meridians as well as several others. Each of the twelve major meridians, or pathways of energy, are connected to different major organs in the body. Each pathway originates in an energy center of the body, or chakra. Acupuncture points, or *tsubos*, are the specific points along the skin where the meridians surface. These are not precisely physical but specific areas of energy. When pressed, these points ache and tingle in a distinctive way from other places in the body.

✦

In the next chapter, we will discuss the modern science of yoga. Some of the ancient claims of yoga's effect on the body and mind correspond to phenomena well described in modern scientific research, and what might be perceived as very asynchronous ideas might actually be similar to the duality of light as being both a particle and a wave. As doctors trained in modern medicine, we believe that you can still hold onto rational thought and science and treat with respect and wonder the ways we understood the mind and body thousands of years ago.

Table 2.2 Traditional Chinese Medicine Meridian System

Meridian / Channel	Type	Path	Extremity	Element	Chakra	Emotion
Heart	Lesser Yin	Heart down to small intestine and branches upward to eye through lung, armpit, inner arm to little finger	Hand	Fire	Chakra Three	Joy/Sadness
Heart Protector	Faint Yin	Center/front of chest to heart and inner organs, branches to armpit, inner arm, middle of palms to tip of middle finger	Hand	Fire	Chakra Three	Joy/Sadness
Triple Heater	Lesser Yang	Tip of ring finger, outer arm, shoulder, pericardium and descends; one branch goes upward to collarbone, ear, eyebrow	Hand	Fire	Chakra Three	Joy/Sadness
Small Intestine	Greater Yang	Outer edge of little finger, outer edge of arm, and branches; one branch down to chest, heart, small intestine; other branch up to face, ear, eye	Hand	Fire	Chakra Three	Joy/Sadness
Lung	Greater Yin	Stomach to large intestine, up through lungs, head, armpit, upper and inside of forearm, ends in thumb	Hand	Metal	Chakra Four	Grief
Large Intestine	Yang Bright	Index finger, back of hand, outside of arm and branches at collarbone; one branch down to large intestine; other branch upwards to side of nose	Hand	Metal	Chakra Four	Grief

(continued)

Table 2.2 Traditional Chinese Medicine Meridian System (*continued*)

Meridian / Channel	Type	Path	Extremity	Element	Chakra	Emotion
Spleen	Greater Yin	Inner edge of big toe, inner edge of foot/ leg to abdomen, chest, throat, tongue; branches to stomach and heart	Foot	Earth	Chakra One	Desire/Worry
Stomach	Yang Bright	Side of nose up to eye; one branch up to forehead; downward exterior and interior branch to spleen, stomach and front of leg to lateral second toe	Foot	Earth	Chakra One	Desire/Worry
Kidney	Lesser Yin	Outer small toe, inside of foot/leg through abdomen and kidneys, lungs, heart, base of tongue	Foot	Water	Chakra Two	Fear
Bladder	Greater Yang	Inner corner of eye to forehead, brain, top of head and then branches down back through kidneys, down to outer edge of small toe	Foot	Water	Chakra Two	Fear
Liver	Faint Yin	Big toe, inside of leg, lower abdomen, liver	Foot	Wood	Chakra Three	Anger
Gallbladder	Lesser Yang	Outer eyebrow to forehead, ear then splits into internal branch to gallbladder and liver and external branch outside of leg to outer toe	Foot	Wood	Chakra Three	Anger

CHAPTER 3

The Modern Science of Yoga

The signs of progress on the path of Yoga are health, a sense of physical lightness, steadiness, clearness of countenance and a beautiful voice . . . a balanced, serene and tranquil mind.

B. K. S. IYENGAR, *LIGHT ON YOGA*

In 1970, Elmer and Alyce Green, preeminent researchers who developed the concept of biofeedback, and their colleagues at the Menninger Clinic studied forty-five-year-old Indian yogi Swami Rama. In their psychophysiology laboratory, Swami Rama was able to change his body temperature by 4 degrees Fahrenheit and increase his heart rate to three hundred beats per minute on command. Noting that it was the most difficult thing that he had learned to do, Swami Rama was able to control the blood flow of his hand to generate an 11 degree Fahrenheit difference between his little finger and thumb on one hand. And he could stop his pulse for seventeen seconds. Even though this level of control takes decades to master, by using your breathing rate and postures, you, too, will notice how you can change your heart rate and blood pressure with just your breath and movement.

Why is it important to be able to change our heart rate and blood pressure with yoga? Because it reflects a stronger connection to a deeper physiological system in our body that is in charge of coping with stress. When you practice yoga, you build a buffer against stress. Your *resilience*—your ability to tolerate physical and mental stress—improves at several levels throughout your body and mind—from molecular DNA all the way up to your brain chemistry levels, and then your muscles, joints, and bones. In this chapter, we will take a closer look at the modern scientific approach to understanding how yoga changes our mind, body, health, and well-being.

Research supports that yoga can improve overall life satisfaction and can motivate you to pursue a healthier lifestyle. In a survey conducted by the National Institutes of Health, more than 40 percent of people who did yoga reported that doing yoga motivated them to eat healthier, and over 60 percent said yoga encouraged them to exercise more. But the most important benefit is the effect of a persistent attitude of being good and valuing yourself. And that attitude is at the center of how yoga changes us.

The Rapid Rise of Scientific Yoga Research

Scientific research on yoga has tripled in the past decade.[1] Between 1975 and 2014, a total of 312 randomized controlled trials of yoga were published from over twenty-three different countries.[2] Most yoga research is done in India and the United States.

Over 90 percent of randomized yoga studies found that yoga made a positive impact on your health.[3] Almost half of the studies (45%) were randomized control trials, which are considered the strongest forms of science within the medical community. This type of study design randomly assigned participants to either an experimental group (yoga) or a control group (no yoga) to analyze whether yoga makes a difference. About a quarter of the studies focused on healthy people; the rest studied how yoga could help different medical conditions. The most commonly

> Over 90 percent of randomized yoga studies found that yoga made a positive impact on your health.

studied medical conditions were breast cancer, depression, asthma, and type 2 diabetes. The median length of study was nine weeks. The sample size in most research studies on yoga was on the smaller side (fewer than 100 people) and did not compare it to other forms of exercise, so larger, more rigorous studies are still needed. Over a third of the studies did not specify the style of yoga used. About 80 percent of the yoga studies used postures, three quarters used breath control, and half used meditation. Only 10 percent used yoga philosophy lectures, though yoga philosophy has been shown to be more advantageous in improving quality of life when integrated in the program. In the meantime, there is a growing body of scientific literature supporting the health benefits of yoga.

But the growth of yoga research is still very promising for many reasons. One, it helps us better understand how yoga helps us. Two, it lends powerful scientific credibility for yoga's health benefits and helps to promote yoga as a tool for people who are already healthy as well as those who have medical issues. The stronger the scientific evidence the better the case for health insurers to cover or reimburse the cost of yoga as a form of preventative health care, giving more people access to yoga.

Researchers over the past decade have been able to show how yoga changes our body through many newer scientific methods—from measuring our biochemical levels in the brain through magnetic resonance spectroscopy, at brain magnetic resonance imaging (MRI), and even by taking a closer look to changes in our DNA.

Now, you're probably wondering how yoga does all this. To understand how yoga works, let's take a step back and take a closer look at something that we've all encountered before—the problem of stress.

The Problem of Stress

Stress and stress-related problems account for up to 90 percent of why people go to see their doctor. It is the third-costliest health-care expenditure in the United States, after only heart disease and cancer. But astonishingly few doctors—only 3 percent—talk to their patients about how to can reduce stress in their everyday lives.

Our body is kept in balance by two branches of the autonomic nervous system: the sympathetic system, which is responsible for our "fight-or-flight" response, and the balancing counteracting parasympathetic system, otherwise known as the "rest and digest" state. Each network has an intricate, interconnected network of nerves running between our brain and organs and communicate through a variety of neurotransmitters, which further signal different chemicals to be released in our blood to change your organ functions. These chemicals regulate the pace of our breathing, our heart rate, the dilation of our pupils, and the function of our gut and bladder.

This is the process behind the fight-or-flight fear, or survival response. When you're feeling threatened or stressed, the emotional alarm center of your brain, the amygdala, interprets this danger and signals distress to another region in the brain, the hypothalamus. The hypothalamus, the command center of your brain, then sends signals through your sympathetic nervous system to your adrenal glands to release adrenaline (also known as epinephrine) into the bloodstream. As a result, your heart beats faster, your breath becomes shallow and rapid, your palms get sweaty, and your stomach tightens and stops digesting food. All this happens to enable you to focus and harness your energy to run away ("flight") or react immediately to the threat ("fight").

Sound familiar? We have all felt this way at some point in our lives—when we have to give a speech in front of a large audience, are stuck in a traffic jam while running late to a meeting, or watch a horror film. Being in this activated state for a little while isn't damaging. Eventually, the stress is removed—the speech is over, the traffic jam clears, the movie ends—and the parasympathetic nervous system kicks in to reset the balance back to normal. Like opening a window when it gets too hot or venting your stove when there's smoke in the air, your parasympathetic nervous system counteracts the fight-or-fight response with its own cascade of chemical signals and calms the body. You're able to cool off, and your heart rate returns to normal. You breathe easier.

But if the alarm stays on for longer and your parasympathetic nervous system doesn't step in, then a second wave gets activated through the hypothalamic-pituitary-adrenal (HPA) axis. This system releases stress hormones, such as cortisol, which circulates through your entire body and shuts down your immune system. This happens when you are stressed for days and weeks without being able to reset yourself, and can lead to anxiety, emotional fragility, or simply feeling worn down. When you are more vulnerable and haven't had a chance to relax or reset, you can end up more easily upset by small problems that wouldn't usually bother you. Once the stress hormone release is activated, you breathe in a pattern suited to emergencies, both shallower and more rapid.

Both your body and mind suffer from this chronic stress. Consistently elevated levels of cortisol circulating in your body leads to long-term physical problems, including a weaker immune system, inflammation, weight gain, sleep problems, heart disease, and stomach issues.

Stress turns on your "fight-or-flight" system, the sympathetic nervous system, and if you're constantly stressed, you end up tired, irritable, and more vulnerable to weight gain and health issues. Your stress hormone levels are supposed to naturally drop after the threat is gone, but if you're constantly stressed, the levels stay high. This imbalance makes you even more sensitive and weakened, leading to a downward spiral of exhaustion that is itself paradoxically difficult to bounce back from.

In a national survey, over 85 percent of people who did yoga felt it helped them reduce stress. Across twenty-five yoga research studies, yoga has reduced symptoms of depression, anxiety, and stress.[4] Yoga has been shown to relieve stress for healthy people as well as people suffering from depression and anxiety.

Yoga stops the negative cycle of stress by turning on your body's relaxation response, a state of deep rest, which is produced by the counterstress parasympathetic nervous system. This system is in charge of reducing physical and emotional stress by releasing chemicals and hormones that relax your muscles and slow your breathing. Meditation, yoga, and other mind-body activities, such as tai chi, all activate the relaxation response. You can experience this by noticing how your heart rate slows down and you feel a sense of calm after a short breathing exercise. It's important to remember that this relaxation response is like a muscle—the more that you do yoga, the more you are able to reach this relaxed state. Consistency is key. The next time you encounter something frustrating or difficult, you can shoulder the burden more easily.

Yoga helps you learn how to diffuse tension and anger. Research studies have shown yoga can decrease chronic stress levels, as measured by daytime stress hormone cortisol levels in the blood, which is important since higher daytime cortisol levels have been linked to worse health outcomes.

Consider: Victorious Breath (page 93), Lion's Breath (page 96), Alternate Nostril Breath (page 94), Breath Meditation (page 241), Body Scan Meditation (page 247), Tonglen Meditation (page 250), Downward Facing Dog Pose (page 122), Low Lunge Pose (page 143), Revolved Low Lunge Pose (page 153), Standing Forward Bend (page 129), Wide-Legged Forward Bend (page 134), Reclining Bound Angle Pose (page 189), Fish Pose (page 181), Legs up the Wall Pose (page 207)

The Mind-Body Connection and Relaxation Response

Yoga has been scientifically proven to fight stress. It does this by switching on your counterstress system so that you can experience a healthier state called the relaxation response, a term coined at Massachusetts General Hospital in the 1970s based on cardiologist Herbert Benson's observations on meditation.

The relaxation response is a physical state of deep relaxation that restores your body back to prestress levels, instills peace, and improves health. There are many ways to turn on the relaxation response, including practices that strengthen the connection between your mind and body, including guided visualization, tai chi, qi gong, and yoga. The result is not binary or rapid, so don't expect to get results on the first try. Rather than its being like a light switch, think instead of the relaxation response as working out a muscle or building a reservoir of drinking water: the more you practice yoga, the more you can strengthen that muscle or deepen the well. This allows you to better access the counterstress response when you need it. When you run into a stressful situation, you're better able to get through it by staying grounded without setting off major alarms. And when alarms are set off, you're better able to turn them off and cool down.

How much yoga do you need to practice to get this relaxation response? You may feel it the first few times that you try yoga, but it's much more likely you'll get a better and better response with practice. Most research studies on yoga find changes to the body with, at minimum, sixty minutes weekly for eight to twelve weeks. More positive results appear when you do yoga at least three to four times a week. If you only have a few free hours each week, it's best to spread out the time throughout the week. Consistency is key. The bottom line is that the more regularly you do yoga, the more likely and stronger the benefits will be.

This effect of yoga is seen at the biological level by lowering your heart rate and blood pressure. Yoga has been linked to a more stable response to stress and lower fight-or-flight response. In other words, by enhancing the connection between your mind and body, you expand your ability to tolerate difficult emotions and challenging situations.

Our ability to withstand stressful situations physically translates into a measure called heart rate variability, or the ability to change our heart rate. For people with heart disease, diabetes, or respiratory problems, heart rate variability is low. If you are healthy, then your heart rate variability is high. Yoga can improve your heart rate variability over months of practice.

Yoga also supplies another important ingredient to our wellness. By bringing together our body and mind, yoga gives us powerful information about ourselves.

Yoga Improves Flexibility and Balance

Yoga helps you increase flexibility gradually over time by loosening and stretching connective tissues and muscles. Yoga also helps improve your balance by building strength and stability. Dozens of studies have found yoga improves a range of measures of balance in healthy people.

Yoga also improves the awareness of where your body is in space as well as when you're moving, a sensory ability called proprioception. Proprioception is crucial for strength, coordination, and avoidance of injury. A month of daily yoga was able to help blind children improve proprioception. Yoga has also been able to help older adults reduce their fear of falling while improving balance, stability, and flexibility.

Yoga Builds Muscle and Bone Strength

Exercise builds bone, joint, and muscle strength and certain types of exercise can slow bone loss that comes with aging. Yoga uses your own body weight and strengthens muscles that support your spine to improve posture. Exercise stimulates bone mass prior to and during puberty. Bone mass plateaus during adulthood and declines during aging, particularly for postmenopausal women due to the drop in estrogen, which plays an important role in stopping bone loss. Osteoporosis, a condition of decreased bone density that makes bones fragile and vulnerable to fracture, and its precursor, osteopenia, or low bone mass, affects one in three women and one in five men older than fifty.

Certain types of exercise, such as walking and running, can be helpful to improve bone mineral density in adults, but other exercises, such as swimming, have not been found to change bone mineral density. One of the major hazards of space travel is the severe bone mass loss caused by the lack of gravity during space missions. It's still unclear exactly what types of exercise are best for keeping bones strong, but most likely moderate weight-bearing and muscle strengthening exercises are helpful. A few small studies provide encouraging evidence that yoga may be able to protect bones by slowing the decline in bone mineral density both for pre- and postmenopausal women.[5] One study found that the more time spent doing yoga directly increased bone formation, even better than walking.[6]

Modified yoga can be a gentle way to exercise for people with osteoporosis, though there is no one-size-fits-all approach in this group. Individual needs and the degree of osteoporosis vary. We will discuss poses that are riskier for people with osteoporosis in Appendix A.

Yoga builds muscle mass and strength as well. When you strengthen your muscles, your joints are also better supported. Moving your joints through a full range of motion in yoga also pumps fresh blood, oxygen, and nutrients to the cartilage in your joints and revitalizes areas that might otherwise be neglected.

Yoga Improves Heart Health

You can get similar cardiovascular benefits from yoga as you can from aerobic exercise. Yoga has been shown to lower blood pressure, heart rate, and cholesterol as much as brisk walking or biking for the same amount of time. Yoga can improve your body mass index (BMI) and total cholesterol levels. In one study, low-density ("bad") cholesterol dropped by 12 mg/dl and high-density ("good") cholesterol rose by 3 mg/dl.[7] Yoga has been shown to lower the resting heart rate, improve oxygen uptake, and the capacity to exercise.

There is also promising evidence that yoga can even help people in cardiac rehabilitation programs. Studies have found that yoga was able to improve exercise capacity, oxygen levels, and quality of life for people with chronic heart failure. Yoga also helped people recovering from coronary bypass grafting surgery by improving their ejection fraction, which measures how well the heart can pump blood with each contraction, and reduced anxiety, depression, and stress, which can often occur after surgery.

Yoga Helps with Weight Management

Yoga can help you maintain a healthy weight. Some forms of yoga, such as hot yoga or fast-moving power yoga, count as moderate intensity exercise, which burns 4 to 7 calories a minute, similar to brisk walking. Yoga also motivates people to do other forms of exercise.

But you don't have to do high-intensity style of yoga to lose weight. Burning calories is only one factor in weight management. An important factor in weight gain that is often ignored is the impact of chronic stress. Constant levels of stress cause high chronic levels of the hormone cortisol, which stimulates appetite and raises insulin levels. This leads to higher levels of glucose production, which is typically converted into fat. Stress-induced weight gain ends up in areas that are particularly sensitive to cortisol, such as the waistline. Reducing your overall stress levels is a really important way to help normalize appetite and weight in a healthy manner.

Have more low-intensity styles of yoga been shown to be effective for people who are overweight? Yes, restorative yoga has been linked with loss of long-term body fat and weight loss that is maintained over time. One study found that a year-long restorative yoga program led to weight loss and less body fat in over-weight women.[8] The benefits in the yoga group were both longer lasting and more prominent compared to the group that performed stretching exercises. The restorative yoga group was able to shed twice the weight and subcutaneous fat at the waistline compared to the stretching group and was able to keep up this weight loss about a year later. One explanation is that restorative yoga is better able to lower stress and chronic cortisol levels.

It is important to remember that your weight is just one measure among many other factors to assess overall health and fitness and can fluctuate day to day. Such physical activities as yoga can help develop muscles in your body, which weigh more than body fat, so the isolated number is not a reliable indicator of health or fitness. Also, for many people, especially those who struggle with body image or eating disorders, it is important to move away from focusing on body weight and image, radical yo-yo dieting, or a negative attitude toward their body. Body self-hating is a culturally driven phenomenon of immense power and can be very toxic to your self-esteem and self-worth, creating a rocky, acrimonious relationship between your mind and body.

Yoga is intended instead to help you connect your body and mind in an accepting and positive way—a form of harmony. The more you are able to let go of weight as a form of self-criticism or judgment, and the more you can do yoga instead to expand self-compassion, then you will notice that your relationship with your body will be more loving and kind.

Yoga Helps You Sleep Better

Yoga and meditation help you get a better night's sleep. A national survey found that over 55 percent of people who did yoga felt it improved their sleep. About 60 percent of studies on mind-body interventions for sleep show benefit on at least one measure of sleep.[9]

Yoga also helps you become more aware of the mental and physical states that prevent sleep. Yoga has helped sleep in people suffering from post-traumatic stress disorder, military veterans, the elderly, and nurses. Yoga also can improve sleep quality in people with physical illnesses, including osteoarthritis, breast cancer, Parkinson's disease, and irritable bowel syndrome. A recent national randomized controlled study found that a yoga program integrating poses, breathing, and meditation improved overall sleep quality and memory in cancer survivors.

One study used focus groups to find out how mindfulness exercises changes sleep. Several people found that mindfulness helped them relax so that they could "just decompress and fall asleep."

One person experienced immediate effects, "[My sleep] was almost immediately, positively impacted though I didn't sleep longer, but I slept better. So, I woke up more refreshed even though I wasn't sleeping more, and that happened for me very quickly."

Mindfulness also increased awareness of disruptions that made it hard to wind down. One person stopped using the phone at night and reported becoming "possessive of my winding down time."

Consistent practice was key, as one person noted:

I couldn't meditate during the vacation. And I noticed that the benefits left me. I came back home and here was the chatter all back again. *I shouldn't have said that. Shouldn't have done that. I said the wrong thing to that person.* It was all back. And as I went to lie down and go to sleep I couldn't get to sleep. And when I do the meditation, that chatter goes away. And I can't even say how it goes away, it just goes away.

Yoga has been shown to improve sleep quality, reduce nighttime awakenings, and reduce the need for sleep medication.

Suggested for sleep: Yoga Nidra, Victorious Breath (page 93), Alternate Nostril Breathing (page 94), Standing Forward Bend (page 12), Wide-Legged Forward Bend (page 134), Reclining Bound Angle Pose (page 18), Legs up the Wall Pose (page 207), Happy Baby Pose (page 204), Body Scan Meditation (page 247)

WHAT IS YOGA NIDRA?

Yoga nidra is a state of deep relaxation, a state of consciousness between sleep and being awake. Nidra sleep can release stress and tension and help you feel restored, especially when it may be difficult to get actual sleep.

This nidra sleep is a promising tool for people who suffer from the effects of trauma both in the months after the event and in the long term. Even though it is a form of in-bed meditation, it can be helpful even if you have found that other forms of meditation do not work as well.

1. Day or night, lie comfortably on your back, your whole body loose, head on a small pillow, fingers interlaced, thumbs together, hands on your navel, eyes gently closed. Breathe normally.

2. Assess your breathing, notice your lungs filling at the top and then gently pushing your belly up against your loosely clasped hands. This is the key step—your belly pushes your hands an inch or two upward (gravitationally upward, away from the floor or mattress). Allow the breath to leave your chest, throat, nose, passively pushed up and out by the weight of your belly and hands.

3. Keep your eyes gently closed, but roll your eyeballs upward toward a point between your eyebrows. They won't stay there, but keep at it, rolling them back while you're pushing your belly up against your hands. Back and forth, it won't be perfect, but keep at it. Try to focus on your eyes and your belly, and gently push out of your mind all the other things that want to intrude.

4. Eventually you'll drift off, not into actual sleep but into nidra sleep, a relaxed meditative state. In it you don't lose the sense of thoughts occurring and emotions present, but they are more distant. Time seems to stop. You come out of it refreshed.

Yoga and Brain Health

You might not realize that even after childhood and adolescence, your brain continues to evolve and change. Some neuronal pathways become stronger while others are pruned, like a bonsai tree—scientists call this process neuroplasticity. What we choose to do influences which pathways gets stronger or weaker. By doing yoga and meditating, you actually are choosing to take part in the development of your mind at a spiritual and physical level.

As we age, our brain also shrinks in size. Every decade after the age of forty, our brain shrinks by 5 percent.[10] Yoga can protect us from this natural aging. The theory is that the size of the brain area is related to the level of function. When that brain area grows, it indicates more rigorous ability for whatever that brain area is in charge of, such as sensory perception. Conversely, areas of the brain that shrink would indicate weaker function.

Yoga is likely *neuroprotective*, meaning that people who do yoga regularly have a brain size that you would expect of a much younger person.[11] Yoga "protects" in particular, the left side of the brain, the side of the brain that is most connected with our parasympathetic nervous system response and positive emotions, such as joy and happiness.

Neuroscientists have also examined the power of meditation on the brain as well through neuroimaging. Experienced meditators have brain sizes that you'd expect of people half their age, particularly in areas of the brain dealing with attention, auditory, and sensory perception as well as memory and decision making.[12] In one study, people who were new to mindfulness took part in an 8-week program. By eight weeks, the participants had more gray matter in brain areas dealing with empathy, compassion, learning, memory, understanding of the self, and emotional regulation.[13] One area of the brain stem that produces many neurotransmitters, the pons, also grew.

In contrast, one area of the brain actually shrank, and that was the amygdala, the center of the brain in charge of emotional reactivity, or your fight-or-flight response. This supports the idea that people who regularly meditate or do yoga build their capacity to tolerate difficult situations, rather than become overwhelmed and paralyzed with fear or anger.

Yoga Changes Neurotransmitters

Yoga measurably changes the levels of circulating chemicals in our brain and throughout our whole body. These brain chemicals, or neurotransmitters, are responsible for many functions in the body, including physical pain, weight, sleep, mood, and concentration. GABA, or γ-aminobutyric acid, is a neurotransmitter that occurs naturally in our body. People with depression, anxiety, and post-traumatic stress disorder have lower levels of GABA in certain brain areas. Researchers at Boston University School of Medicine looked at how twelve weeks of yoga changed GABA levels in the part of the brain called the thalamus and also compared yoga with walking for the same amount of time.[14] Yoga improved anxiety and mood better than walking and also boosted GABA levels in the thalamus, specifically in the left thalamus, which is linked with the parasympathetic nervous system.

Yoga also helps increase proteins that help with neuron growth. Yoga leads to more of a growth factor called brain-derived neurotrophic factor (BDNF), which helps neurons survive longer, encourages growth of new neurons, and helps long-term memory. The impact of yoga is not just in the brain though—it is throughout your entire system.

Yoga Boosts Natural Antioxidants

Yoga also protects our body from the toxic process of oxidative stress, or damage from free radicals, chemicals that circulate through our blood and attack DNA, cells, and tissues. Our cells and tissues are constantly exposed to free radicals from such environmental toxins as pollution, ultraviolet rays, or the natural by-products of processing energy in our body. Oxidative stress has been linked to health problems, such as heart disease, cancer, and even eye problems, such as glaucoma.

Our ability to mop up and deactivate free radicals and fix this damage is through a group of biochemicals called antioxidants. Antioxidants come in many forms. Some are naturally produced by our body and others come from outside sources, such as fruits and vegetables. Antioxidants include vitamin C, vitamin E, and beta-carotene, as well as such minerals as selenium and manganese. The list of antioxidants is long and diverse, including proteins, enzymes, and such substances as glutathione, coenzyme Q10, lipoic acid, flavonoids, phenols, polyphenols, and phytoestrogens.

Eating foods rich in antioxidants, such as olive oil, nuts, fruits, vegetables, and even chocolate, has been linked with better memory, heart health, and reduced rates of cancer. You may be familiar with antiaging, antiwrinkle creams' containing antioxidant vitamin E or C, which helps combat wrinkles and skin damage caused by the sun and aging. Now you can add yoga to your list of natural "antioxidants."

Researchers found that twelve weeks of yoga, including breathing and meditation, at least four times a week, boosted the body's natural antioxidants and enhanced the immune system.[15] Our body has natural antioxidant defense systems that combat oxidative stress. Yoga was able to increase these natural antioxidants in the body, including boosting levels of the protein glutathione and an enzyme called glutathione peroxidase. Glutathione levels went up for both the yoga group and the regular exercise group, but *much more so in the yoga group*. In fact, yoga more than doubled the presence of glutathione in the body. Yoga beat running, cycling, and jumping rope for lowering levels of harmful free radicals.

Yoga Reduces Inflammation, Strengthens Your Immune System

Another source of harm to your body comes in the form of inflammation. Inflammation is a process in the body that you're all too familiar with if you've ever gotten acne, poison ivy, sinus infections, allergies, arthritis, or even the common cold. Your body sends out white blood cells and a variety of immune cells to protect your body and fight the harmful invader, such as bacteria or a virus. In the case of a toe wound, the inflammatory process leads to an irritated, hot, swollen, red, and painful toe. Inflammation is also your body's attempt to get rid of the harmful irritant and start healing. But if there is no clear invader to fight off, for example, in such diseases as arthritis, inflammation ends up causing more harm than good by damaging your tissues and leading to fatigue, pain, and poor sleep and appetite. Many other diseases that you might not think of as inflammatory, because there isn't a visible wound, have been linked to low-grade but chronic inflammation, including obesity, heart disease, cancer, and even depression.

The anti-inflammatory power of yoga helps explain why yoga helps with such a broad range of illnesses, including ones related to "invisible" inflammation. Yoga postures one hour weekly led to higher levels of anti-inflammatory proteins apolipoprotein A1 (ApoA1) and adiponectin after only six weeks.[16] Apolipoprotein A1 is part of "good cholesterol," a high-density lipoprotein (HDL) complex that helps clear cholesterol and fats from artery walls and is anti-inflammatory. ApoA1 protects against heart disease and possibly even Alzheimer's disease. Adiponectin is an anti-inflammatory protein hormone that that helps with blood sugar control and is lower in adults who are overweight or develop diabetes.[17]

There is another group of protein "messengers" called cytokines, which you can imagine as the UPS or FedEx delivery agents of your bloodstream. Different types of cytokines can either signal stopping or starting inflammation. Yoga decreases cytokines that call for more inflammation (proinflammatory), and increases cytokines that stop inflammation (anti-inflammatory). Yoga strengthens your immune system by lowering the stress hormone cortisol and helps produce more of the proteins that defend your body.

How does yoga change the amount of various agents in the body? Researchers have demonstrated that yoga changes a process called gene expression.

Our cells contain DNA, which are the genetic blueprints to make various proteins and molecules that our body needs. Our cells produce proteins and agents based on transcribing specific DNA sections, but not every section needs to be transcribed at all times. Gene expression is similar to how you adjust the flame of your stove or the audio volume on your speakers—sections of your DNA can be turned on or off to produce more or less protein product. This is regulated through a category of molecules called transcription factors, which bind to our DNA and are the traffic controllers of our genome, in charge of turning certain genes on or off.

In one of the largest studies of yoga, researchers found that two hundred breast cancer survivors who did yoga for three months had much lower levels of a specific transcription factor called nuclear factor kappa B.[18] This transcription factor is responsible for turning on parts of the genome that leads to inflammation. This means that yoga is anti-inflammatory because at a molecular level it's changing what genes are turned on and off.

The process seems to be astonishingly rapid. One study found that one sitting of eight hours of meditation could turn off the expression of genes associated with inflammation. This was the first study of its kind.[19]

Yoga Protects Our DNA

Science shows that this protection from stress and aging occurs even at the molecular DNA level. Yoga keeps our cells safe from the wear and tear of natural aging. The tips of our chromosomes are protected by areas called telomeres, which act as bumpers or caps to prevent DNA from unraveling, like the plastic tips at the ends of shoelaces. As we endure physical and mental stress and natural aging, our telomeres erode. Once telomeres are gone, DNA unwinds, leading to cell death.

In a 2015 randomized control study, published in the journal *Cancer*, researchers found that yoga and meditation helped breast cancer survivors maintain telomere length. The study found that breast cancer survivors who went through eight weeks of yoga and meditation maintained their telomere length. In contrast, the group that did a supportive seminar had shortened telomeres. Scientists have also found that meditation twelve minutes a day for eight weeks also increases telomerase, an enzyme that helps maintain telomere length and protects cells from aging. In a small study by Harvard Medical School, blood samples from fifteen meditators who practiced compassion meditation had longer telomeres compared to people who didn't meditate.

When you regularly practice yoga in all its forms—breathing, meditation, and postures—you strengthen your body and your mind. Yoga has an extraordinary ability to help you bounce back physically and mentally, and we are continuing to understand the science behind these changes. Now that you understand the science behind how yoga works, let's introduce you to some fundamental concepts in yoga.

PART II

Getting Started: Yoga Fundamentals

CHAPTER 4

Build Your Foundation

Waking up this morning, I smile. Twenty-four brand new hours are before me. I vow to live fully in each moment and to look at all beings with eyes of compassion.

THÍCH NHẤT HẠNH

Find a comfortable seated position and close your eyes. Take a deep breath in through the nose and focus only on your breath, counting up to five. Exhale and release your breath for five counts. Continue to breathe in and out, listening to your breath and noticing how it feels in your chest, throat, and nose. Notice how your breath sounds.

While you're breathing, you might notice distracting thoughts, such as *What am I going to eat today?* or *What project needs work?* Let those thoughts come and go without entangling yourself with them or following them too closely. If you start to notice critical thoughts, such as "I'm not doing this right," or "should" thoughts, such as *I should be breathing deeper* or *I shouldn't be so distracted*, just notice it, and move on. You don't need to get caught up in them. Even if you do, just gently remind yourself to return your focus back to your breath and don't get down on yourself.

It's a little like being a bystander on a road watching the traffic of thoughts and feelings in your mind pass by. So, don't try to run into traffic or stop or redirect the cars. Just bring your attention back to your breath. And notice and watch.

What did you notice about this experience? Was it difficult and, if so, how? Was it relaxing?

Well, you've just done some yoga.

You may think of yoga as primarily a physical exercise to get your body into certain shapes, but yoga actually encompasses a lot more than that. One of the essential transformative powers of yoga begins with this foundation of what we call awareness, or being nonjudgmental. We will explain these cornerstones of yoga in this chapter; they are fundamental to how we encourage you to approach our 8-week program of yoga breathing, poses, meditation, and self-reflection.

You might notice that many of these foundational concepts in yoga overlap with an approach known as mindfulness. A common definition of mindfulness, as defined by Jon Kabat-Zinn, founder of Mindfulness Based Stress Reduction (MBSR), is "paying attention in a particular way: on purpose, in the present moment, and nonjudgmentally."[1] Mindfulness and yoga have a lot in common because they are rooted in many of the same ancient Eastern traditions.

Here are some important ideas that can help you build a strong and healthy yoga practice.

Awareness: Be Aware

The ability to pay attention to what is happening now and not try to change, escape, or judge is at the heart of yoga. Becoming more aware of your body, mind, and situation is a unique benefit of yoga over just stretching or workouts. It's also an important way to prevent yourself from getting hurt in yoga, as we'll discuss in Chapter 5. This might mean paying attention to your body when poses aren't comfortable and stopping when you feel pain.

After a difficult week, a client asked me, "Do you get how unhappy and frustrated I am?"

What she was asking was whether I could see and acknowledge her suffering. Part of the therapeutic effect of yoga is that it *allows us to acknowledge our own experience, whether it is suffering or joy, fear or hope, uncertainty, or fulfillment.* Yoga gives us the space to experience and sit with ourselves.

The concept of sitting still with our emotions or pain is often all too unfamiliar in the modern age since we are so used to rushing from one event to another, one day to the next. We automatically react by trying to get rid of negative emotions or states. This is the mental equivalent of physiological "flight." We drink coffee when we are tired; take ibuprofen if we have a headache; or might turn to unhealthy ways, such as overeating, drinking, or mindlessly browsing the Internet, to escape difficult situations. Sometimes these coping mechanisms are healthy and work well. But sometimes there are difficult situations that don't get better through distraction or avoidance. Yoga offers a different approach. Yoga isn't trying to distract you or immediately solve your problems. Instead, yoga helps you learn to *just be* and tune into your experience and remind you that it's really important to be kind to yourself.

While these changes sound promising, a skeptic might ask, "Does practicing yoga make actual physical changes beyond better blood pressure and stronger muscles?"

Science brings us proof that yoga can change us on a level that is deeper than just the muscles and joints. The power of awareness has been studied for over a century. Researchers studied progressive muscle relaxation, a technique where you focus and notice muscle tension, in the early 1900s and throughout the 1920s and 1930s. In the 1950s, scientists used electrodes over muscles to show people through visual and auditory feedback when small areas of muscles fired. They found that people could become aware of and voluntarily set off specific microscopic muscle fibers. Throughout the next decades, researchers developed techniques using various instruments to give people biofeedback—from muscle tension to skin temperature to heart rate—to help them address such medical issues as headache, anxiety, and high blood pressure. At the heart of biofeedback was the idea that when you become more aware of your body, you are better able to control it. As a result, biofeedback has been called a form of "Westernized" yoga.

The beauty of yoga is that you don't need to be hooked up to outside instruments to get this information about your body. By becoming connected to and aware of your breath, body, thoughts, and movement, you act as your own instrument. In 1975, Chandra Patel and W. R. S. North published a study of yoga with biofeedback in the top British medical journal, the *Lancet*. They found that yoga with biofeedback lowered blood pressure in people who had high blood pressure. Decades later, these results have been duplicated for people with high blood pressure who do yoga without formal biofeedback as well.

Nonjudgmental Attitude:
Let Go of Self-Judgment, Self-Criticism, and Perfectionism

Yoga helps us become attuned to our individual needs—body and mind—while making room for accepting exactly where we are, without judgment.

The purpose of yoga is not to get your body to twist and bend into a perfect shape.

The fundamental philosophy of yoga encourages you to let go of trying to be "perfect" or "right." There are already so many ways in which we naturally question being "enough," whether at work or at home in our personal lives—questions of being "good enough," "effective enough," "skinny enough," or "attractive enough." In the process of understanding and accepting your body and mind, yoga aims to help you. It's important to note that you always have the option to substitute or skip certain techniques or poses. If a specific pose or breathing exercise is painful, then *don't do it.*

The Present Moment:
Pay Attention to What's Happening *Now*

A concept in yoga and mindfulness is called the present moment. All that means is that you stay attuned to what is happening now around you (such as sounds, smells, sights) or within you, meaning your thoughts, feelings, and reactions. It's really easy for your mind to wander to other times—an argument yesterday with a friend or the work you have on your to-do list for tomorrow. Bringing your attention back to what is going on right now improves your focus as well as prevents feelings that can arise from looking too far into the future (anxiety) or too far into the past (depression).

Self-Compassion:
Practice with Kindness and Patience Toward Yourself

Yoga is built on a foundation of empathy and compassion—and that starts with self-compassion—being able to be generous to yourself first. Notice whether you are holding on to harsh thoughts. Try to weave self-acceptance through your practice. This might mean letting go of the idea of perfection, competition, or the self-critical voice that worries whether you're doing something right. Yoga is not about climbing a ladder to reach the top. It's not about achievement or accomplishment or performance. Instead, when you're feeling frustrated, give yourself compassion and nourish yourself with kindness. This helps you figure out where in your practice you are getting stuck.

A Beginner's Mind: Remain Curious and Open

Sometimes people who are really good at competitive sports can find it challenging to be a beginner. For everyone, even for the most experienced, it is helpful to approach yoga with a beginner's mind. Curiosity and openness are encouraging attitudes so you don't weigh yourself down with competition, achievement, or goals. Simply let your practice be what it is. Be curious, and don't judge yourself for it. No matter how advanced or athletic you are, keep a beginner's mind.

Intentions: Set Your Intention

Setting an *intention* at the beginning of a yoga session helps build awareness, helps bring attention to how you're feeling physically or mentally. What would feel good for your body today? Are you feeling overwhelmed? Are you tired and craving more energy? Do you feel flighty and want to feel more grounded? Stop a moment and reflect on your intention.

> Curiosity and openness are encouraging attitudes so you don't weigh yourself down with competition, achievement, or goals. Simply let your practice be what it is. Be curious, and don't judge yourself for it.

Intentions can be about other people as well. You can form an intention directed toward others, such as dedicating your practice to another person or event. Do you feel sadness for a friend that is going through a hard time? Use your yoga to tune into these feelings and just be with them. Setting an intention gives you the opportunity to use yoga as a way to connect to people or situations around you.

You may want to use setting an intention off the yoga mat, too. For example, when you wake up, think of your intention for the day. How would you like your day to go? Are you hoping to feel more connected or satisfied? If we can imagine our days filled with our individual sense of fulfillment and meaning, we become more open to and aware of experiences that nourish us.

Expectations: Let Go of Expectations

Expectations and intentions are not quite the same thing. Expectations are beliefs that you should or must achieve something. Expectations create anxiety, fear of the future, or disappointment if things don't happen. In contrast, intentions are about creating a sense of focus or purpose. As you prepare for practice, it is good to let go of the belief that you *should* achieve anything in particular or anything at all.

Resilience: Use Challenges
as Opportunities to Practice, and Be Resilient

No journey is ever 100 percent smooth. It's normal to find certain poses challenging. Maybe meditation feels like your kryptonite. If yoga were not challenging, it would not be interesting or an avenue for constant growth. How you approach and handle challenges is more important. Yoga helps you learn to be more mentally flexible and continue to move through unexpected blocks to build resilience.

Trust: Have Courage and Trust Yourself

If yoga is just being aware of how things are now, then will you just be okay with whatever happens and never change or grow? Will you become lazy by being content? Yoga doesn't make us passive in situations that aren't good for us. It puts us in touch with our needs, our feelings, our current situation and gives us the courage to respect and listen to our own voice. Awareness empowers our ability to act in a way that is good for us. When we become more aware that a pose is painful, then we have a choice to be kind to ourselves and free ourselves gently from it. This is true for areas of our lives beyond the mat, too.

Yoga encourages us to be able to hold onto what can seem like two contradictory ideas at once—to become more comfortable with exactly where and who we are and to expand our ability to work toward finding what is right for us. Yoga helps us tolerate the inevitable paradox of being alive, then over time even to welcome life's paradoxes.

Self-Acceptance: Work with Your Body Just as It Is
(a.k.a. There's No Such Thing as a Perfect Yoga Body)

It's really common for certain thoughts to stop you from doing yoga: *What if I'm not flexible? What if I can't do headstands or those challenging balance or twisting poses? Do I need to lose weight first?* Everyone's body is different and unique. Yoga poses can safely be adapted to feel comfortable for a whole range of body shapes, sizes, and levels of flexibility and strength. There are alignment guidelines to help keep poses safe, but poses can and should be tailored to the individual. Props, such as blocks, straps, and blankets, chairs, or the wall, can help you find a version of the pose that is right for *you*.

Your Personal Path:
Continue to Discover What Is Right for You

There is no one-size-fits-all approach in yoga. Yoga embraces our own growth and individuality. While we provide a framework to help you learn yoga in a structured way, our book is by no means the one "right" way to do yoga as there are hundreds of ways of practicing yoga. We provide you with the tools and structure to build your own practice and hope you will continue to discover what is right for you.

Everyone's body is different and unique. Yoga poses can safely be adapted to feel comfortable for a whole range of body shapes, sizes, and levels of flexibility and strength.

CHAPTER 5

How to Prevent Yoga Injuries

> When you are practicing a pose in yoga, can you find the delicate balance between taking the pose to its maximum extent, and taking it beyond that point so that there is too much effort creating wrong tension in the body?
>
> B. K. S. IYENGAR, *THE TREE OF YOGA*

Yoga is generally a safe and healthy way to improve muscle strength, endurance, flexibility, and balance. In a 2015 review of yoga studies from 1975 to 2014, yoga was found to be as safe as walking or stretching exercises, even for people with a wide variety of health issues.[1] That said, it is possible to injure oneself doing yoga. In this chapter we'll look at some basic precautions you can take to limit the likelihood of sustaining an injury while doing yoga.

Most problems that occur during or after yoga, such as muscle soreness or lightheadedness, are not serious and resolve with time, rest, and hydration.[2] The most common injuries in yoga are musculoskeletal soreness or strain, which can be prevented by using many of the principles that we describe in this chapter—warming up, going easy on the body, using proper "alignment," and being careful not to overdo a pose. In Table 5.1, we have summarized these guidelines to help you prevent injuries from yoga.

General Tips to Prevent Injuries

Avoid anything painful—and stop if you feel pain.
If you experience any pain during a pose or exercise, stop immediately and gently shift your body out of that pose or stop the exercise.

Table 5.1 Yoga Safety Guidelines

Preparation Before Practice

1. Avoid eating a large meal before practice; wait at least 2 hours.
2. Hydrate adequately before, to prevent dizziness.
3. Avoid alcohol or other substances before or during practice.
4. Select sequences based on your intention (for instance, whether you want a stimulating or calming effect).
5. If you have a medical condition, consult your physician to find out whether yoga is right for you.

During Practice

1. Warm up with gentle poses.
2. Let go of the idea of perfection.
3. Stay attentive to both body and mind.
4. Check your alignment through bodily awareness and by looking at yourself.
5. Explore different modifications to find the right fit.
6. Use props, such as blankets, blocks, or straps, to modify the pose and protect your joints.
7. Don't continue **anything** painful. If you feel pain during a pose or breathing exercise, **stop**. If it's painful, gently ease your way out of the pose.
8. If you're taking sedative or pain medications, be careful not to go past your limit in poses or stay in a pose too long.

After Your Practice

1. Notice how you feel—both body and mind.
2. Hydrate with water and electrolytes.
3. Practice with consistency.
4. Don't be hard on or judge yourself.

Warm Up Your Body

You should warm up your muscles and joints to prevent injuries. Gentle warm-up exercises let you gradually pump up your heart rate, increase body and muscle temperature, and improve blood flow to your muscles. This means you feed more oxygen to your muscles so that you can process energy better and keep your joints and muscles limber. When you warm up, you can go into deeper poses later without overstretching your muscles.

Your muscles have a reflex that protects them from overstretching. There are stretch receptors in your muscles that have evolved to send feedback to your brain. The more forcefully and rapidly you stretch, the more the muscle contracts to resist the stretch and protect itself. The stretch reflex responds to both force and acceleration. The inverse stretch reflex is an opposite reflex that releases your muscle contraction to protect tendons from being damaged from over-contraction.

These two sets of reflexes balance each other. You can stretch more safely and effectively when you slowly ease into a pose and hold it for at least ten seconds, so that your muscles don't resist you. Transitions between poses should also be gradual and fluid.

Stay Hydrated

You've probably felt lightheaded at some point when you stood up suddenly. If you experience lightheadedness when changing positions in yoga, such as from forward bends to standing poses, this could be caused by a sudden drop in blood pressure that doctors call orthostatic hypotension. This can be worse with dehydration or if you're on certain medications, such as diuretics. So, be sure to stay hydrated before, during, and after yoga. Let your blood pressure adjust more gradually by slowly changing positions.

Take Breaks

It's important to give your body a break from yoga when you're feeling tired or need to rest your muscles. Slow down if you need to. Rest between other poses in Child's Pose (page 112) or a seated pose, such as Hero Pose (page 111).

Pay Attention

If a pose or a breathing exercise or meditation isn't working for you, then stop. What does your body or mind need right now?

We call this important process "being aware" and the adjustments that you make, "listening to yourself." When you pay attention—and then adapt based on what you discover, you prevent injuries.

Are you daydreaming about what you want to eat after yoga? Is your mind wandering to what happened yesterday? With each breath, gently bring your mind back to your pose, breathing, or meditation. If you stop paying attention and become distracted or don't listen to your body's warning signs, then this can lead you to overstretch and hurt yourself.

Use Proper "Alignment"

Alignment, which we will discuss in more detail in Chapter 7, is an important principle to keep yoga poses safe. Alignment is the ideal position of the body in yoga postures that keeps the body stable and safe, especially for your joints and muscles. Alignment is not about perfection, however, and there are many proper variations of alignment for every pose, depending on your individual body. These options help you safely adapt poses to your body, rather than adapting your body to the pose.

Check Your Physical Alignment

Where is your knee in relation to your foot? Are your shoulders creeping up toward your neck?

Physical awareness comes from a combination of proprioception, coordination, and sensory input—that makes up somatic intelligence. There are two ways to check your alignment so as to prevent wear and tear on your muscles and joints.

The first way to check your alignment is simply by looking at your body. Examine how you hold parts of your body relative to one another and where you place your body. For example, you can check where your knee is relative to your ankle in Warrior I Pose or glance back at your arm and hand behind you in Warrior II Pose to make sure they are parallel to the floor. But what if you can't see parts of your body, such as your spine or your shoulders?

The second way of checking alignment is through a sensory skill known as proprioception. Close your eyes and point to the front of the room. Draw a circle with your finger in the air and then touch your nose with your finger. How were you able to know where you finger and nose were without seeing either of them? Through proprioception, your mind internally senses the position of parts of your body relative to one another. Receptors in your muscles and joints send your brain data about your body's position, and its movement and integrates this information with data from your vestibular system in your inner ear so that you can coordinate movement and balance. You can use both visual checking and proprioception to check your alignment throughout your practice. The more you listen to your body, the more your awareness of your body, your somatic intelligence, grows.

Everyone has a different amount of flexibility, and flexibility also varies with each body. One person may be very flexible in the shoulder joint but very tight in the low hamstrings. Some people who are naturally more flexible from loose tendons and ligaments should also be careful, because overstretching can lead to unstable joints, leading to injuries. Every person is different, so it's important to know your own limits to prevent straining or tearing muscle tissue.

Keep a Relaxed Attitude

A relaxed attitude that focuses on what's best for your body is key in yoga, because many yoga teachers have found that being overly competitive or determined to complete a challenging pose, are two of the most common reasons that students hurt themselves while practicing yoga. So, it's important to keep a relaxed attitude that isn't about reaching a certain "level" in yoga. Trying your very hardest to show off in yoga isn't the point.

That attitude can result in injuries if your body isn't ready for the pose or if you go beyond what is safe for your body. Instead, if you're willing to become aware of and acknowledge what feels right for your body, you are making more progress, even if it doesn't look like an "advanced" pose.

> If you're willing to become aware of and acknowledge what feels right for your body, you are making more progress, even if it doesn't look like an "advanced" pose.

Acting from pride or perfectionism leads to injury. A study of over a thousand yoga teachers found that overzealousness was one of the top reasons people hurt themselves in yoga. So, the first important step to make yoga safe is to let go of perfection and loosen your focus on outward appearance or competition for "perfect" form. When you act and move from a place of learning and compassion toward yourself, you're using far more effective and safe tools of yoga, rather than trying to achieve perfection or worry about comparing your pose to how they look in magazines or on social media.

Experiment and Find the Right Modifications for You

It's easy to fall into routine and just try to "get through" a practice. Our body changes from day to day, so today's Downward Facing Dog Pose is not the same one you did yesterday. Don't do the same pose the same way every time just because it's familiar and routine. Experiment to see what different versions of the same pose work best for you in that moment. You can use props, such as blocks, straps, and blankets, to modify poses or cushion your joints. Styles of yoga that emphasize the use of props for proper alignment include Iyengar and restorative yoga.

> Our body changes from day to day, so today's Downward Facing Dog Pose is not the same one you did yesterday. Don't do the same pose the same way every time just because it's familiar and routine. Experiment to see what different versions of the same pose work best for you in that moment.

Select Versions of Poses Based on Your Individual Flexibility and Strength

Your own needs can vary from day to day. Pick a sequence, intention, or version of the pose. For example, if you feel that you have been very self-critical, your intention can be to focus on being gentle toward yourself. Or if you have been feeling sluggish and heavy, your intention may be to have a stimulating practice. If you feel adrift, you may want a calming and grounded practice. You can also combine both energizing (*brahmana*) and calming (*langhana*) elements of yoga to achieve a balancing (*samana*) effect.

Consistency Is Key

Practicing regularly, even in shorter sessions, can help protect your body from injuries because your body awareness and flexibility will improve and you will be less likely to push yourself too far in one session. Shorter, regular sessions are more valuable to build strength, flexibility, and your relaxation response compared to doing yoga for a long period of time intensely but infrequently.

Know What Poses Are Risky When You're Just Starting Out

In a 2013 review of scientific case reports and yoga studies, researchers found that the most commonly cited yoga practices that result in what scientists call adverse events, which includes injuries, are forceful breathing and the poses Lotus, Shoulder Stand, and Headstand.[3] For this reason, we recommend that you work with an experienced certified yoga teacher when first learning those practices or just avoid those practices if you're just starting yoga. There are plenty of other poses to learn—such as the ninety-five poses we have in this book!

Poses such as Plow (Figure 5.1), Shoulder Stand (Figure 5.2), and Headstand (Figure 5.3) pose can be particularly risky for your head and neck area.

We don't teach these poses in our book for this very reason and instead teach alternative Inversion poses with the same effect, such as Supported Shoulder Stand (page 206) or Legs up the Wall (page 207).

Lotus Pose (Figure 5.4) and Double Pigeon Pose (Figure 5.5) can strain your knee and hip joints and require a lot of flexibility of the hip joint. It's not safe to try these poses without first warming up your body. Don't force the pose if you're not flexible enough for it. We don't teach these two poses in our book, and you can get the same effect with other Hip Opener Poses (pages 185–194).

In Table 5.2 we have listed some additional poses that have been associated with injuries.

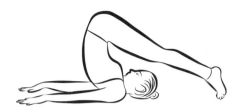

Figure 5.1   Plow Pose.

Guidance from an experienced yoga teacher is recommended for this pose, given risk of strain or injury to neck and shoulders.

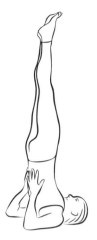

Figure 5.2 Shoulder Stand Pose.

Guidance from an experienced yoga teacher is recommended for this pose, given risk of strain or injury to neck and shoulders.

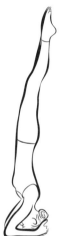

Figure 5.3 Headstand Pose.

Guidance from an experienced yoga teacher is recommended for this pose, given risk of strain or injury to the neck and shoulders.

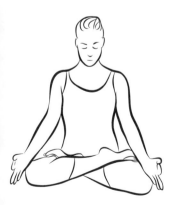

Figure 5.4   Lotus

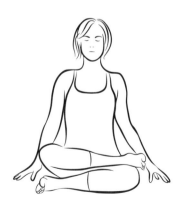

Figure 5.5   Double Pigeon

Table 5.2 Areas of Injury with Associated Poses

Areas of Injury	Associated Poses
Wrist, Hand	Downward Facing Dog, Low Plank, Side Plank, Handstand
Neck	Headstand, Shoulder Stand, Plow, Extended Side Angle, Extended Triangle
Shoulder & Rotator Cuff	Low Plank, Downward Facing Dog, Side Plank, Bow, bound arm variations
Upper Thoracic Spine, Rib Cage	Twists (Revolved Lunge, Revolved Fierce, Revolved Triangle, Revolved Side Angle, Seated Spinal Twist), Backbends (Camel, Upward Facing Dog), Shoulder Stand, Plow, Standing and Seated Forward Bend, Headstand, Handstand
Lower Back, Sacrum	Standing Forward Bend, Seated Forward Bend, Revolved Fierce, Revolved Triangle, Revolved Lunge, Upward Facing Dog, Seated Spinal Twist
Knee	Warrior I, Warrior II, Extended Triangle, Lotus, Half Pigeon, Hero
Hip	Extended Triangle, Half Moon, Warrior I, Warrior II, Half Pigeon, Yogi Squat, Goddess, Lizard, Twists
Groin	Extended Triangle, Goddess, Yogi Squat, Wide-Legged Forward Bend, Low Lunge, Bound Angle, Reclining Bound Angle
Hamstring	Seated Forward Bend, Standing Forward Bend
Lower Leg, Ankle, Foot	Warrior I, Warrior II, Warrior III, High Lunge, Balance (Tree, Eagle, Extended Hand to Big Toe, Revolved Hand to Big Toe), Hero, Lotus
During Pregnancy	Twists (Revolved Triangle, Revolved Side Angle), Inversions, jump-backs, backbends (Camel, Bow, Locust), intense abdominal work, rapid or forceful breathing, breath retention
Eyes	Inversions, (Headstand, Handstand), Standing Forward Bend
Cardiac	Inversions, hot or rapid vinyasa, rapid or forceful breathing
Fall Risk	Headstand, Handstand, Balance (Tree, Eagle, Extended Hand to Big Toe, Revolved Hand to Big Toe)

You may wonder whether Balance Poses (pages 158–168) put you at greater risk of injuries from falling. There are single cases of fall-related injuries during yoga, but they are pretty rare. And one study found that doing yoga regularly doesn't increase your risk for falls or fall injuries.[4] It's also helpful to remember that yoga can help protect people from falls since it improves balance, movement, and coordination.

Diversify Your Yoga and Fitness Routine

It's important to diversify your routines to prevent developing repetitive strain injuries from yoga, which can develop from doing the same movement or sequence over and over or from overuse. So, if you find that you're doing yoga every day for months, it's important to diversify your sequence and try out other forms of exercise, such as biking, running, swimming, or walking. When you build strength in other ways, you're helping prevent injuries from repetitive movements in yoga.

How to Protect Your Joints

According to a survey of yoga teachers, areas of the body most commonly injured are lower back, shoulder, knee, and neck and hamstrings, and less commonly, wrists, hands, hips, and groin. Here are specific ways to help protect your joints in yoga.

Neck

Think of your neck as an extension of your spine. It's important to protect the neck from injury in backbends and inversions. In backbend or "heart opener" poses, such as Cobra, Camel, and Upward Facing Dog Pose (pages 172, 177, and 174), a common mistake is to thrust your head back too far in a misguided effort to shape the pose, but this actually puts unnecessary pressure on your vertebrae. More extreme curvature is not better form. People mistakenly think that a sharper angle in the neck or spine is better. The point is to stretch out these areas so as to bend them, not to bend them so as to stretch them. Protect your neck by focusing on the arch of your thoracic spine instead and focus on broadening the chest by drawing your shoulder blades down and toward each other. This maneuver will help to "open your heart," rather than crunch the cervical vertebrae in your neck. Also, proper sequence is important for backbends. Start with gentler backbends (e.g., Baby Cobra and Cobra Pose, pages 173 and 172) first as a warm-up before moving on to more advanced backbends (e.g., Upward Facing Dog or Camel Pose). For example, Camel Pose should be generally performed only after significant warm-up with prior backbends. Camel Pose can be modified by placing your hands on the lower back or onto your heels with your toes tucked under.

Other poses that can strain your neck are Extended Side Angle Pose (page 146) and Extended Triangle Pose (page 148), so it's important to adjust the neck to a position that doesn't feel strained. We also discuss at the end of this chapter such poses as Plow Pose, Shoulder Stand, and Headstand, which can pose a rare but serious injury related to neck strain.

Wrists

Protect your wrists by making sure your entire hand—palm and fingers—is pressing on the ground in such poses as Downward Facing Dog Pose (page 122) or Side Plank Pose (page 166). Spread your fingers wide to ensure that pressure is distributed evenly on your hands and to take the weight off your wrists. If you have wrist injuries or conditions, such as carpal tunnel syndrome, you can modify such positions as Downward Facing Dog Pose to your forearms, which is Dolphin Pose (page 125), to avoid bearing weight on your wrists. Again, a particular pose is not a "better" pose.

Shoulders

Externally rotate your shoulders in Downward Facing Dog Pose (page 122) to strengthen your external rotator cuff muscles. Make sure your hands are shoulder width apart and that your elbows are not sticking out toward the sides—this places weight unevenly on the inner parts of your hands. Instead, *externally rotate your shoulders so that your elbows creases face forward*, which allows weight to be more evenly distributed between all your fingers on your hand. This also activates your external rotators of your shoulders to help strengthen your rotator cuff and helps prevent future rotator cuff injury.

Release tension in your shoulders: Melt your shoulders away from your ears. Chronic tension can lead to your shoulders creeping up toward your ears. Check your shoulders in such poses as Warrior I Pose (page 140), Warrior II Pose (page 141), or Upward Facing Dog Pose (page 174) to make sure that your shoulders are not hunched or shrugged. Draw your shoulder blades down and toward each other to release tension in your shoulder and neck muscles.

Elbows

Tuck your elbows in toward your ribs when lowering down from High Plank Pose (page 126) to Low Plank Pose (page 127). Don't let your elbows buckle outward. If this does not feel comfortable, try lowering your knees during Low Plank Pose to build your core strength and support your elbows.

When you jump back from Standing Half Forward Bend (page 132) to Low Plank Pose (page 127), make sure your elbows are bent when landing in order to lessen the impact on your elbow and shoulder joint. Avoid landing on a fully extended elbow (i.e., don't jump back and land in High Plank Pose).

Spine and Lower Back

Forward bends, especially twisted forward bends, can be hard on your spine and lower back. It is important, particularly for people with low bone density, to avoid pulling excessively forward with your hands.

First check whether you are able to bend your legs more than 90 degrees toward your torso in Reclining Hand to Big Toe Pose (page 196). If you are not able to bring your legs past 90 degrees toward your torso in this pose comfortably, then you should not try to bend at your hips more than Staff Pose (page 198), such as in Seated Forward Bend (page 199).

Don't use your arms as numb tools to bend your body—they should be sensing and purposeful along with the rest of your body. Instead, first make sure that your tailbone is pointing to the floor.

Do not use yours hands to pull you forward. This can cause your back to round and put severe strain on the spine. Instead, consider keeping your knees soft or bent and focus on the middle of your chest drawing forward toward your thighs so that your torso can rest on your thighs.

In Seated Forward Bend (page 199), try sitting on a folded blanket to tilt the pelvis forward toward the legs. Or broaden the space between your thighs to help prevent excessive flexion of your lumbar spine. The focus should be bending at the hip joint rather than curving your spine.

Knees

When your front knee is bent in standing poses, such as Warrior I Pose (page 140), Warrior II Pose (page 141), or High Lunge Pose (page 145), your knee should be vertically in line with your ankle so that it forms a 90-degree angle. *It's important that your knee is not leaning in toward your ankle.* When your knee is in the knock-kneed position, then your anterior cruciate ligament (ACL) in your knee is more vulnerable and at risk of injury.

Choose modifications for poses to avoid putting strain on your knees. If Half-Pigeon Pose (page 193) feels uncomfortable on your knee, then substitute Reclining Pigeon Pose (page 192).

Cushion your knees if needed. If pressing your knee into the mat for certain poses, such as Low Lunge Pose (page 143), causes pain, use a folded towel or blanket to cushion your knee.

Do not directly apply pressure onto a joint. In such positions as Tree Pose (page 163), avoid pressing directly on your knee with your other foot. Instead, place your foot along either your thigh or your shin.

Hips

In hip opener postures, support your hips with blocks and modifications, particularly if you have tight hips, which is more common in men, or prior hip injuries.

In Lizard Pose (page 190), place blocks under your hands or forearms to help you avoid sinking too deeply into your hips.

In Half Pigeon Pose (page 193), place blocks underneath the thigh of your back leg and your bottom/pelvis to support your hips if they are not able to reach the ground.

In Reclining Bound Angle Pose (page 189), if your knees don't reach the ground, add blocks (or cushions) beneath both bent knees in order to avoid straining your hips.

Jaw Joint

Release your jaw joint: When you are in difficult yoga poses, notice if you are clenching your jaw tightly (this is common!). Chronic stress can cause you to clench your jaw joint and lead to such problems as teeth-grinding and pain in the jaw joint. Loosen your jaw by opening and letting it relax, or flutter your lips to make noise in forward folding poses, such as Standing Forward Bend (page 129) or Wide-Legged Forward Bend (page 134).

What If I Have an Active Medical Condition?

If you are taking a yoga class, it is important to let your yoga teacher or yoga therapist know about any active or recent injuries or medical conditions. If you suffer from medical conditions or are over the age of seventy, then you may be at higher risk of injuries from yoga, and it's important to discuss yoga with your doctor first. As with any activity, it's important to weigh your risks versus benefits to see whether yoga is right for you.

Some medical conditions can make certain poses more risky (see Appendix A for precautions for specific medical conditions), but it really depends on the individual case, so it is important to consult your doctor, physical therapist, or other health professional to see whether yoga or a particular yoga style is the right fit for you and consider working with a yoga therapist who will work with you individually.

Rare but Serious Injuries

In terms of serious injuries from yoga, most are musculoskeletal—ligament tears, fractures, or joint injuries. A less common type of injury during yoga can involve the eye, in people who already have glaucoma, a medical condition of increased pressure within the eye (we describe in Appendix A what to avoid if you have glaucoma). Another uncommon but serious injury is nerve damage to peripheral nerves, leading to weakness, numbness, or tingling. These occur if positions are held for too long, usually because people have fallen asleep accidentally from sedating medications or drugs, but this kind of problem usually does not cause permanent damage.

There are also reports of extremely rare but very serious injuries. The medical literature documents isolated cases of bleeding in the abdominal muscle,[5] a collapsed lung,[6] and three cases of stroke after yoga, which may be due to carotid artery dissection.[7] People with high blood pressure or who smoke are at higher risk for carotid artery dissection. Given the very few cases, more research is needed to find out the risk of stroke during yoga. Poses that may strain the neck in the area of the carotid artery include Plow Pose (Figure 5.1), Shoulder Stand (Figure 5.2), and Headstand (Figure 5.3), where the neck bears much of your body weight in a forward flexed position.

For these reasons, we do not teach these poses in our program (we teach a modified version of Shoulder Stand [page 68] that puts far less pressure on the neck). If you are interested in these poses, we encourage you to work in person with a certified yoga teacher.

✦

These guidelines aim to help you prevent any injuries in yoga. We encourage you to come back to these guidelines regularly to remind yourself of how to prevent injuries as you build your practice.

PART III

Build Your Yoga Practice

CHAPTER 6

Breathe More, Breathe Better: Yoga Breathing (Pranayama)

Smile, breathe and go slowly.

THÍCH NHẤT HẠNH

Pranayama is the heart of Yoga. Yoga is lifeless without Pranayama.

B. K. S. IYENGAR

The quality of our breath expresses our inner feelings.

T. K. V. DESIKACHAR

Think back to the last time you felt frustrated, upset, or overwhelmed. Were you holding your breath? Did you feel like you had stopped breathing, or that your breath was "taken away"? When you feel overwhelmed, frustrated, scared, or angry, your breath becomes fast and shallow, seeming out of control. Breath is the pulse of the mind. Tuning in to the sound of our breath calms the feeling of chaos and frenzy and slows the wheels of churning negative thoughts. When we observe and listen to our breath, we start to create some space around our fear and frustration. Breath is an important cornerstone to connecting with our body and grounding our mind.

According to many yoga traditions, breath is an essential part of yoga and is associated with life force or energy, called *prana*. Breathing techniques in yoga are called *pranayama* in Sanskrit. *Prana* is breath or vital energy in the body, and *ayama* means to stretch, extend, stop, expand, or lengthen. The root word *yama* means to rein or drive and has also been translated as "control." Different yoga breathing techniques can be heating or cooling, energizing or relaxing, rapid or slow. Changing your breath with intention and attention is sometimes called "disciplining" or "controlling" the breath, but those words can imply force, struggle, or dominance. Instead, think of these breathing exercises as a way of *directing* or *expanding* your breath. Breath should begin self-compassion and self-acceptance.

It may be surprising that breath is such an important part of yoga. Much of yoga in the United States focuses on fitness and postures, leaving breath as an aside. But yoga breathing has been an important part of yoga for thousands of years. In yoga traditions across the world, breath is at the center of yoga practice. Breath is considered *the* path toward self-reflection, self-transformation, and self-realization.[1] In such traditions as Iyengar and Ashtanga yoga, breathing is taught only after familiarity with postures.

Breath has an inextricable relationship with energy. Inhalation is metaphorically seen as drawing energy in and exhalation is a release of energy. Yoga breathing can be energizing or relaxing, heating or cooling, depending on the type of breath. You can choose which breathing techniques you want to do, based on how you feel day to day. If you find that you are tired in the morning, do breathing exercises that energize the body. If you are having difficulty falling asleep at the end of a long day, try breathing exercises that relax the body.

You can use your breath several ways in yoga. Breath can connect your movement with meditation by creating a focus for your energy. You can use your breath to deepen postures and keep them active. You can use breath to ease into poses more gently and to pace Sun Salutation or sequence of posture. Your breath awareness helps prepare your mind for meditation. You can do breathing techniques in separate daily sessions. Regardless of how you choose to practice yoga breathing, the more you practice, the more your attention and awareness of your breath will grow. Physiological studies suggest that healthy people need to practice, at minimum, ten weeks of breathing techniques to be able to make a noticeable improvement in their lung capacity, and longer sessions are more helpful in improving lung function.[2]

Models of Yoga Breathing

Historically, there are two main models of yoga breathing. In classical yoga, outlined in Patanjali's *Yoga Sutras*, yoga breathing is the fourth limb of the eight limbs of yoga. Whereas earlier levels of breathing techniques are more controlled, the goal of breathing practice in classical yoga is to achieve a more natural way of breathing.[3] The purpose of yoga breathing is to calm the fluctuations of the mind. In this model, you allow yourself to follow your breath.

A second model comes later from hatha yoga, a tradition of yoga described by Svatmarama Yogindra in the *Hatha Yoga Pradipika* (Light on Forceful Yoga). In the *Hatha Yoga Pradipika*, the breath is important to prepare and steady the mind, "When the breath is steady or unsteady, so is the mind, and with it the yogi. Hence, the breath should be controlled."[4] Breathing as a way to gather and direct energy among the chakras in the body—you guide your breath.

Yoga Breathing Components

Your breath has four components: (1) inhalation ("in-breath"), (2) a pause after inhalation, (3) exhalation ("out-breath"), and (4) a pause after your exhalation. The pauses between your inhalation and exhalation are called "retention" or "suspension" (*kumbhaka* in Sanskrit). The number of times of breathing cycles is called *samkhya*.

Just as there is a pause at the end of a pendulum's arc, there is a natural pause between the in-breath and the out-breath, and between the out-breath and the in-breath. The pause after inhalation is sometimes referred to as being at the top of your breath, while the pause after exhalation is called being at the bottom of your breath. Retention occurs naturally and can also be prolonged on purpose; for example, during rhythmic yoga breathing exercises. Our exercises gradually extend the pause after inhalation, since prolonging the pause after exhalation is more challenging. Over time, the more you practice breath control, the longer your total breath cycle naturally expands. Your respiratory rate becomes slower. Some yoga traditions believe that the whole science of yogic breath control is learning breath retention.

Table 6.1   Parts of the Breath

Breath Part	Inhalation	Pause after inhalation	Exhalation	Pause after exhalation
Sanskrit	*Puraka*	*Antara Kumbhaka*	*Rechaka*	*Bahya Kumbhaka*
Action	Even, continuous breath through the nose	Breath retention	Smooth, continuous exhalation through the nose	Suspension, or holding the breath out
Also known as	In-breath	"Top of the inhale"	Out-breath	"Bottom of the exhale"
Energy Theory	Absorption of energy	Union of the universal and individual self	Surrender of energy	Union of the individual and universal self

In yoga, breath has a location and direction in your body. Since breath imbues energy or life force, your breath can conceptually direct energy or your life force *prana* throughout your body. You can in your mind "send your breath" to a specific area of the body, which also helps you focus attention on parts of your body. Using your breath to direct your energy intentionally throughout your body is a key part of breathing as a form of meditation.

Breaths can be cooling or warming, calming or energizing.

Breathing is also a form of free expression—an unblocked, uncensored, and liberating way to express yourself, which is represented by the throat chakra. As you try different yoga breathing techniques, you will discover how breathing affects your mood, body, and mind.

Breaths can be cooling or warming, calming or energizing. Does it make you calmer or more energized? Does it heat or cool your body? Do you feel more grounded or airy?

Breathing is another method in yoga that helps us connect our body and mind, build more awareness, assess, and honor our individual needs. The style of your breath, whether you keep your mouth closed or open, its rhythm, and its effects on your body and mind will vary based on the breathing technique. As you begin

Using your breath to direct your energy intentionally throughout your body is a key part of breathing as a form of meditation.

to feel the effects of different yoga breathing techniques on your body and mind, you will then be able to select breathing techniques based on how you feel and what you seek. Breathing exercises also help you be more aware of your facial muscles. Notice whether you are frowning, grimacing, or furrowing your brow. Try to relax your facial muscles during breathing exercises.

If you're a very goal-directed person, it may be challenging to feel that there is a value in just breathing. As with much of yoga, the value of breathing practice requires a bit of a leap of faith and requires consistent, regular practice to experience its effects over time. Modern science continues to provide evidence that supports the power of breath to improve our health and wellness.

The Science of Breath

In *A Treatise on the Yoga Philosophy* published in 1851, N. C. Paul observed that yogis practiced in a cave, or *gupha*, and lined the entrance of the cave with clay, grass, or cotton, sealing themselves off during practice like a hibernating bear. He noted that in the confined space of a cave, the yoga practitioner exhaled less carbon dioxide compared to fresh air, creating a shift in respiratory gases in the body. Modern-day scientists have confirmed Paul's theory. Hibernating animals build up carbon dioxide in their bodies in a den and subsequently slow their metabolism. Similarly, practicing yoga breathing in a cave would lead to a rise in carbon dioxide levels. Higher levels of carbon dioxide cause our blood vessels to dilate, leading to an increase in blood flow and oxygen delivery throughout the body, including our brain and muscles. This probably explains why it can feel oddly more "refreshing" to practice in a closed, small, crowded yoga studio compared to doing yoga alone on an open beach with fresh air, though that has a separate appeal.

Yoga Breathing Raises Carbon Dioxide Levels, Which Is (Surprisingly) Good

This carbon dioxide model contradicts a common myth in yoga that yoga breathing is good because we breathe in more oxygen. Our natural breathing rate is generally determined by the amount of carbon dioxide in our bloodstream. At rest, healthy adults breathe between ten and twenty cycles a minute. The effect of yoga breathing is not actually from increasing oxygen in our body, since our regular levels of oxygen saturation are already very high. If we are healthy, our hemoglobin, which carries and transports oxygen, is saturated between 95 and 100 percent. Small fluctuations in oxygen do not account for the effects of yoga breathing. Breathing techniques don't change our oxygen consumption, which is instead increased by such activities as cardiovascular exercise. Rapid and slowed yoga breathing does, however, change our *carbon dioxide* levels. When we intentionally speed up or slow down our breathing, we are actually manipulating our carbon dioxide levels, which in turns either constricts or expands our blood vessels.

Slowed yoga breathing, such as Victorious Breath, which for advanced yogis can be ten times slower than the normal breath, doubles our carbon dioxide levels. This, in turn, dilates our blood vessels, so that our brain can receive more blood flow and more oxygen. As early as the 1930s, Kovoor T. Behanan studied the effect of yoga breathing, specifically Victorious Breath, on mental processes.[5] He found that slowed yoga breathing caused the mind to become slowed, even slowing math calculations.

In contrast, rapid yoga breathing, such as Breath of Fire and Bellows Breath, drops carbon dioxide levels, since we're rapidly replenishing ourselves with fresh air that contains very little carbon dioxide. When our carbon dioxide levels drop quickly, our blood vessels contract, leading to a drop in oxygen to the brain. In other words, what we commonly know as hyperventilation can lead to lightheadedness, dizziness, blurry vision, and even fainting.

Yoga Breathing Lowers Blood Pressure

Slow and deep breathing ("paced breathing," similar to rhythmic breathing exercises) has been shown to lower blood pressure in people with high blood pressure in several studies.[6] Slowed, deep techniques of yoga breathing directly affects our heart rate and blood pressure by stimulating the vagus nerve. The vagus nerve, named for its wandering "vagrant" branches, is the longest cranial nerve, starting at the base of the brain and branching into several nerves that run through your neck, chest, and abdomen. The vagus nerve connects your brain to your heart, lungs, liver, stomach, and kidneys and is responsible for your parasympathetic "rest and digest" nervous system. It is in charge of relaxing and calming your body, lowering your heart rate and blood pressure, and relaxing muscles, such as your larynx. This explains why, when you're really nervous, your throat closes up, your chest tightens, your stomach churns, and you feel as if you can't speak.

One way to measure how well your body handles stress, or how "toned" your vagus nerve is, is by measuring your heart rhythm in terms of *heart rate variability*. Heart rate variability is the ability of your heart to change beat to beat. If you are healthy, when you breathe in deeply, your heart rate naturally speeds up. When you exhale, your heart rate naturally slows down. *High* heart rate variability is healthy. It means that your body is resilient in responding to the demands of stress or changes in your environment. On the other hand, people with diabetes or heart disease, as well as people who smoke, have lower heart rate variability compared to healthy people. Lower heart rate variability has been linked to higher rates of sudden death.

Yoga, including yoga breathing, has been found to *increase* heart rate variability—indicating that yoga breathing boosts our ability to handle stress in a healthy manner. Yoga breathing practiced routinely for six to eight weeks has been shown to reduce stress, fatigue, and sadness as well as improve feelings of social connectedness and gratitude.[7]

Yoga Breathing Energizes or Calms

What about such techniques as alternate nostril breathing or one-nostril breathing? According to ancient yoga texts, the right nostril is associated with the sun (*surya*), whereas the left nostril is associated with the moon (*ida*): Airflow through your right nostril is activating and energizing, whereas airflow through your left nostril is calming. Uninostril (one-nostril) yoga breathing shifts your breath through only one nostril—right or left—depending on your intended effect. Is there science behind why breathing through right or left nostrils would make a difference? Alternate nostril and one-nostril breathing can sound like superstition or pseudo-science, but, again, there are modern research studies that lend some scientific support for this ancient theory.

As background, we don't breathe evenly through our nostrils. Our breath naturally has a dominant nostril, which can shift and alternate every few hours. Want to figure out which nostril is dominant right now? Take a pocket mirror, and hold it under your nose. (You can refrigerate the mirror for a few minutes to make sure it's cool enough to form condensation.) Exhale through your nose onto the mirror so that condensation forms on the mirror under both nostrils. The side of condensation that disappears last is the dominant nostril at that time. Repeat this in the morning, noon, and night to find out how your dominant nostril varies throughout the day.

In a 2014 study, researchers in India compared two groups of healthy young adults—daily for one hour for six weeks, one group did left nostril breathing, while another group did right nostril breathing.[8] At the end of six weeks, the group who did right nostril breathing had *higher* resting heart rates and blood pressure as well as signs of a more activated fight-or-flight stress system, or sympathetic nervous system, compared to when the group first started. In contrast, the left nostril breathing group had *lower* resting heart rates and blood pressure after six weeks. In other words, right nostril breathing did activate the nervous system, even when people were not actively practicing the breathing technique, and left nostril breathing was more calming—exactly what ancient yoga theory predicts. Alternate nostril breathing, which is a calming yoga breath, has also been linked to lower blood pressure and heart rate in normal healthy people as well as people with high blood pressure.[9]

Why would your body react to right and left nostril breathing so differently? Scientists don't have an anatomical or physiological explanation yet. One possibility is that breathing through one nostril activates different parts of the brain. Researchers have use different methods, including infrared spectroscopy and electroencephalography (EEG) to look at what part of the brain becomes more active during right and left nostril breathing. In one spectroscopy study, researchers found that right nostril breathing increased oxygenation and blood volume in the left prefrontal cortex of the brain, whereas left nostril breathing and breath awareness did not. In EEG studies, right nostril breathing activates the left hemisphere.[10] Another possibility may be that forced breathing through right or left nostrils activates your vagus nerve differently because of its asymmetrical anatomy.

Yoga Breathing Protects Brain Size

What we do know is that regular yoga breathing practices, along with postures and meditation, have been shown to protect our brain from the natural decline in brain size due to aging. Our brain and nervous system are malleable and trainable, even in adults. It's what scientists call *neuroplasticity*, or the ability of our brain to form and strengthen new neural connections throughout our life. Yoga strengthens areas of your brain associated with such emotions as joy, self-awareness, and relaxation. Meditation studies—and breath is a form of meditation—have shown that with meditation, brain areas related to fear and anxiety shrink.

Yoga Breathing Releases Tension and Stress

You have probably also noticed that it can feel good to sigh, and this can be integrated in yoga while seated or during such postures as forward folds. Sighs are deep, long breaths that can express sadness, relief, or being tired. But sighing is not merely expressive; it is critical to life and based on reflexes and neuronal circuits[11] that exist from a very early age—even newborns have the reflex to sigh. When we breathe in the same pattern for too long, our lungs get stiff and less efficient. Sighs occur spontaneously every few minutes as a way to loosen—to stretch and reinflate—the tiny balloonlike air sacs in our lungs. Sighs instill a sense of relief. Lion's Breath, which is effective to release tension and stress, is a more forceful and intense version of sighing and can be used in a variety of poses or while seated. But you can also simply sigh in between your yoga breathing exercises to find some relief.

Cautions for Yoga Breathing

Yoga breathing, particularly the calming techniques, is generally safe for healthy people. Most yoga breathing techniques engage your diaphragm and abdominal muscles, so it's best to practice on an empty stomach before meals. It's important to note that yoga breathing should not be painful. If you feel pain, stop immediately.

If you have a cold or nasal congestion, wait to practice yoga breathing until you've recovered. If you feel lightheaded or dizzy during yoga breathing, you should also stop because you may be hyperventilating and should allow your breathing to return to normal.

If you are pregnant, you should avoid breath retention and any rigorous, forceful, or rapid breathing exercises, such as Bellows Breath and Breath of Fire. People with panic disorder or high levels of anxiety, including chronic post-traumatic stress disorder, should be careful when practicing deep or rapid breath techniques. Such breathing exercises may cause your body to be overstimulated, which can, in turn, trigger a panic attack or worsen anxiety. If you have respiratory illnesses, such as asthma or emphysema, or cardiovascular conditions, such as high blood pressure, check with your physician first before trying yoga breathing and review our chapter on yoga safety.

Now, with that long introduction behind us, let's begin, shall we?

Seated Posture

Breathing techniques should be done in a comfortable seated position. If you are able to sit on the floor, sit in Easy Pose or Hero Pose to prepare yourself for yoga breathing. If you have tight hips, you can sit on folded blankets or a block so that your knees are even or lower than your hips. You can also place blankets underneath your knees in Easy Pose to support your hips. In Hero pose, you can sit on a block. If you have discomfort from these poses from groin or knee injuries, try sitting upright in a chair.

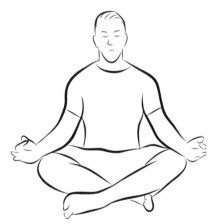

Figure 6.1

Easy Pose for Breathing Exercises

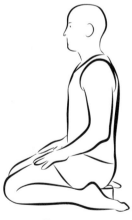

Figure 6.2

Hero Pose modified with block for Breathing Exercises

In your seated posture, your spine should be tall and erect so that your head is positioned directly over your shoulders. Your head, neck, and trunk are aligned so that there is a central line from the base of your pelvis to the crown of your head. Your chest and rib cage are gently lifted. Finally, relax your shoulders away from your ears. If you have difficulty maintaining this alignment, you can use a wall for support for your back.

A word here about Lotus Pose: Lotus Pose is the pose everyone associates with yoga, in which you sit cross-legged on the floor, with your feet resting on the top of your opposite thighs. It is an advanced posture that requires a lot of hip flexibility, is often uncomfortable for many people, and has been associated with a higher rate of injuries compared to other poses, so it is not recommended unless you have comfortably done it before. For some, Lotus Pose can take on a kind of status symbol, a sign you're "doing it right" or even excelling. But this kind of thinking comes from the ego, and there's no evidence that Lotus Pose leads to "better" yoga. We encourage finding a comfortable posture. Sit up tall. Pay attention to six points in your body before you get started: your bottom, legs, hands, neck and spine, jaw, and your eyes. All of them should feel stable and comfortable. You can choose to close your eyes or gaze softly straight ahead.

Yoga Breathing Techniques

After you get used to paying attention to your breath, you are now ready for breathing techniques that intentionally direct and expand your breath. Full breathing includes awareness of all four stages of the breath and can relax the entire body. These breathing techniques engage your diaphragm, the large, dome-shaped muscle in your abdomen that draws the lungs open to allow us to breathe. On the inhalation, the diaphragm drops lower in the abdomen and creates space for your lungs to expand. When you exhale, the diaphragm rises and pushes air out from your lungs. By engaging your diaphragm, rather than just your chest and rib cage muscles, you get a fuller breath. The fundamental underlying principle of yoga breathing is to help focus your awareness of your mind and body—it is not about getting perfect rhythms or ratios or trying to hold your breath the longest that you can. In general, if you're looking to feel more active, expand your inhalation. If you're looking to calm down, lengthen your exhalation.

A common misconception of "deep" breathing is that you must do it with a severe intensity or extreme effort for it to "work." Sometimes people will breathe in so deeply or with so much force that the exercise can be uncomfortable or even painful. This ends up stimulating your body's fight-or-flight response and you'll feel more anxious and upset, which runs counter to the point of calming types of breathing exercises. The techniques for calming and stress relief are not intended to activate your fight-or-flight response, so if you're uncomfortable or in pain, relax and ease your breath, regardless of whether you've made it to the "right" number of counts or the "right" depth of breathing.

There are several types of yoga breathing techniques, many of which you can do at home on your own. If you are new to yoga breathing, we recommend seeking a yoga teacher before trying more advanced yoga breathing, since such techniques as Breath of Fire and Bellows breath are safer when done with supervision and guidance.

Awareness Breaths

These breaths help you mentally focus and feel your breath physically. These breaths are useful to help you improve your concentration, reduce distraction, and settle your mind. Use them at the beginning of your separate breathing sessions or before you do yoga postures.

Simple Breath Awareness

Let's start with an exercise that develops breath awareness. In this exercise, you do not have to intentionally change or manipulate your breath—just pay attention to it. When we tune into our breath, our attention alone can smooth our breathing. Breath awareness is a form of simple meditation.

Three-Part Breath (Dirga Swasam Pranayama)

Three-part breath is expansive, calming, and reduces stress and anxiety. It's useful to do at the end of the day to wind down. This simple breath exercise is good for beginners.

Lie down on your back in Corpse or Reclining Bound Angle Pose. If you feel lower back tension, you can place your feet close to your tailbone hip distance apart. Keep your spine long and relaxed on the ground. You can relax your arms alongside your torso or place one hand on your chest and the other on your abdomen. As you inhale, imagine the breath filling up your lungs from your abdomen, to your rib cage, and then upward to your chest. As you exhale, visualize your breath being released from the top of your lungs, all the way down to your abdomen. You should feel the rise and fall of your chest and abdomen with each breath, like gentle waves on an ocean.

Table 6.2 Yoga Breathing (*Pranayama*) Techniques

Level (1 to 3)	Breath	*Sanskrit Name*	Purpose	Used with Poses	Avoid With
Expanding Awareness					
1	Breath Awareness	•	Awareness, focus	Easy, Hero, Corpse	Generally safe
1	Three-Part Breath	*Dirga Swasam*	Awareness, mind-body connection	Easy, Hero, Corpse	Respiratory conditions
Grounding					
1–3	Rhythmic or Ratio Breathing Even Breathing Uneven or Irregular Breathing	*Savitri Sama Vrtti Visama Vrtti*	Focus, awareness, relaxation	Seated (Easy, Hero)	Respiratory conditions
1	Victorious, a.k.a. Ocean	*Ujjayi*	Focus, attention, heating energy in the body, connecting movement and postures	Resting and during transition of poses	Respiratory conditions
Calming					
1	Humming Bee	*Bhramari*	Calming	Seated	Respiratory conditions
2	Alternate Nostril Breath	*Nadi Shodhan*	Calming	Seated (Easy, Hero)	Sinus and upper respiratory conditions
2	Left Nostril Breath	*Chandra Nadi*	Calming	Seated (Easy, Hero)	Sinus and upper respiratory conditions
1	Lion's Breath	*Simhasana*	Release energy tension in face/neck	Seated, Reclined Hero, Downward Facing Dog, Reverse Plank, Camel	Respiratory conditions
Cooling					
2	Tongue Hissing	*Shitali*	Cooling	Seated	Respiratory conditions
2	Teeth Hissing	*Sitkari*	Cooling	Seated	Respiratory conditions
Energizing					
3	Breath of Fire* Skull Shining Breath*	*Kapalabhati*	Heating	Seated, Yogi Squat, Goddess	Pregnancy, anxiety, asthma, respiratory issues, hernia, glaucoma, high blood pressure, epilepsy
3	Bellows Breath*	*Bhastrika*	Activating	Seated, Yogi Squat, Goddess	Pregnancy, anxiety, asthma, respiratory issues, hernia, glaucoma, high blood pressure, epilepsy

*Do these breathing techniques with guidance of a yoga teacher, for safety reasons.

Table 6.3 Simple Breath Awareness

Simple Breath Awareness
1. Sit in a comfortable position or lie down.
2. Close your eyes and let your body relax, summoning self-acceptance.
3. Start to notice your breath. What does your breath feel like? Is it rushed or calm? Is your breath loud or soft? Does it feel warm or cool?
4. As you inhale through your nose, say to yourself "Breathing in, I observe breathing in."
5. As you exhale through your nose, say to yourself "Breathing out, I observe breathing out."
6. Continue to follow your in-breath and out-breath. Let your breath deepen.
7. After observing your breath for a five to ten cycles, your breath will automatically become slower, smoother, and feel more natural.
8. You can continue for as long as you feel comfortable, anywhere between a few minutes to half an hour.

Table 6.4 Three-Part Breath

Three-Part Breath
1. Sit in a comfortable position or lie down on your back. This technique may be easier when lying on your back in such poses as Corpse or Reclining Bound Angle.
2. Close your eyes and let your body relax, summoning self-compassion.
3. Place one hand on your abdomen and the other in the center of your chest. You can also keep your arms relaxed alongside your torso as well.
4. Focus your attention on a point a few fingers below your navel.
5. Begin to notice your breath.
6. Breathe in softly and feel your abdomen expand.
7. Continue to inhale, filling your abdomen, to your rib cage, and up to your chest. As you inhale through your nose, say to yourself, "I breathe in, filling up with breath."
8. Breathe out slowly and relax the chest naturally. Continue to exhale downward, feeling your rib cage and then your abdomen relax and sink inward. As you exhale through your nose, say to yourself, "I breathe out, emptying out breath."
9. Rest for a few seconds and continue the next cycle of breath.
10. Continue to follow your in-breath and out-breath for 10 more cycles, noticing the natural expansion and contraction of your abdomen and chest muscles.

Grounding Breaths

Rhythmic (Savitri) or Ratio (Vrtti) Breathing

Rhythmic, or ratio, yoga breathing deliberately paces and sets the length of your inhalation, retention, and exhalation. In these exercises, inhale and exhale through your nose. Ratio breathing can be divided into two types: even breathing (*sama vrtti*), in which the length of each part of the breath is the same, or uneven breathing (*visama vrtti*), in which inhalation and exhalation vary.

You will keep count of your inhalations and exhalations by counting or by repeating syllables or phrases. In Table 6.5, we also offer some examples of phrases that you can repeat in your mind to pace yourself during rhythmic breathing exercises. Breathing counts can also be combined with other techniques, such as alternate nostril breath.

If you are a beginner, start with even breathing, keeping inhalations and exhalations the same count without adding a pause in between (e.g., 4 seconds inhalation, 4 seconds exhalation). Continue even breathing cycles and continue to expand your breath for longer periods of time.

Once you are comfortable with even breathing for longer breaths, try introducing uneven breathing by gradually extending your exhalation so that it's longer than your inhalation. After this becomes comfortable, add breath retention after inhalation. Over the course of several months and even years, you can gradually advance your rhythmic breathing by extending each part of the breath, and add parts of the breath, such as the retention after inhalation and then retention at the end of exhalation. Make sure that you do what feels comfortable for your body.

The primary goal of this yoga breathing exercise is not to develop a certain length or ratio of breathing, or even to slow the breath, but to allow the mind to be aware and focused on the breath. In our breathing exercise ratios, we do not specify how long to hold the breath out since adding suspension after exhalation is traditionally considered more difficult and advanced. Instead, resume your inhalation for the next breathing cycle when you feel ready—how long you wait between cycles of your breath is up to you and what feels comfortable.

The traditional notation for rhythmic breathing counts uses punctuations like dashes or colons. Dashes typically indicate the numbers of counts or seconds for each part of the breath: inhalation ("in-breath"), retention (a pause "at the top of the breath" with lungs filled), and exhalation ("out-breath"). For example, 1-4-2 means to inhale for 1 second, pause and retain the breath for 4 seconds, then exhale for 2 seconds. Colons between indicate the ratio of each part of the breath. For example, 1:4:2 is a ratio of parts of the breath (inhalation: retention: exhalation), such as 2 seconds inhalation, 8 seconds retention, and 4 seconds

Table 6.5   Rhythmic (*Savitri*) or Ratio (*Vrtti*) Breathing Exercises

Rhythmic or Ratio Yoga Breathing	Ratio of Inhale *Retention: Exhale: Optional Retention*	Instructions (s = seconds)	Variations (s = seconds)	Example Phrases to Repeat in Your Mind
Beginner Level 1	1:0:1	Inhale 4s, exhale 4s	3s in, 3s out (easier) 6s in, 6s out (harder)	"I breathe in, I breathe out."
Beginner Level 2	1:0:1.5	Inhale 4s, exhale 6s	3s in, 5s out (easier) 6s in, 9s out (harder)	"I breathe in, I breathe out and let go."
Beginner Level 3	1:0:2	Inhale 4s, exhale 8s	3s in, 6s out (easier) 5s in, 10s out (harder)	"I am breathing in. I am breathing out and letting go."
Beginner Level 4	1:0.5:1	Inhale 4s, hold 2s, exhale 4s	3s in, 1s hold, 3s out 5s in, 2s hold, 5s out 6s in, 3s hold, 6s out	"I breathe in to fill with breath. I retain my breath. I breathe out to empty my breath."
Beginner Level 5	1:1:1	Inhale 4s, hold 4s, exhale 4s	3s in, 3s hold, 3s out 5s in, 5s hold, 5s out 6s in, 6s hold, 6s out	"I breathe in, observing my breath. I retain my breath to focus. I breathe out, observing my breath."
Intermediate Level 1	1:1:2	Inhale 4s, hold 4s, exhale 8s	3s in, 3s hold, 6s out 5s in, 5s hold, 10s out	"Breathing in, I calm my mind. Pausing, my mind and body become one. Breathing out, I calm my mind and release any negative energy."
Intermediate Level 2	1:2:1	Inhale 4s, hold 8s, exhale 4s	3s in, 6s hold, 3s out 5s in, 10s hold, 5s out	"Breathing in, I fill up with breath. Pausing, I retain my breath and connect my body and mind. Breathing out, I empty my breath."
Intermediate Level 3	1:2:2	Inhale 4s, hold 8s, exhale 8s	3s in, 6s hold, 6s out 5s in, 10s hold, 10s out	"Breathing in, I let go. I retain my breath to concentrate my body and mind. Breathing out, I let go and am aware of my whole body and mind."
Advanced Level 1*	1:2:2:1	Inhale 4s, hold 8s, exhale 8s, pause 4s	5s in, 10s hold, 10s out, 5s pause	"Breathing in, I feel calm and peaceful. I pause to observe my whole body and mind. Breathing out, I feel calm and peaceful. I pause to connect with my body and mind."

*These levels should be done with the guidance of a yoga teacher.   *(continued)*

Table 6.5   Rhythmic (*Savitri*) or Ratio (*Vrtti*) Breathing Exercises (*continued*)

Rhythmic or Ratio Yoga Breathing	Ratio of Inhale *Retention: Exhale: Optional Retention*	Instructions (s = seconds)	Variations (s = seconds)	Example Phrases to Repeat in Your Mind
Advanced Level 2*	1:2:2:2	Inhale 4s, hold 8s, exhale 8s, pause 8s	5s in, 10s hold, 10s out, 10s pause	"I inhale and free my mind. I retain my breath, letting feelings or thoughts pass. I exhale and free my mind completely."
Advanced Level 3*	1:3:2	Inhale 4s, hold 12s, exhale 8s	3s in, 9s hold, 6s out	"Breathing in, I feel joy. I retain my breath and concentrate my whole body and mind. Breathing out, I feel joy."
Advanced Level 4*	1:4:2	Inhale 4s, hold 16s, exhale 8s	3s in, 12s hold, 6s out	"I breathe in and fill with peace. I retain my breath to concentrate, calm, and connect to my body and mind. I breathe out and free my mind and observe letting go completely."
Advanced Level 5*	1:4:2:2	Inhale 4s, hold 16s, exhale 8s, pause 8s	3s in, 12s hold, 6s out, 6s pause	"Breathing in, I observe a feeling of peace and joy. I retain my breath and feel peace and joy. Breathing out, I observe emptying my breath. I keep my breath emptied and observe feeling whole."

*These levels should be done with the guidance of a yoga teacher.

10-MINUTE DAILY BREATHING EXERCISE

1. Start with Simple Breath Awareness (Table 6.3) for 5 cycles.
2. Do Three-Part Breath (Table 6.4) for 5 cycles.
3. Next, do 10 cycles of even breathing (Table 6.5) at a ratio that you are comfortable with, such as 1:0:1.
4. Then, do 10 cycles of uneven breathing (Table 6.5), such as 1:0:2.
5. Return back to Simple Breath Awareness for 5 cycles.

exhalation. For more advanced breathing, the fourth part of the breath, or retention after exhalation, is added. The four-part breath ratio notation of 1:4:2:1 means 2 seconds inhalation, 8 seconds retention, 4 seconds exhalation, and 2 seconds retention at the end of your exhalation. (Why is it not written as 2:8:4:2? Because we always reduce to the lowest common denominator.)

Breath awareness and rhythmic breathing techniques can be combined in a single session of yoga breathing for as little as ten to fifteen minutes a day.

Victorious (Ocean) Breath (Ujjayi)

Victorious Breath is commonly used during yoga postures and should fill your room with the sound of the ocean. This breath is slow, calming, and quiets the mind. It should be loud enough that people next to you would hear your breathing. When you listen to your breath, you will also find that it can drown out the distracting thoughts in your mind. Victorious Breath also stirs energy in the body, keeps the mind focused when you hold yoga poses, and can be used to pace the flow in a sequence of poses.

Victorious Breath can also be combined with *bandhas* or muscle contractions: root lock (*Mula Bandha*) and abdominal lock (*Uddiyana Bandha*). This means that on the inhalation, the pelvic floor and abdominal muscles are drawn inward and upward, directing your breath into the upper chest. But wait to add these muscle locks in after you are more comfortable with Victorious Breath. (Chapter 8 is devoted to Muscle Locks.)

Table 6.6   Victorious (Ocean) Breath (*Ujjayi*)

1.	Sit in a comfortable position.
2.	Close your eyes and let your body relax, summoning self-acceptance.
3.	Inhale through your nose slowly and smoothly by expanding the lower chest first, then the middle rib cage, and finally the upper chest.
4.	Exhale through your nose and keep your mouth closed while gently constricting the back of your throat, or glottis, as if you are saying the word *home*.
5.	Your exhalation should pass through the back of your throat so that it sounds like a distant ocean wave or Star Wars' Darth Vader.
6.	Continue the next cycle of breath when you are ready.
7.	Continue to follow the sound of your breath for 10 cycles.

Table 6.7 Humming Bee Breath (*Bhramari*)

1.	Sit in a comfortable position.
2.	Close your eyes, cultivating self-acceptance.
3.	Inhale through both your nostrils deeply and slowly for 5 to 8 counts, depending on your comfort level.
4.	Keep your mouth closed and exhale with the sound of a bee buzzing, like "hmmmmm," for 6 to 12 counts. As you exhale, imagine your body releasing negative energy and stress.
5.	Pause gently at the end of your exhalation to relax your neck and shoulders and observe whether your body feels more grounded.
6.	When you are ready, start your next slow inhalation.
7.	Continue this breathing technique for 10 cycles, gradually increasing your inhalation and exhalation breath count each cycle.

Calming Breaths

Humming Bee Breath (Bhramari)

Humming Bee Breath helps you release stress, anger, and frustration.

Alternate Nostril Breath (Nadi shodhana)

Our breathing is naturally more dominant through one nostril or the other and can vary throughout the day. Alternate Nostril Breath balances your breath between your nostrils. This breath is a cooling and calming breath and should not be forceful or effortful. You can use rhythmic breathing ratios to vary the number of breath counts for your inhalation, retention, and exhalation.

Left Nostril Breath (Chandra Nadi)

Left Nostril Breathing is calming and relaxing. The left nostril is associated with the moon—feminine, soft, and relaxing.

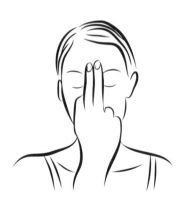

Figure 6.3
Alternate Nostril Breath
(front view)

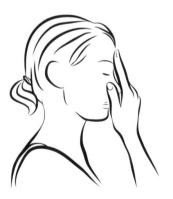

Figure 6.4
Alternate Nostril Breath
(side view)

Table 6.8   Alternate Nostril Breath (*Nadi shodhana*)

1.	Sit in a comfortable seated position, perhaps with your back supported by a wall.
2.	Close your eyes reminding yourself not to judge anything you're doing.
3.	Take a few slow breaths in and out.
4.	Rest your left hand on your left knee.
5.	Fold your ring finger and little fingers toward the palm on your right hand.
6.	Place the index and middle fingers of your right hand in the middle of your forehead, between your eyebrows. You can also curl your index and middle finger toward your palm and rest them on your forehead if that feels more stable.
7.	Exhale slowly through your nose, allowing your lungs to empty completely.
8.	Close your right nostril with your thumb.
9.	Inhale gently and slowly through your left nostril for 5 counts.
10.	Press and close your left nostril with your ring and little fingers. Hold for 2 counts.
11.	Lift your thumb to release your right nostril, and exhale slowly through your right nostril for 5 counts. Stay empty for 2 counts.
12.	Inhale gently and slowly through your right nostril for 5 counts.
13.	Press and close your right nostril with your thumb. Hold for 2 counts.
14.	Release your left nostril, and exhale through your left nostril for 5 counts. Stay empty for 2 counts.
15.	Start another cycle by inhaling through your left nostril. Continue this pattern for 10 cycles. After you exhale from one nostril, remember to breathe in from that same nostril before switching.
16.	Optional: You can change the lengths of inhalation, breath retention, and exhalation using rhythmic breath ratios to pace your breath.

Table 6.9   Left Nostril Breath (*Chandra Nadi*)

1.	Sit in a comfortable position.
2.	Close your eyes, focusing on self-acceptance.
3.	Take a few deep, calm breaths through both nostrils.
4.	Fold the ring and little fingers of your right hand toward your palm.
5.	Place the index and middle fingers of your right hand in the middle of your forehead, between your eyebrows. You can also curl your index and middle fingers toward your palm and rest them on your forehead if that feels more stable.
6.	Use your thumb to press and close your right nostril.
7.	Inhale gently and slowly through your left nostril for 5 to 8 counts, depending on your comfort level.
8.	Exhale slowly through your left nostril for 5 to 8 counts.
9.	Keep your right nostril closed, and continue to inhale gently and slowly through your left nostril for 10 cycles.
10.	Optional: You can add breath retention after inhalation or exhalation. Use the different ratios of rhythmic breath to pace your breath.

Table 6.10   Lion's Breath (*Simhasana*)

1. Kneel on the floor in Hero Pose. If this pose is uncomfortable, you can sit in a chair.
2. Press both palms against your thighs, spreading your fingers wide, summoning courage and strength.
3. Close your eyes and focus your mind on the spot between your eyebrows.
4. Take a deep inhalation through your nose.
5. Open your mouth wide, stick out your tongue toward your chin, and exhale loudly with the sound "ha," as if you are fogging up a mirror. Your breath should pass through the back of your throat.
6. You can repeat this breath cycle 3 to 5 times.
7. Optional: You can keep your eyes open during Lion's Breath, and on the exhale, focus your eyes or gaze (*drishti*) on either the middle of your eyebrows (*bhru madhya drishti*) or at the tip of your nose (*nasa agra drishti*).

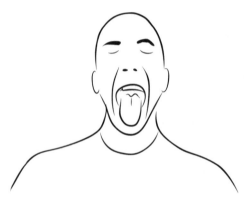

Figure 6.5   Lion's Breath

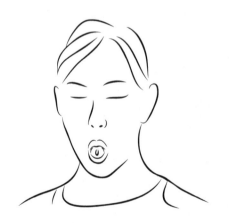

Figure 6.6   Tongue Hissing Breath

Lion's Breath (Simhasana)

Lion's Breath releases tension when done alone or when done in such postures as forward folds.

Cooling Breaths

These cooling breaths are useful to improve attention and cool yourself when you're feeling overheated, anxious, angry, or scattered.

Tongue Hissing Breath (Sitali)

Tongue Hissing Breath is a refreshing breath with a cooling sensation as air passes over your tongue during inhalation. If you are not able to roll your tongue into the shape of a straw, you can try Teeth Hissing Breath instead for the same effect.

Teeth Hissing Breath (Sitkari)

This cooling breath is useful for people who are not able to curl their tongue for Tongue Hissing Breath.

Table 6.11 Tongue Hissing Breath (*Sitali*)

1.	Sit in a comfortable position. Keep your spine long and tall.
2.	Close your eyes, and imagine the cooling sensation of water.
3.	Breathe slowly in and out through your nose for a few cycles.
4.	Open you mouth and form an O shape with your lips.
5.	Stick out your tongue and roll it into the shape of a straw, using your lips to shape it.
6.	Inhale slowly for 5 to 7 counts, allowing air to pass through your tongue, as if you are sipping through a straw, and feel your lungs expand.
7.	After inhalation, withdraw your tongue and let it relax as you close your mouth.
8.	Exhale slowly through your nose, keeping your mouth closed. Imagine releasing heat or any angry thoughts.
9.	Repeat this pattern of inhalation and exhalation for 10 cycles.
10.	Optional: You can combine this breath with alternative nostril breath by exhaling through only one nostril. On the next cycle of breath, exhale through the other nostril. Alternate nostrils with each cycle of breath.

Table 6.12 Teeth Hissing Breath (*Sitkari*)

1.	Sit in a comfortable position.
2.	Close your eyes, and imagine the cooling sensation of water.
3.	Place your tongue tip to the roof of your mouth behind your upper teeth.
4.	Gently press your upper and lower teeth together and open your lips so that your teeth are exposed.
5.	Inhale slowly through your mouth, letting air pass through your teeth for 5 to 7 counts. This should produce a hissing sound.
6.	Close your mouth and relax your tongue and lips.
7.	Exhale slowly through your nose, keeping your mouth closed.
8.	Repeat this pattern of inhalation and exhalation for 10 cycles.
9.	Optional: You can combine this breath with alternative nostril breath by exhaling through only one nostril. On the next cycle of breath, exhale through the other nostril. Alternate nostrils with each cycle of breath.

Energizing Breaths

These cleansing breaths give you more energy and are considered purifying breaths. Since these breaths engage your diaphragm and abdomen, avoid doing them on a full stomach—wait at least two hours after eating. Because these activating breaths are more forceful and intense, we recommend doing them with supervision from an experienced yoga teacher. Avoid these breathing techniques if you are pregnant or have medical conditions, including high blood pressure, glaucoma, epilepsy, panic disorder, gastric ulcer, hernia, or vertigo. Be cautious if you have lung disease and check with your doctor before trying these activating breathing exercises. You'll notice that right nostril breathing is not included, even though it is an energizing breath, because regular practice of right nostril breathing can increase blood pressure and sympathetic nervous system, and the long-term health effects are uncertain.

Breath of Fire, or Skull Shining Breath (Kapalabhati)

Breath of Fire is a rapid cleansing breath that has passive inhales and rapid, short, forceful exhales. These powerful exhalations require using your diaphragm and abdominal muscles.

Table 6.13   Breath of Fire (*Kapalabhati*)

1. Sit in a comfortable position.
2. Close your eyes, and focus on strength and energy.
3. Inhale through your nose for 5 to 6 counts.
4. Exhale through your nose in short, forceful breaths. With each exhalation, snap your abdominal muscles inward and upward.
5. Continues these exhalations with a steady rhythm at a pace of 1 exhalation per second for 10 to 15 exhalations (or less if you are feeling uncomfortable).
6. Once you are done with your cycle of exhalations, let your breath return to normal.
7. You can repeat for up to 3 sets of 10 to 15 exhalations as long as it feels comfortable.

Bellows Breath (Bhastrika)

Bellows Breath consists of forceful diaphragmatic inhales and exhales. It clears the mind and is stimulating.

Table 6.14   Bellows Breath (*Bhastrika*)

1. Sit in a comfortable position.
2. Close your eyes, and focus on feeling strong and filled with energy.
3. Take a few breaths in and out through your nose.
4. Inhale through your nose for 6 to 7 counts to fill with breath.
5. Exhale forcefully through your nose to empty your breath completely.
6. Inhale steadily with short, forceful inhalations at a pace of 1 inhalation per second for 10 breaths. The rate of in-breath and out-breath are identical.
7. Let your breath return to normal.
8. You can repeat for up to 3 sets of 10 to 15 exhalations as long as it feels comfortable.

Common Problems with Yoga Breathing

Yoga breathing typically has immediate and pleasant effects. You may encounter some issues when starting out, so we address some of the challenges you might experience here.

I Feel Dizzy or Lightheaded During Yoga Breathing

Some breathing exercises can cause dizziness or lightheadedness, especially rapid breathing techniques or if you hold your breath for too long. If you become dizzy, stop and let your breath return to normal so that your body can equilibrate. Breathe naturally until you feel comfortable again. Try slowed yoga breathing techniques instead. The key is not to force yourself to push through discomfort.

It Feels Painful When I Do Deep Breathing

Yoga breathing should not be painful. Everyone's lung capacity volume is different, so you should not go past what is comfortable for your inhalations, retention, and exhalation breath counts. If you feel pain during yoga breathing, stop. You may be pushing yourself too hard, or the exercise just may not be a good fit for you. You might feel pain in your chest when breathing deeply if you are inhaling rapidly or with a lot of force, causing your rib cage muscles to suddenly stretch. You may feel pain in your abdomen area or tightness in your chest if you are holding your breath for too long.

The bottom line is that the calming yoga breathing techniques are not intended to set off your body's fight-or-flight response. Even energizing breaths, such as Breath of Fire and Bellows Breath, are not supposed to be painful. If you have continued pain, even after stopping the breathing exercise, it's important to seek medical attention. There have been a few cases of medical issues occurring after yoga breathing; they are rare but can be serious. People with respiratory or lung diseases should be especially careful with yoga breathing and check with their doctor first.

I Can't Hold My Breath for That Long

Focus first on just becoming aware of your breath at your normal pace. See whether you can sit up a little taller so that your lungs have more room to expand. Once breath awareness is familiar and comfortable, focus on lengthening your exhalation gradually. Once your exhalation expands comfortably, begin to focus on lengthening your inhalation. When both your inhalation and exhalation are comfortable, work on adding retention after inhalation. With retention, release when you feel ready. Do not continue to hold past your discomfort. The purpose of such exercises like as rhythmic or ratio breathing is not to achieve a specific ratio or number of breath counts, but to improve your awareness and concentration on the breath, so don't be discouraged when pacing your breath. The extension of your breath and breath retention will come naturally with regular practice. Continue to experiment with different ratios and work gradually.

I Don't Feel Motivated to Do Breathing Exercises Because Breathing Isn't Going to Do Anything

Many people think that breathing exercises will not change their body—but science continues to prove otherwise. Just twenty minutes of yoga breathing can decrease stress-related inflammation in the body.[12] Breathing exercises can immediately change your heart rate, blood pressure, and stress levels, and when practiced regularly, produce long-term effects. Breathing turns on activity in specific areas of the brain related to awareness. Breathing sessions also improves your ability to cope with stress and improves your attention.[13]

It's Impossible for Me to Sit Still and Just Focus on Breathing

Sitting still can be difficult for a lot of people for a variety of reasons, whether it's restless mental or physical energy, chronic lower back pain, or injuries. If the source of your restlessness is mental distractions or feeling fidgety, you can practice sitting daily for very short periods of time—for only a few minutes or as long as you feel comfortable—and then gradually extend those times by a few minutes a day. If sitting is painful or challenging from physical limitations, try standing in Mountain Pose for your breathing exercises.

You can also try combining breathing techniques with walking, similar to a walking meditation. Use your steps as a way to count your breaths. Inhale for five steps, retain your breath for two steps, and then exhale for five steps. Depending on how fast you are walking, tailor your breath count to keep your breath relaxed and smooth. Movement coordinated with breath can help you relax and feel calmer so that sitting might become an option over time. Another option is to combine breathing techniques, such as Victorious Breath or Lion's Breath, with yoga postures. Focusing on your breath while moving will also make it easier to focus on your breath when sitting still.

I Don't Have Time to Do Breathing Sessions

Breathing exercises are quick, portable, and easy to do. You can do them for as little as five minutes a day, during your commute, on a plane, or taking an elevator. You don't need a lot of time, and you don't need any equipment. Even if it feels as if you don't have time, try focusing on your breath while you're waiting in line at the grocery store next time or while riding the elevator. All you have to do is find a comfortable place to sit or stand. Consistent practice is key, even if it's just a few minutes of breath awareness daily.

CHAPTER 7

Roll Out Your Mat: Yoga Poses (Asanas)

Body is the bow, asana is the arrow, and the soul is the target.

B. K. S. IYENGAR

What we're trying to do in yoga is to create a union, and so to deepen a yoga pose is to actually increase the union of the pose, not necessarily put your leg around your head.

RODNEY YEE

Yoga poses, or *asanas* in Sanskrit, are what most Americans think of when they hear yoga. They are considered the third path in the eight paths of yoga described by Patanjali. Although many people try yoga to improve health, tone muscles, or strengthen their body, the purpose of poses in the yoga tradition is not actually about the body. The aim of poses is to calm our mind and prepare us for meditation, which is why yoga sequences are often referred to as "movement in meditation."

Poses improve our flexibility, balance, and strength. But there are many additional effects that make yoga unique and quite different from fitness activities. Yoga poses help us develop body awareness. Unless we are trained as dancers or fitness gurus, most of us don't really work with our body on a daily basis. Through yoga poses, we get to know our body better. Poses also enhance our mind-body connection. Our body and our moods are intimately connected. When we're tired, we have a tendency to slump. When we're stressed, our stomach and shoulders tense. We can tap into this connection of the mind and body by using yoga poses to shift our mood and energy.

There are dozens of yoga poses and hundreds of modifications. Due to the higher risk of injuries with certain poses, we have left out poses, such as Headstand, Shoulder Stand, Plow, Wheel, and Dancer Pose, that require guidance and supervision from a certified yoga teacher. But just because a pose is included in this chapter does not mean that it is safe on your particular body.

One of the fundamental principles to ensure the safety of yoga is listening to your body in all its individuality, not forcing a pose, and modifying it, which can mean avoiding the pose, based on your individual body. We can't say this enough. Listen to your body. Don't be macho about yoga. It shouldn't hurt!

One of the fundamental principles to ensure the safety of yoga is listening to your body in all its individuality, not forcing a pose, and modifying it, which can mean avoiding the pose, based on your individual body. We can't say this enough. Listen to your body. Don't be macho about yoga. It shouldn't hurt!

Core Principles of Yoga Poses

Here are some important guidelines for doing poses that go beyond just the physical setup and anatomy of the body and make yoga a unique mind-body practice.

Form an intention. The first step before beginning your practice is to form an intention. Setting an intention means focusing on a quality or theme that you would like to be at the center of your poses. Your intention can focus on enhancing virtues, such as patience, self-compassion, forgiveness, or gratitude. You can choose to focus on accepting yourself or others, and practice being nonjudgmental. Other intentions can be physical, such as deciding to focus on your breath, build strength and stability, or cultivate peacefulness and restfulness. You can form an intention whether in a comfortable seated pose or in Mountain Pose.

Listen to your body. Being able to follow your intention requires mind-body attunement. This means you just observe what is happening in your body and mind without any judgment. The first step in the process is "listening" to your body. This holistic awareness of mind, body, and self is critical. Without this awareness, you can accidentally stretch your joints or muscles too far in the pose, or your ego may force your body to stay in a challenging position for too long.

Table 7.1 Core Principles of Yoga Poses

Core Component	Core Principles
Intention	Intention is bringing awareness of a quality or focus that you would like to concentrate on during your practice.
Mind-Body Attunement	Mind-body attunement is awareness of both the mind and body during yoga. It's important to listen to your body or mind, assess its state, and determine its needs. Attunement also recognizes that our needs vary from person to person, hour to hour, and day to day.
Individualization	Individualization is doing what's right for your body and mind. It is the process or ability to "listen" to your body and select or change poses based on mind-body attunement. You can individualize poses by choosing, modifying, or avoiding certain poses.
Alignment	Alignment is how you hold your body relative to itself. Proper alignment gives you guidelines to help keep your body stable and safe so as to help prevent musculoskeletal injury or strain. You can check your alignment by looking at your body or by using your body awareness, known as proprioception.
Proprioception	Proprioception is the sensory skill of body awareness and has two parts: (1) the ability to be aware of where your body is in space and (2) the awareness of where your body is relative to itself.
Modification	Modification is one method of individualizing a pose for your body and needs. This can mean providing more support through props, such as blocks, blankets, or using the wall, or changing the shape or position of the pose.
Breath	Use your breath to focus your energy in poses and synchronize your movement between poses. In general, exhale when you draw your body toward itself (e.g., go from Mountain Pose to Standing Forward Bend). In general, inhale when you extend your body away from itself (e.g., Standing Forward Bend to Mountain Pose).
Energy	There are two types of energy in poses: (1) energizing energy, or *brahmana* in Sanskrit, similar to yang; and (2) calming and soft energy, or *langhana* in Sanskrit, similar to yin.
Muscle Lock (*bandha*)	Muscle locks (Chapter 8) are specific muscular contractions that help you breathe and focus energy in the body.
Gaze (*drishti*)	The yogic gazing technique uses the specific direction of the eyes to focus and control attention, concentration, and energy in a pose.
Pace	The pace of poses—how fast one stays in and transitions to other poses—develops a rhythm and can be used to build energy or calm the body.
Balance	Balance can exist literally in a pose, your physical balance, but the term also refers to the balance of energy in a pose or the pacing of poses. A pose can be done in a way that emphasizes its energizing (*brahmana*) or calming (*langhana*) qualities.
Ego	A healthy ego can help motivate and improve yourself. But when ego as a sense of self-importance or pride drives the pose, you risk pushing yourself too far and hurting your body.
Nonjudgmental Attitude	Observing our feelings, thoughts, and emotions without labeling them as "good" or "bad," or "right" or "wrong."
Meditation	Postures are traditionally done to prepare the mind for meditation and are also referred to as "meditation in action" or "meditation in movement."

Avoid pain. Once you gain mind-body attunement and self-assessment, the next step in "listening" to yourself is making decisions for your poses that feel right for you. For example, you may select or avoid certain poses, perform poses in a gentler way with props, or modify them to build more strength. You may decide to stay longer or shorter in a pose. You can always change your mind during a pose, because you should be constantly observing and reassessing your needs. Our body is ever changing, requiring us to be aware constantly of our needs and experience. The saying "no pain, no gain" does not apply in yoga. At no point should the pose be painful.

Get to know the poses. Poses offer different types of energy. In the yoga tradition, quieting energy is *langhana* and exciting and expanding energy is called *brahmana*, similar to yin and yang. Your mind-body attunement will tell you whether to dial your energy up or down. Every pose has aspects of both types of energy, but, depending on type of pose and how you choose to do the pose (e.g., modifications), you can stimulate *brahmana*, creating more energy and vitality, or cultivate *langhana*, leading to more calming effects. Each pose has balance of energizing or calming qualities and some poses tend to be more of one or the other. For example, forward bend poses are useful to wind down at the end of a long day. Standing, twisting, or backbend poses build up more energy. The more you do yoga, the more you can notice how different poses affect your energy.

Watch your alignment. Alignment, or the position of your body relative to itself in a pose, is important to helping you do poses as safely as possible. While individualization of poses is important, poses do have general guidelines in terms of what keeps the body safe and healthy. Check your alignment visually by looking at your body, or use a sensory skill called proprioception, which is the ability to know where our body is in space, even with our eyes closed. The human body has receptors throughout its muscles and joints that send information to the brain about body position and movement.

Individualize the poses for *your* body. Yoga poses can be individualized. Keep a safe alignment, but also fine-tune poses, using different pose modifications or staying in them for the number of breaths that feels right for your body. You are the orchestra conductor of your body or the driver in the driver's seat. You can choose which poses to do and avoid, or to speed up or slow down the tempo. You determine how long to hold poses. You decide whether and how to use modifications, such as props to support the body or deciding to do alternative variations of the same pose. An important part of yoga is exploring and figuring out what works for you with a gentle and compassionate mind-set toward your mind and body.

Connect and reconnect with your breath. Breathing is a very active and essential component of doing yoga poses. Actively breathing helps you maintain strength and flexibility in a pose. If you find that you have lost track of your breath in certain poses, return to a resting pose such as Child's Pose or Downward Facing Dog to reconnect with your breath. Breath can also be used to remain active and deepen the pose, such as in twisting poses, a principle commonly referred to as "breathing into a pose." A common saying in yoga is that "asana is at the bottom of the breath." This means that the full pose occurs during exhalation. When you are in a delicate balance between being active and relaxed and are neither straining to "hold" the pose nor fully being lax, this is the fulfillment of the pose.

Use your gaze to sharpen your focus. Where you look with your eyes during a pose is an active part of your pose called gaze (*drishti*). Use your gaze to sharpen your focus in each pose. In the Ashtanga yoga tradition, there are eight specific gazes, or *drishtis*.

Quiet your inner critic. Yoga poses are also an opportunity to practice nonjudgment, or the ability to let go of the critical, negative internal voice that often follows us around. You want to stay alert and active, but not force yourself past what is safe or comfortable. When you are engaged in a pose, you might find yourself thinking thoughts such as *I am not flexible enough* or *I want to do a perfect pose*. In yoga classes, you might find yourself comparing yourself to others who are doing a pose

Table 7.2   Gazes (*Drishti*)

Gaze	Sanskrit	Direction	Sample Poses
Tip of Nose	Nasagrai Drishti	End of the nose	Upward Facing Dog, Standing Forward Bend, Wide-Legged Forward Bend
Third Eye	Naitrayohmadya or Broomadhya	Forehead between brows	Meditation, Fish Pose
Navel	Nabi Chakra Drishti	Belly button	Downward Facing Dog
Hand	Hastagrai Drishti	Hand	Extended Side Angle, Extended Triangle, Warrior II
Sideways	Parsva Drishti	In the direction of the twist	Seated Spinal Twist
Upward	Urdhva Drishti	Upward to the sky	Fierce, Warrior I
Toes	Pahayoragrai Drishti	Big toe	Seated Forward Bend
Thumb	Angusta Ma Dyai Drishti	Thumbs	Upward Salute

that looks more advanced. Yoga is not about perfection. Yoga encourages *letting go* of perfection and the ability to free yourself from judgment. Often judgment comes in the form of "should" statements. *I should get this pose right.* Or *I should be able to be more flexible.* If you find yourself thinking such thoughts, just notice them and let them go. And try not to judge yourself if you slip into judging. Nonjudgmental attitude does not mean that you must avoid experiencing any judgments or negative emotions. It just means being able to observe and let go of these negative thoughts when they do happen and not to become entangled with labeling them "good or bad" or "right or wrong."

When you practice all of these principles together, you are doing yoga in a way that builds your mind-body connection and allows you to practice "meditation in action" or "meditation in movement." The traditional intention of yoga poses and breathing exercises is to prepare your body for meditation, which we will discuss in Chapter 9.

Equipment

You don't need a lot of equipment for yoga. You don't need to spend a lot of money on the right clothing. It's really fairly basic. Here is a short list of the equipment you'll want to have in order to get started with yoga poses. You can find yoga equipment in many kinds of stores: specialty stores, yoga studios, sporting goods stores, big-box stores, department stores, and online.

Yoga mat. Practicing your poses on top of your mat gives you some cushion, which makes them less stressful to your body.

Two yoga blocks. Blocks generally bring the ground closer to you and can be used for support or to extend poses. They come in different materials, including cork, foam, or wood, and are usually 4 by 6 by 9 inches. Different materials offer different advantages. Foam blocks are lighter and softer when used to support the body, whereas cork or wooden blocks are firmer and can stay in place better since they are heavier. Because of their shape, yoga blocks also offer three different heights.

A yoga blanket or thick towel. A folded thick towel or blanket can be useful to put under your knees or back in certain poses to provide cushion or a little added height. For example, in Camel or Low Lunge Pose, you may want to place a folded blanket underneath your knees for more padding.

Yoga strap. A yoga strap is used as an extension of your hands to assist your reach in such poses as forward bends.

How to Get Started

There are many ways to do yoga poses, including a few poses at a time. You can also build your own sequences. We provide you a general outline for how to build your own basic sequences in Chapter 10 (see pages 255–257).

We suggest you start by following our 8-week program (see page 260). You will learn about ten poses a week, starting with simpler, foundational poses and building up toward more complex poses.

For each of these poses, we recommend starting off in the pose for less than a minute, about 5 to 6 steady breaths. Use your natural breath as your metronome or timer. When you are in the pose, look steadily in the direction of the recommended "gaze," or you have the option to close your eyes (see Table 7.2). As you build up your practice, you will be able to stay in the poses for longer, building up to 8 breaths, and eventually even to 10 breaths. The important part of yoga is not to rush yourself. And, as we've mentioned before, yoga shouldn't hurt. If so, stop and gently get out of the pose.

✦

And now, let's begin.

Starting Poses

Starting poses give you a chance to center yourself. They build a strong foundation of calm, focus, and awareness and are good poses to bring together your body, mind, and breath, also known as integration poses. Use these starting poses to settle your mind and combine them with yoga breathing exercises. They are also useful for meditation, particularly the seated starting poses, Easy and Hero Pose.

Table 7.3   Starting Poses

English Name	Sanskrit Name	Gaze	Modifications	Cautions & Contraindications
Easy, or Cross-Legged, Pose	Sukhasana	Eyes closed or forward	Sit on block	Knee and ankle injury
Hero Pose	Virasana	Eyes closed or forward	Sit on block between your shins	Knee and ankle injury
Child's Pose	Balasana	Eyes closed or upward toward Third Eye	• Arms behind you alongside torso • Hands on blocks or fingertips tented • Widen knees	Shoulder injury Widen knees for tight hips or during pregnancy
Mountain Pose	Tadasana	Eyes closed or forward	Block between thighs	Ankle, knee, or hip injury

Easy Pose (Sukhasana)

Easy Pose is a seated pose that can be used at the start of practice. Easy Pose is also used for seated meditation or breathing exercises.

1. Sit on the mat or ground.
2. Cross your shins and fold your legs in toward your pelvis. Your shins and thighs should form a triangle. There should be a gap between your feet and your pelvis.
3. Relax the feet so that their outer edges are on the ground. You can sit on a folded thick blanket or on the edge of a block so that your hips are even with or slightly above your knees.
4. Your neck, shoulders, and hips should be aligned above one another so that your spine is tall and erect.
5. Lengthen your tailbone toward the ground.
6. Your hands can be on your knees, palms up or down, or in separate mudras, such as Wisdom or Consciousness Mudra (page 220), or in your lap in Meditation Mudra (page 223).

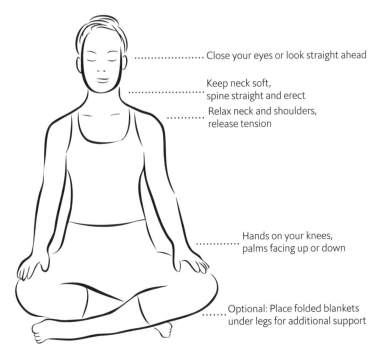

Close your eyes or look straight ahead

Keep neck soft, spine straight and erect

Relax neck and shoulders, release tension

Hands on your knees, palms facing up or down

Optional: Place folded blankets under legs for additional support

Figure 7.1   Easy Pose

Hero Pose (Virasana)

Hero Pose is a seated pose that can be used at the start of practice to become aware of your body and mind. Hero Pose is also used for seated meditation or breathing exercises.

1. Kneel on the ground with your thighs perpendicular to the ground.
2. Bring your knees together.
3. Slide your feet apart, and untuck your toes so that the tops of your feet are on the ground.
4. Roll your calf muscles outward with your thumbs to create space, and then sit down between your feet. This can require a lot of flexibility in your knee joint, hip flexors, and ankles. If you start to feel discomfort or strain, place one or two blocks under your seat to raise and support your spine.
5. You can support your knees and calves with a rolled blanket so your ankles and feet are off the back edge of the blanket to relieve some of the pressure on the tops of your feet.
6. Widen your chest and lift your sternum.
7. Place your hands on your thighs either palms up, if you are seeking more energy, or down, if you would like to feel more grounded. You can also use other hand mudras (pages 220–227).

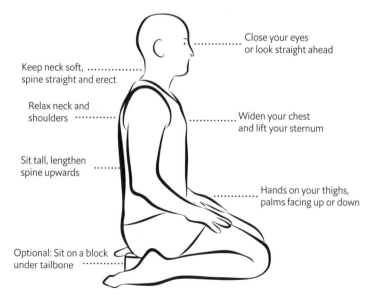

Close your eyes
or look straight ahead

Keep neck soft,
spine straight and erect

Relax neck and
shoulders

Widen your chest
and lift your sternum

Sit tall, lengthen
spine upwards

Hands on your thighs,
palms facing up or down

Optional: Sit on a block
under tailbone

Figure 7.2   Hero Pose

Child's Pose (Balasana)

Child's Pose is a restful pose used at the beginning of your practice or in the middle of your practice to take a break, especially if you've lost track of your breath. Don't be afraid to go into Child's Pose when you feel that you need a break.

1. Kneel with your knees about hip width apart, or wider if you have tight hips, and bring your feet together.
2. Untuck your feet so that the tops of your feet, where your shoelaces would be, rest on the mat.
3. Sit with your hips back onto your feet. Let your torso rest on your thighs.
4. Rest your forehead on the mat, close your eyes, and focus on your breath.
5. Extend your hands toward the top of the mat, palms facing down. Reach your fingertips forward and press into the mat.
6. Let your shoulders relax away from your ears.
7. Mentally focus on the point between your eyebrows, which is called an "internal" gaze, or the Third Eye. Rock your head back and forth to massage your forehead on the ground.

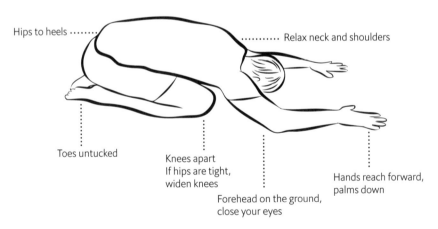

Hips to heels

Relax neck and shoulders

Toes untucked

Knees apart
If hips are tight,
widen knees

Forehead on the ground,
close your eyes

Hands reach forward,
palms down

Figure 7.3 Child's Pose

If your neck and shoulders are tight, tuck your arms behind you, alongside your torso, and let them relax and be heavy. If you have tight hips, keep your knees wide, to the edge of the yoga mat.

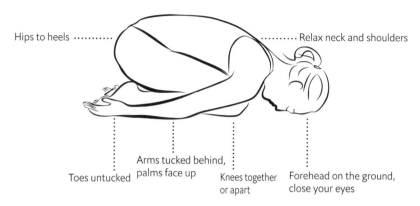

Hips to heels ⋯⋯⋯⋯

⋯⋯⋯⋯ Relax neck and shoulders

Toes untucked Arms tucked behind, palms face up

Knees together or apart

Forehead on the ground, close your eyes

Figure 7.4   Child's Pose Arms Back

If you have injuries that make it difficult to bend your knees, keep your thighs perpendicular to the ground and your hips above your knees. Extend your arms forward for Extended Child's Pose, also known as Puppy Pose, allowing your chest to relax toward the ground. This stretches your shoulders and chest.

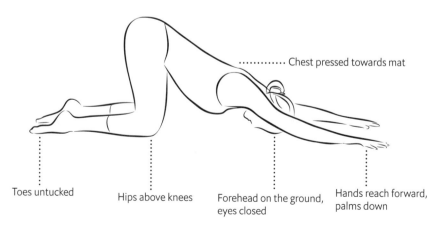

⋯⋯⋯⋯ Chest pressed towards mat

Toes untucked

Hips above knees

Forehead on the ground, eyes closed

Hands reach forward, palms down

Figure 7.5   Puppy Pose

Mountain Pose (Tadasana)

Mountain Pose is typically used to start standing poses and is useful to feel grounded and centered. Use this pose to create more awareness, stability, and acceptance in your body.

1. Stand with your big toes touching, with a small space between your heels, so that your feet are parallel.

2. Shift in different directions, like oil coating a pan, and explore how it feels to move weight between your feet and from front to back.

3. Imagine that there are four corners to each foot and that you are evenly sealing all four corners onto the ground firmly. This firmness in your feet requires you to engage your thighs and use them to lift your kneecaps. You should feel a line of energy from the inner arches of your feet to your upper inner thighs and groin and a slight internal rotation of your upper thigh. If it is difficult to feel this energy, then place the narrow width of a block between your upper thighs and press your thighs into the block.

4. Lengthen your tailbone downward. Stand tall to keep your neck long and above your pelvis.

5. Widen your collarbones to expand your chest.

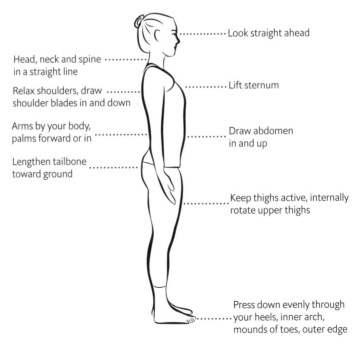

Look straight ahead

Head, neck and spine in a straight line

Lift sternum

Relax shoulders, draw shoulder blades in and down

Arms by your body, palms forward or in

Draw abdomen in and up

Lengthen tailbone toward ground

Keep thighs active, internally rotate upper thighs

Press down evenly through your heels, inner arch, mounds of toes, outer edge

Figure 7.6   Mountain Pose

6. Draw your shoulder blades together and down, and relax your shoulders away from your ears.

7. Relax your facial muscles. Let your arms hang alongside your torso, or spread your fingers wide, and spin your thumbs outward so they point to the sides of the room.

8. Look straight ahead, focusing on the feeling of being rooted into the ground.

Warm-up Poses

Warm-up poses prepare your body for more strenuous stretching and movement and are important to prevent injury. Warm-up poses are less intense but still build body awareness and the mind-body connection. Continue to use your breath through all your warm-up poses to heat up the body. Using your breath helps you flow from one pose into another, as you'll see.

Table 7.4 Warm-up Yoga Poses

English Name	Sanskrit Name	Gaze	Modifications	Cautions & Contraindications
Tabletop Pose	Goasana	Between hands or slightly in front of hands	Blanket underneath knees, hands into fists	Knee or wrist injury
Cat Pose	Marjariasana	Navel	Blanket underneath knees	Back injury
Cow Pose	Bitilasana	Tip of nose	Blanket underneath knees	Back injury
Thread the Needle Pose (Revolved Child's Pose)	Parsva Balasana	Side	Blanket underneath knees or shoulders	Shoulder, neck, or back injury
Upward Salute	Urdhva Hastasana	Thumbs	Block between thighs	Shoulder, neck, or back injury
Sidebending Mountain Pose	Parsva Tadasana	Straight ahead	Block between thighs	Shoulder, neck, or back injury

Tabletop Pose (Goasana)

Tabletop Pose offers stability and integration with body, mind, and breath. Tabletop Pose is useful to warm up the body, especially paired with Cat and Cow Poses.

1. Kneel with your thighs perpendicular to the ground and hips above your knees. Your knees should be hip width apart.
2. Place your palms on the ground with your hands directly beneath your shoulders, so that your shoulders, elbows, and wrists are in line with one another and perpendicular to the ground.
3. Spread your fingers, pointing forward.
4. Press into your hands so your shoulders can relax away from your ears.
5. Your back should neither be rounded nor arched but in a neutral and comfortable position.
6. Your neck should be a natural extension of your spine, and reach forward with your sternum.
7. Keep your gaze on the ground between your hands or slightly in front of them.
8. If your wrists feel too much pressure, then make your hands into fists. You can also cushion your knees with a folded blanket.

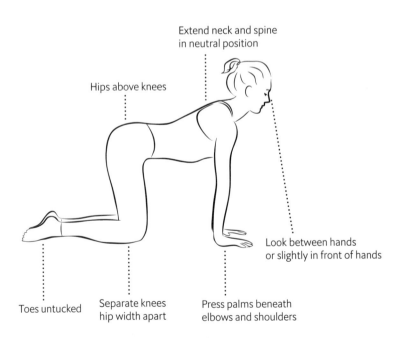

Extend neck and spine
in neutral position

Hips above knees

Look between hands
or slightly in front of hands

Toes untucked

Separate knees
hip width apart

Press palms beneath
elbows and shoulders

Figure 7.7   Tabletop

Cat Pose (Marjariasana)

Cat and Cow Pose can be paired together to warm-up your back and stretch the neck and torso.

1. Start in Tabletop Pose, and take in a deep breath.
2. Exhale as you draw your abdomen in and up, drawing your navel to your spine.
3. Round your back toward the sky, careful not to be too forceful.
4. Let your head and neck be relaxed toward the ground.
5. Your knees should stay directly under your hips, and your shoulders stay above your elbows and wrists.
6. Inhale and return to Tabletop Pose, moving on to Cow Pose.

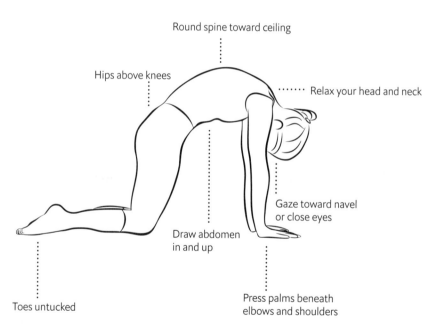

Round spine toward ceiling

Hips above knees

Relax your head and neck

Gaze toward navel or close eyes

Draw abdomen in and up

Toes untucked

Press palms beneath elbows and shoulders

Figure 7.8   Cat

Cow Pose (Bitilasana)

1. From Tabletop position, inhale and lift your chest upward, letting your stomach drop toward the ground slowly.

2. Your shoulders should stay in line with your elbows and wrists. Keep your hips above your knees.

3. Lift your head gently to look forward.

4. Exhale and return to Tabletop position. Do 5 cycles of Cat and Cow Pose with your breath to warm up your back and torso.

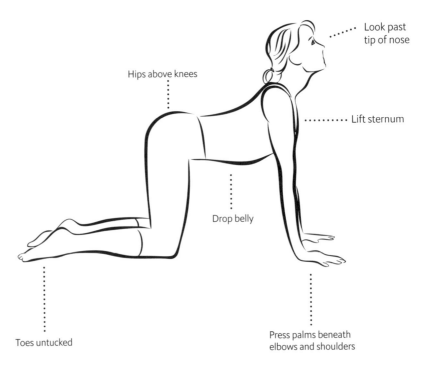

Figure 7.9   Cow

Thread the Needle Pose (Parsva Balasana)

Thread the Needle releases neck and shoulder tension and has a gentle twist. It invigorates the upper torso.

1. From Tabletop Pose, inhale and reach your right hand toward the sky to stretch your shoulder.
2. Slide your right hand, palm upward, underneath your left shoulder through the space between your left knee and hand.
3. Keep your hips above your knees.
4. Continue to slide your arm until your right shoulder and right side of your head reaches the ground.
5. Relax your shoulder and head on the ground to release your neck, shoulder, and upper back muscles.
6. Close your eyes, or look to the side.
7. Breathe in and out for 5 breaths. Extract your arm and lift your chest back into Tabletop Pose, and repeat on the other side.

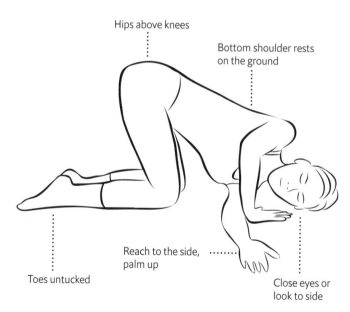

Hips above knees

Bottom shoulder rests on the ground

Reach to the side, palm up

Toes untucked

Close eyes or look to side

Figure 7.10   Thread the Needle

Upward Salute (Urdhva Hastasana)

Upward Salute is a standing gentle backbend pose that is often done after Mountain for a warm-up and is used in Sun Salutation sequences.

1. Stand in Mountain Pose.

2. Turn both thumbs outward, so that they point backward.

3. Inhale and sweep wide, as if you are a flying bird, to bring your palms together above your head. If you have tight shoulders, keep your palms separate but facing each other, so that your arms are parallel. Otherwise, continue to reach until the base of your palms press against each other.

4. Without compressing your neck, look up at your thumbs and continue to reach your arms upward.

5. Stay rooted firmly in both feet, and lift your sternum as you continue to breathe deeply. This is a gentle backbend. Lengthen your tailbone toward the ground.

6. Keep your abdominal muscles contracted in and up, drawing your navel toward your spine, to prevent your lower back from arching.

7. Breathe for 5 breaths. Exhale as your sweep your arms downward, and release your arms alongside your torso.

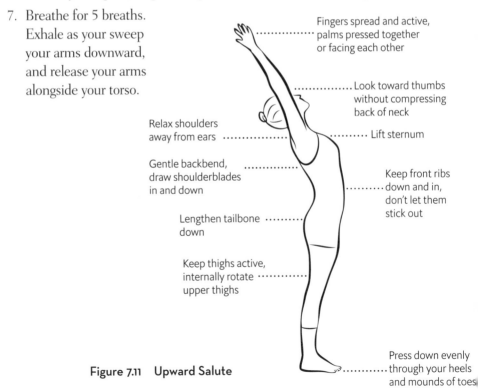

Fingers spread and active, palms pressed together or facing each other

Look toward thumbs without compressing back of neck

Relax shoulders away from ears

Lift sternum

Gentle backbend, draw shoulderblades in and down

Keep front ribs down and in, don't let them stick out

Lengthen tailbone down

Keep thighs active, internally rotate upper thighs

Press down evenly through your heels and mounds of toes

Figure 7.11   Upward Salute

Sidebending Mountain Pose (Parsva Tadasana)

Sidebending Mountain is a gentle warm-up pose that stretches the intercostal muscles between your ribs and abdominal muscles to give you more room to breathe. It also stretches the hips and thighs.

1. From Mountain Pose, inhale and raise your arms to interlace your fingers above your head. Reach your arms toward the sky.

2. Keep your hands interlaced and spin your palms to the sky. Reach to the right and gently bend and lengthen the side of your body. You can also take your right hand and clasp it around your left wrist and gently stretch your left side of the body. Do not pull your wrist.

3. Press down firmly on both feet, so that you are rooted into the ground as your reach toward the sky.

4. Continue to feel the side stretch of your body and breathe for 5 breaths.

5. To exit, exhale as you come back to center with your arms. Release your arms alongside your torso as you return to Mountain Pose. Repeat on the other side.

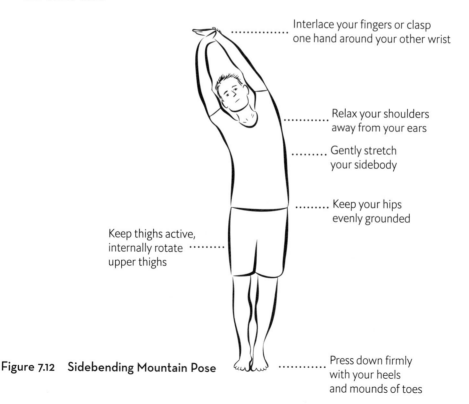

Interlace your fingers or clasp one hand around your other wrist

Relax your shoulders away from your ears

Gently stretch your sidebody

Keep your hips evenly grounded

Keep thighs active, internally rotate upper thighs

Press down firmly with your heels and mounds of toes

Figure 7.12   Sidebending Mountain Pose

Arm Support Poses

Arm support poses are basic poses that place weight on both your arms and legs. They can be done on their own or as part of the Sun Salutation sequences. They are important to develop your body awareness as well as improve your core strength.

Table 7.5   Arm Support Poses

English Name	Sanskrit Name	Gaze	Modifications	Cautions & Contraindications
Downward Facing Dog Pose	Adho Mukha Svanasana	Navel or between thighs, knees, or ankles	• Hands on blocks • Knees soft	Wrist injuries, carpal tunnel syndrome
Dolphin Pose	Ardha Pincha Mayurasana	Navel or between thighs, knees, or ankles	• Interlace fingers	Shoulder or neck injury
High Plank Pose (High Push-up)	Kumbhakasana	Tip of nose, forward and down	• Knees down on ground or blanket for more support • Forearm plank for wrist injuries	Wrist or shoulder injuries, carpal tunnel syndrome
Low Plank Pose (Low Push-up, Four-Limbed Stick)	Chaturanga Dandasana	Tip of nose, forward and down (to the floor about 6 inches in front)	• Knees down on ground or blanket for more support	Wrist or shoulder injuries, carpal tunnel syndrome

Downward Facing Dog Pose (Adho Mukha Svanasana)

Downward Facing Dog can be done on its own and as a starting "integration" pose used to connect your mind, body, and breath. It is an important pose in the traditional Sun Salutation A and B sequences. Downward Facing Dog is also a more active version of resting pose to catch your breath between other poses, instead of Child's Pose.

1. Start from Tabletop Pose. Make sure that your shoulders are above your wrists and your knees are below your hips.
2. Press yours hands firmly down and forward on the ground shoulder width apart. Your index fingers should be parallel to each other or slightly externally rotated.

3. Turn your toes under and exhale as you lift your knees and sitting bones toward the sky. Keep your knees gently bent, particularly if you have tight hamstrings or if it's the first pose of the day.

4. Spread your fingers widely with enough force that if someone tried to pick up your fingers, they would stay firmly on the ground.

5. Press your heels toward the ground, but your heels do not need to reach the ground. Do not lock your knees. Your feet should be hip width apart (on average, 6 to 8 inches).

6. Continue to lift your hips high, and roll your inner thighs inward. Draw your shoulder blades in and toward the tailbone to widen your collarbone. This should help relax your shoulders away from your ears.

7. Traditionally, your gaze is directed toward your navel, but for most people, it's easier to look at the space between your thighs, knees or ankles, at the back edge of the mat. Keep your neck long. Your back should not be rounded or arched.

8. Stay for 5 breaths, and then bring your knees to the ground for Child's Pose or step forward to Standing Forward Bend.

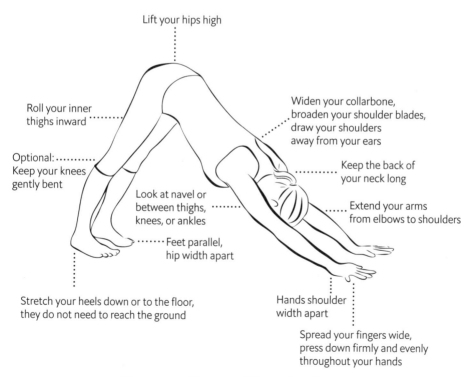

Lift your hips high

Roll your inner thighs inward

Optional: Keep your knees gently bent

Look at navel or between thighs, knees, or ankles

Feet parallel, hip width apart

Stretch your heels down or to the floor, they do not need to reach the ground

Widen your collarbone, broaden your shoulder blades, draw your shoulders away from your ears

Keep the back of your neck long

Extend your arms from elbows to shoulders

Hands shoulder width apart

Spread your fingers wide, press down firmly and evenly throughout your hands

Figure 7.13 Downward Facing Dog Pose

You can modify Downward Facing Dog by placing blocks underneath your hands, which is helpful for people who are tall. If you have tight shoulders, try rotating both hands slightly outward so that your thumbs and forefingers of both hands make the shape of a *W*. If you have difficulty with keeping your legs active or inner thighs rolled in, then place a block between your upper thighs.

Another modification for those with hand or wrist issues is Half Dog Pose against the wall. The pose releases lower back tension and stretches your arms and backs of your legs.

1. Stand in Mountain Pose facing the wall with distance between you and wall about the length of your legs.

2. Place your hands at your shoulders height and press actively forward with your entire palm and fingers against the wall.

3. Keep your neck long and in line with the spine. Your ears are between your upper arms. Look down at the ground as you stretch your spine.

4. Continue to press forward for 5 breaths, and release to Standing Forward Bend, or inhale to rise back to Mountain Pose.

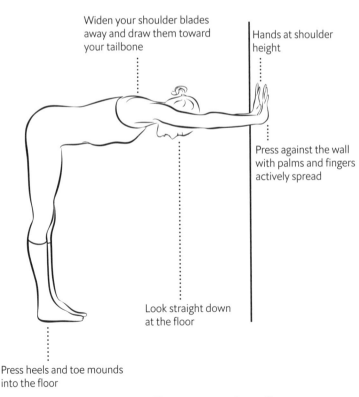

Widen your shoulder blades away and draw them toward your tailbone

Hands at shoulder height

Press against the wall with palms and fingers actively spread

Look straight down at the floor

Press heels and toe mounds into the floor

Figure 7.14   Half Dog against the wall

Dolphin Pose (Ardha Pincha Mayurasana)

Dolphin Pose strengthens your shoulders and upper body. Dolphin Pose puts less pressure on your wrists and can be used as an alternative to Downward Facing Dog. It is also a pose that prepares you for Headstand.

1. Start from Tabletop position.
2. Bring your forearms down to the ground so that they are parallel to each other and shoulder width apart. For more upper body support, you can also interlace your fingers together, keeping your elbows shoulder width apart, so that your forearms form the top of a triangle. Firmly press your palms and forearms into the ground.
3. Curl your toes under and lift your knees up as you exhale. Continue to lift your sitting bones up, keeping your knees gently bent. Widen your shoulder blades and draw them toward your tailbone.
4. Your neck should be long so that your head is between your upper arms. Straighten your knees and press your heels toward the ground without rounding your back. To avoid rounding your back, you can keep your knees bent and heels lifted to preserve the length of your spine.

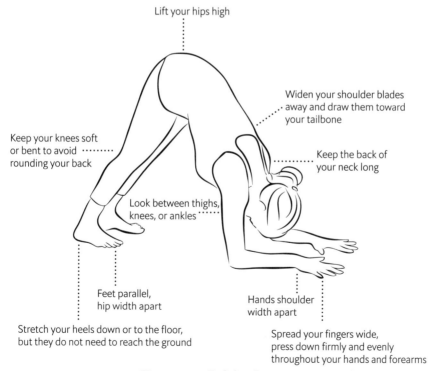

Lift your hips high

Widen your shoulder blades away and draw them toward your tailbone

Keep your knees soft or bent to avoid rounding your back

Keep the back of your neck long

Look between thighs, knees, or ankles

Feet parallel, hip width apart

Hands shoulder width apart

Stretch your heels down or to the floor, but they do not need to reach the ground

Spread your fingers wide, press down firmly and evenly throughout your hands and forearms

Figure 7.15   Dolphin Pose

High Plank Pose (Kumbhakasana)

High Plank or Plank Pose builds strength in your core muscles, or the deep abdominal and torso muscles that surround and stabilize your lower back. This pose is also known as High Push-up. It is an important part of the Sun Salutation series.

1. Start in Downward Facing Dog.

2. Inhale and shift your torso forward until your arms are perpendicular to the ground. Your shoulders should be directly above your elbows and wrists. Press actively into the palms and fingers.

3. Lengthen your tailbone to your heels and firm your thighs as if your heels were pressed against a wall behind you. Firm and rotate your thighs inward, as if you were holding a block between your thighs. Your core muscles should be active so that your back should be neither rounded nor arched. You can rock back and forward on your toes to feel the strength of your core muscles.

4. Keep your neck long and soft, and look forward and down at the ground in front of your fingertips. Breathe deeply with 5 Victorious Breaths in this pose. If you find that your hips are dipping toward the ground or your back is rounded to the sky or if you just feel like having more support, bring your knees down to the ground. Remember to be self-compassionate and offer yourself the version of the pose that works best for you.

5. When you are done, return to Downward Facing Dog or Child's Pose.

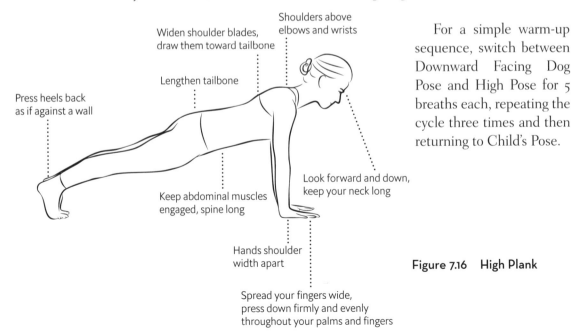

Shoulders above elbows and wrists

Widen shoulder blades, draw them toward tailbone

Lengthen tailbone

Press heels back as if against a wall

Keep abdominal muscles engaged, spine long

Look forward and down, keep your neck long

Hands shoulder width apart

Spread your fingers wide, press down firmly and evenly throughout your palms and fingers

For a simple warm-up sequence, switch between Downward Facing Dog Pose and High Pose for 5 breaths each, repeating the cycle three times and then returning to Child's Pose.

Figure 7.16   High Plank

Low Plank Pose (Chatturanga Dandasana)

Low Plank builds core strength and is an important part of the Sun Salutation series. This pose is also known as Low Push-up or Four-Limbed Staff. This pose can require significant core strength, so allow yourself to bring your knees down for support if needed.

1. Start from High Plank, and exhale as you reach your sternum forward as you lower your torso and legs so they are parallel to the ground. Draw your elbows in toward your torso so they are not buckled outward.

2. Continue to draw your lower abdominal muscles up and in, drawing your navel to your spine.

3. Widen your shoulder blades and continue to press on your palms and fingers firmly. Lift your sternum as you look at the ground about 6 inches in front of you. Keep your neck soft and long.

4. Your body is a long line of energy from the top of your head to your heels. If your lower back sags to the ground or your bottom is up in the air, bring your knees down for support.

5. Breathe for 5 Victorious Breaths and then lower gently to the ground. Or, for more heat and challenge, lift from Low Plank right back into High Plank.

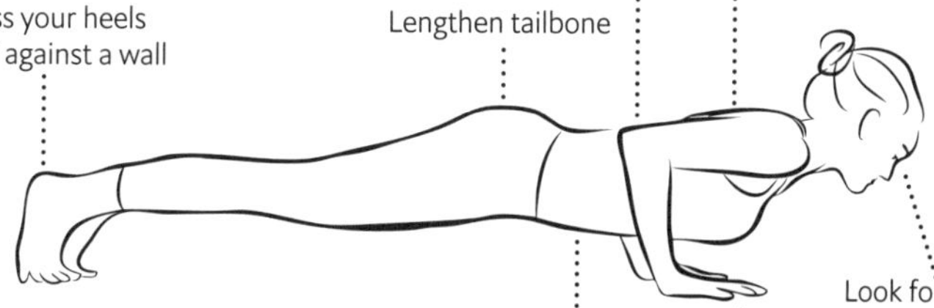

Elbows above wrists, draw elbows in toward torso

Widen shoulder blades, draw them toward tailbone

Press your heels as if against a wall

Lengthen tailbone

Look forward and down, keep your neck long

Keep your abdominal muscles engaged, spine long so there is a long line of energy from the top of your head to your heels

Spread your fingers wide, press down firmly and evenly throughout your palms and fingers

Figure 7.17   Low Plank

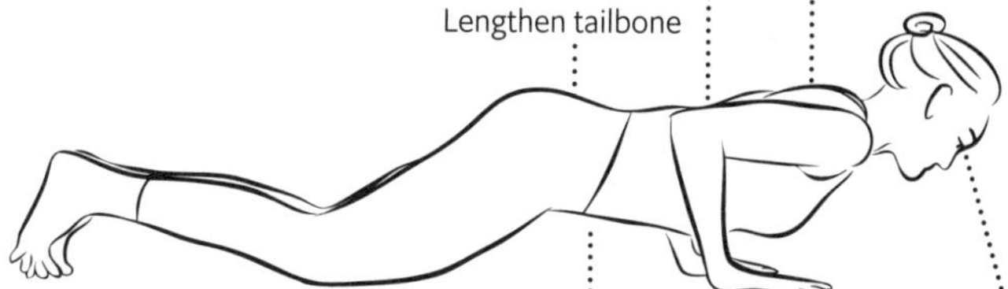

Elbows in line with wrists, draw elbows in toward torso

Widen shoulder blades, draw toward tailbone

Lengthen tailbone

Look forward and down, keep neck long

Toes tucked

Rest knees on the floor

Keep abdominal muscles engaged, spine long

Spread fingers wide, press down firmly and evenly throughout palms and fingers

Figure 7.18   Low Plank modification with knees down

Forward Bend Poses

Forward bends are calming poses that relieve stress, release head and neck tension, and promote sleep. Standing forward bend poses can be used at the beginning of classes to integrate body, mind, and breath and also between standing sequences as resting poses. Seated forward bends are useful for the end of class to wind down and are included in the cool-down section. In standing forward bends, you can gently nod and shake your head to loosen tension in your head and neck.

Table 7.6   Forward Bend Poses

English Name	Sanskrit Name	Gaze	Modifications	Cautions & Contraindications
Standing Forward Bend	Uttanasana	Eyes closed, or tip of nose	• Fingers clasped behind head • Hands to opposite elbows • Knees bent • Hands clasped behind lower back with arms extending away	Neck or lower back injury
Standing Half Forward Bend	Ardha Uttanasana	Floor in front of feet	• Hands to shins or on blocks	Neck or lower back injury
Big Toe Pose	Padangusthasana	Eyes closed, or tip of nose	• Hands on shins	Neck or lower back injury
Wide-Legged Forward Bend	Prasarita	Eyes closed, or tip of nose	• Fingers in line with toes • Hands to blocks below shoulders • Hands clasped behind lower back and reaching forward • Hands grabbing big toes	Neck, lower back, or hip injury
Pyramid Pose	Parsvottonasana	Eyes closed, or tip of nose	• Hands to blocks	Hamstring or back injury

Standing Forward Bend (Uttanasana)

Standing Forward Bend lengthens hamstrings and releases neck and shoulder tension. This pose relieves stress, fatigue, and anxiety and can improve headaches or insomnia. It can also be a resting pose between standing poses.

1. Stand in Mountain Pose with your hands on your hips.

2. Exhale as you bend forward at the hip joints, lifting your tailbone to the sky.

3. Keep your torso long and spine extended. Press your heels firmly into the ground, and notice a slight rotation of your thighs inward. If it is difficult to find this inner rotation of the tops of the thighs, place a block between your thighs.

4. Bring your palms or fingertips to rest on the ground in front of you or beside your feet, underneath your shoulders. Do not pull yourself forward with your hands to reach the ground. Do not round your back or strain to reach the ground with your hands. If it is difficult to reach the ground, rest your fingertips or palms on blocks. The purpose of the pose is to lengthen your back and hamstrings, not to get your hands to reach the ground.

5. Close your eyes. Let your neck relax and head be heavy in this pose. Do not lift your head to look forward. Avoid locking your knees. Stay in the pose for 5 breaths. To come out of the pose, put your hands on your hips, press your tailbone down, and rise up on inhalation, while keeping your torso long and straight.

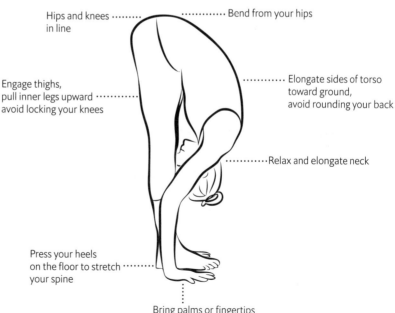

Hips and knees in line

Bend from your hips

Engage thighs, pull inner legs upward avoid locking your knees

Elongate sides of torso toward ground, avoid rounding your back

Relax and elongate neck

Press your heels on the floor to stretch your spine

Bring palms or fingertips to the floor or on blocks, arms shoulder width apart

Figure 7.19   Standing Forward Bend

There are many variations of your arms in Standing Forward Bend. For Ragdoll variation, cross your arms and hold onto your forearms.

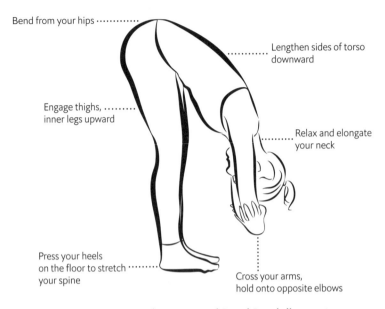

Bend from your hips

Lengthen sides of torso downward

Engage thighs, inner legs upward

Relax and elongate your neck

Press your heels on the floor to stretch your spine

Cross your arms, hold onto opposite elbows

Figure 7.20   Standing Forward Bend Ragdoll variation

If you have tight hamstrings or hips, bend your knees so that your torso is supported by your thighs.

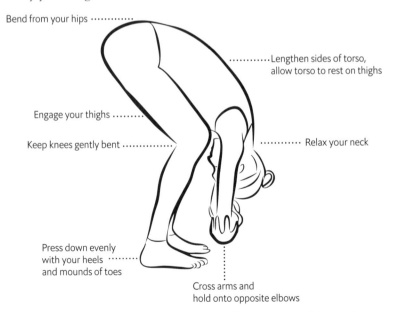

Bend from your hips

Lengthen sides of torso, allow torso to rest on thighs

Engage your thighs

Keep knees gently bent

Relax your neck

Press down evenly with your heels and mounds of toes

Cross arms and hold onto opposite elbows

Figure 7.21   Standing Forward Bend Ragdoll variation with knees bent

To stretch your shoulders, you can interlace your fingers together at your lower back, keep your arms straight, and extend your clasp away from your lower back.

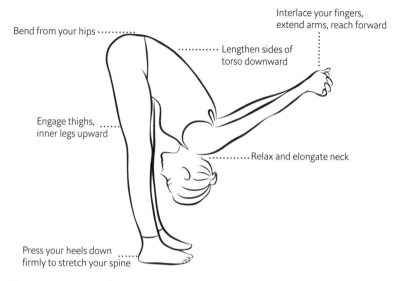

Bend from your hips ....

Interlace your fingers, extend arms, reach forward

.... Lengthen sides of torso downward

Engage thighs, ... inner legs upward

.... Relax and elongate neck

Press your heels down ...... firmly to stretch your spine

Figure 7.22   Standing Forward Bend variation with shoulder stretch

Keep your neck soft. For an additional release of neck muscles, interlace your fingers, clasp your hands behind the base of your head, and let the natural weight of your hands keep your head heavy.

Standing Half Forward Bend (Ardha Uttanasana)

Standing Half Forward Bend strengthens your back and loosens the muscles up and down the back of your body, including hamstrings and calves. It helps improve your pose and stretches your front torso. The pose is also used in Sun Salutation series or during transitions from Standing Forward Bend to High Plank position.

1. Start in Standing Forward Bend. Press your fingertips or palms on the ground. If it is difficult to reach the ground, place your hands on your shins or on two blocks on the ground in front of you.

2. Inhale and straighten your elbows as you lift your torso away from your thighs and press down with your hands.

3. Raise your sternum away from the ground and forward as you lengthen your front torso and the space between your navel and pubic bone.

4. Look forward and down without compressing the back of your neck. Your back should be fully extended and straight. After 5 breaths, return to Standing Forward Bend.

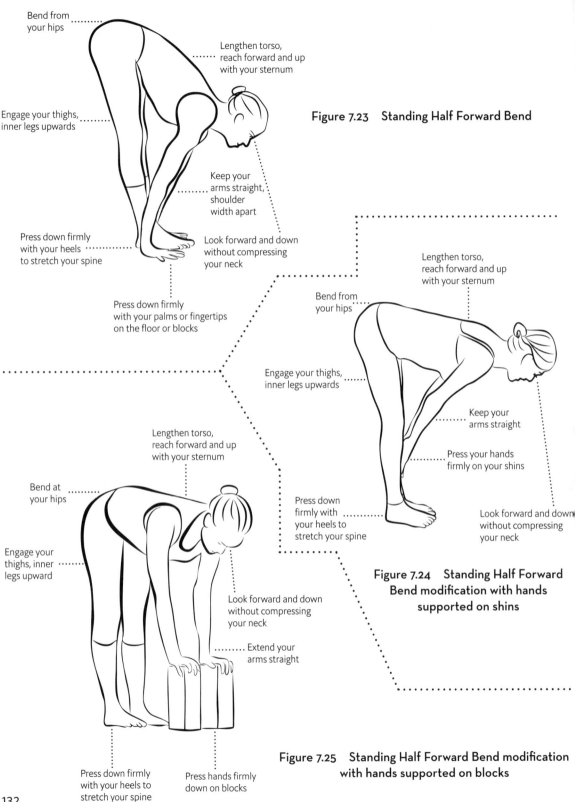

Bend from
your hips

Lengthen torso,
reach forward and up
with your sternum

Engage your thighs,
inner legs upwards

Figure 7.23   Standing Half Forward Bend

Keep your
arms straight,
shoulder
width apart

Press down firmly
with your heels
to stretch your spine

Look forward and down
without compressing
your neck

Press down firmly
with your palms or fingertips
on the floor or blocks

Lengthen torso,
reach forward and up
with your sternum

Bend from
your hips

Engage your thighs,
inner legs upwards

Keep your
arms straight

Press your hands
firmly on your shins

Press down
firmly with
your heels to
stretch your spine

Look forward and down
without compressing
your neck

Lengthen torso,
reach forward and up
with your sternum

**Figure 7.24   Standing Half Forward
Bend modification with hands
supported on shins**

Bend at
your hips

Engage your
thighs, inner
legs upward

Look forward and down
without compressing
your neck

Extend your
arms straight

Press down firmly
with your heels to
stretch your spine

Press hands firmly
down on blocks

**Figure 7.25   Standing Half Forward Bend modification
with hands supported on blocks**

Big Toe Pose (Padangusthasana)

Big Toe Pose is a forward bend that can be used as a resting pose between poses and when you have already warmed up your body a few times with Standing Forward Bend.

1. Stand in Mountain Pose with your feet parallel at hip distance apart.

2. Exhale to bend forward at your hips moving your torso and head downward together.

3. Wrap your index and middle finger in the space between your big toe and your second toe. Wrap your thumb around your big toe. Press your toes down firmly on the ground. If you are not able to reach your toes, place a strap underneath the balls of both feet and hold onto the ends of the strap with your hands.

4. Inhale and lift your torso slightly upward, lengthening your back.

5. Exhale and bend your elbows out to the sides, as you fold deeper. Lift your sitting bones higher and grip your big toes, lifting them with your fingers. Keep the front torso long and stretch your hamstrings, but avoid rounding your back or straining to reach the ground. Stay in the pose for 5 breaths and then release your big toes.

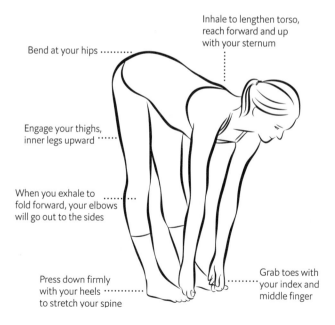

Inhale to lengthen torso, reach forward and up with your sternum

Bend at your hips

Engage your thighs, inner legs upward

When you exhale to fold forward, your elbows will go out to the sides

Press down firmly with your heels to stretch your spine

Grab toes with your index and middle finger

Figure 7.26 Big Toe Pose

Wide-Legged Forward Bend (Prasarita)

Wide-Legged Forward Bend is a calming forward bend that is often used at the end of standing sequences when the hamstrings and hips have already been warmed up. The pose relaxes the spine and stretches the groin and hips. It can be used to prepare for Headstand variations.

1. Stand in Mountain Pose. Step your right foot back so that your body is facing the long edge of the mat. Place your hands on your hips and bring your feet wide, about 3 to 4 feet apart. Keep your feet parallel to each other.

2. As you inhale, push your hands on your hips to lift your torso and chest toward the sky to lengthen your front torso. Exhale and bend forward at the hips. Keep the length in your torso and bend with your head and torso as one unit.

3. When your torso is parallel to the ground, place your hands or fingertips, facing forward, on the ground or blocks below your shoulders in line with your toes. Bend your elbows as you continue to bend forward, lowering your head and torso toward the ground.

4. Rest the top of your head on the mat, if possible. If your head doesn't touch the mat, place a block underneath to support your head or let your neck be relaxed. Do not strain your back to reach the ground. Press your hands or fingertips to the ground or blocks as you lift your sitting bones to the sky.

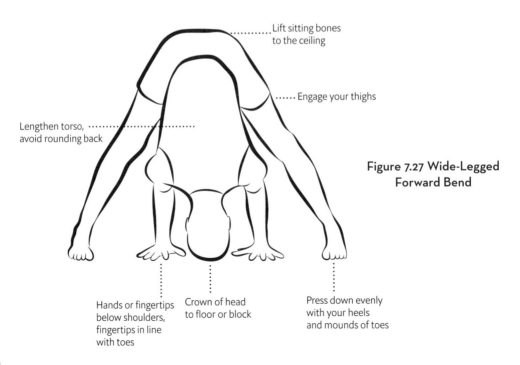

Lift sitting bones to the ceiling

Engage your thighs

Lengthen torso, avoid rounding back

Figure 7.27 Wide-Legged Forward Bend

Hands or fingertips below shoulders, fingertips in line with toes

Crown of head to floor or block

Press down evenly with your heels and mounds of toes

There are many variations of your hands in this pose. You can place your hands onto blocks beneath your shoulders to keep your torso long and not rounded. You can grab onto your big toes, or reach your hands straight back between your legs.

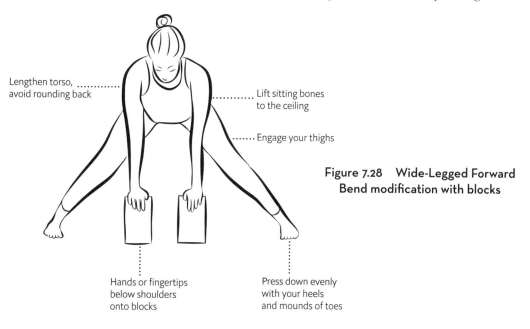

Lengthen torso, avoid rounding back

Lift sitting bones to the ceiling

Engage your thighs

Hands or fingertips below shoulders onto blocks

Press down evenly with your heels and mounds of toes

Figure 7.28   Wide-Legged Forward Bend modification with blocks

For a shoulder stretch, you can interlace your fingers behind your back. Lift your arms away from your lower back, and keep your arms extended.

5. Stay in the pose for 5 breaths. To exit, place your hands below your shoulders. Straighten your arms as your lift your torso and head. Place your hands at your hips, and inhale as you bring your torso up and draw your tailbone down.

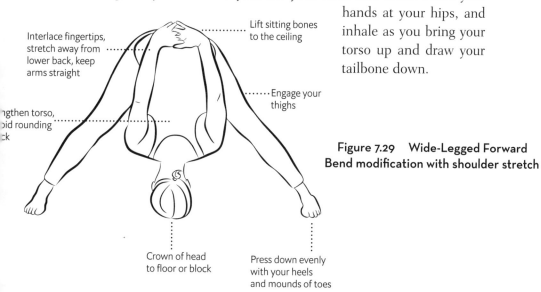

Interlace fingertips, stretch away from lower back, keep arms straight

Lift sitting bones to the ceiling

Engage your thighs

ngthen torso, oid rounding ck

Crown of head to floor or block

Press down evenly with your heels and mounds of toes

Figure 7.29   Wide-Legged Forward Bend modification with shoulder stretch

Pyramid Pose (Parsvottonasana)

Pyramid, or Intense Side Stretch, stretches your hamstrings and calves as well as your shoulders. The pose helps prepare your body for deeper forward bends as well as twists. Pyramid Pose is often paired with Low Lunge.

1. Start in Mountain Pose. Step your right foot back about 3½ to 4 feet, keeping your back heel on the ground.

2. Place your hands at your hips. Your hips should be squared and facing forward evenly. Your feet remain hip width apart, not directly behind each other, to create stability in your legs. Point your front foot forward, and turn your back foot (right foot) about 45 to 60 degrees out from your midline.

3. Inhale and raise your sternum as you lengthen your torso. Shift onto your back leg and press into its heel.

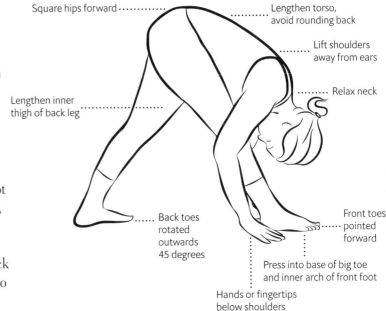

Square hips forward

Lengthen torso, avoid rounding back

Lift shoulders away from ears

Relax neck

Lengthen inner thigh of back leg

Back toes rotated outwards 45 degrees

Front toes pointed forward

Press into base of big toe and inner arch of front foot

Hands or fingertips below shoulders

Figure 7.30   Pyramid Pose

4. Exhale and fold your torso over your front leg without rounding your back.

5. Place your hands or fingertips onto the ground directly below your shoulders. If it is difficult to reach the ground, place your hands or fingertips on blocks.

6. Press inner edge and ball of your front foot firmly into the ground, and pull your front groin and thigh up. Lengthen the inner thigh of your back leg.

7. Release and relax your neck, and close your eyes. Stay for 5 breaths. When you are ready to come out of the pose, place your hands at your hips. Inhale as you lift your torso and head together, keeping your torso long and extended. Switch your feet to do your other side for the same amount of time.

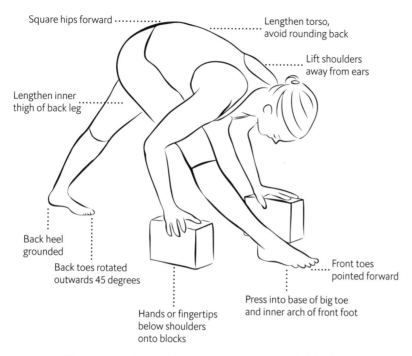

Square hips forward ··········

Lengthen torso,
avoid rounding back

Lift shoulders
away from ears

Lengthen inner
thigh of back leg ·······

Back heel
grounded

Back toes rotated
outwards 45 degrees

Front toes
pointed forward

Hands or fingertips
below shoulders
onto blocks

Press into base of big toe
and inner arch of front foot

Figure 7.31   Pyramid Pose modification with blocks

Standing Poses

Standing poses build strength and heat in the body. A series of standing poses builds focus, concentration, and stability in both the body and mind. Physically, these poses lengthen your spine and firm your legs while your upper body lifts. In many of these standing poses, the directions of energy run in opposite directions from one another. For example, in Fierce Pose, you press downward into your heels to be stable in your legs, but also lift upward through the torso with your arms, so you envision energy running both up and down. In Warrior II Pose, your feet both are drawing energy in toward each other while your arms are extended outward. Some of the poses also give you a gentle side stretch, such as in Reverse Warrior, Extended Side Angle, and Extended Triangle Poses.

Table 7.7 Standing Poses

English Name	Sanskrit Name	Gaze	Modifications	Cautions & Contraindications
Fierce (Chair) Pose	Utkatasana	Upward at thumbs	• Hands pressed together in front of chest • Block between thighs	Shoulder injury
Warrior I Pose	Virabhadrasana I	Straight ahead or upwards	• Hands at hips • Hands pressed together in front of chest • Hands clasped at lower back	Groin injury
Warrior II Pose	Virabhadrasana II	Straight ahead, over middle finger of front hand	• Hands at hips	Groin injury
Reverse Warrior Pose	Viparita Virabhadrasana	Third Eye	• Back hand on hip instead of thigh	Neck or shoulder injury
Low Lunge Pose	Anjaneyasana	Straight ahead or upward	• Back knee up • Back knee down on ground or blanket • Hands on blocks	Knee injury
High Lunge Pose	Alanasana	Straight head or upward	• Hands at hips • Hands pressed together in front of chest	Ankle or foot injury
Extended Side Angle Pose	Utthita Parsvakonasana	Thumb of raised hand	• Lower elbow on thigh • Lower hand on block or ground inside or outside front foot • Upper hand extended forward • Upper hand reaching upward • Upper hand on hip	Neck injury
Extended Triangle Pose	Utthita Trikonasana	Thumb of raised hand	• Upper hand on hip • Lower hand on shin • Lower hand on block inside or outside front foot • Lower hand grabs big toe	Neck injury

Fierce Pose (Utkatasana)

Fierce Pose, shaped like a lightning bolt, is also referred to as Chair Pose, but it is anything but resting in a chair. Fierce Pose is fiery and energizing. Imagine that you are a lightning rod receiving energy from the fingertips rushing down through the bottoms of your feet. Or imagine electric energy flowing the other direction, from the ground up through your fingertips.

1. Stand with your feet together in Mountain Pose.

2. Inhale and sweep your arms to reach the sky so that they are fully extended and straight. Spread your fingers and press your palms together. Or keep your hands shoulder width apart, with palms facing inward, and little fingers spinning in toward each other. If you have shoulder injuries, keep your hands pressed together in front of your chest in Salutation Seal Mudra (page 223).

3. Exhale and bend your knees as you shift your weight into your heels, bringing your hips closer to your heels.

4. Inhale deeply to extend and lift your arms higher. Relax your shoulders away from your ears and draw your shoulder blades in and down.

5. Exhale and sit deeper so that your thighs are as close to parallel to the ground as possible without straining. Draw your tailbone toward the ground and keep your spine straight. Relax your facial muscles.

6. Look upward. Take 5 breaths in this pose, sitting deeper with each exhalation. On the last exhalation, release your arms and fold forward into Standing Forward Bend or straighten your knees to return to Mountain Pose.

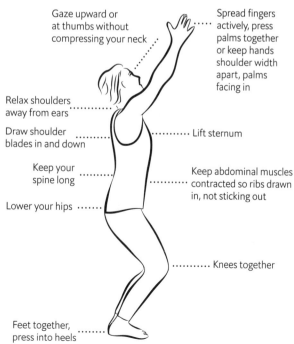

Gaze upward or at thumbs without compressing your neck

Spread fingers actively, press palms together or keep hands shoulder width apart, palms facing in

Relax shoulders away from ears

Draw shoulder blades in and down

Lift sternum

Keep your spine long

Keep abdominal muscles contracted so ribs drawn in, not sticking out

Lower your hips

Knees together

Feet together, press into heels

Figure 7.32   Fierce Pose

Warrior I Pose (Virabhadrasana I)

Warrior I Pose strengthens your legs, back, and your upper body. The pose stretches your shoulders, neck, chest, groin, thighs, calves, and ankle muscles. Warrior I can be done on its own or is a part of the Sun Salutation B sequence.

1. Stand in Mountain Pose. Widen your stance to about 3½ to 4 feet apart with your right foot at the top of your mat and left foot behind you.

2. Point your front foot forward, and rotate your back foot so it points 45 to 60 degrees to the left top corner of the mat. Your feet should be positioned on two separate tracks so that your hip points can face forward. Check to see whether your hips are facing forward by placing your hands at your hip points.

3. Inhale as you reach your hands toward the sky, so that your arms are straight and perpendicular to the ground. Spread your fingers with your palms facing each other or rotate your little fingers in toward each other. Lift your rib cage away from your pelvis.

4. Exhale and bend your front knee so that it is in line with your ankle and your front thigh is parallel to the ground. If your front knee goes past your ankle, then widen your stance between your feet. Your thigh and shin should be at a 90-degree angle. Lengthen your tailbone toward the ground.

5. Press on the outer edge of your back left foot and heel.

6. Relax your shoulders away from your ears. Gaze straight ahead or upward. Breathe for 5 counts. Step forward to return Mountain Pose and switch your feet to do the other side for the same amount of time.

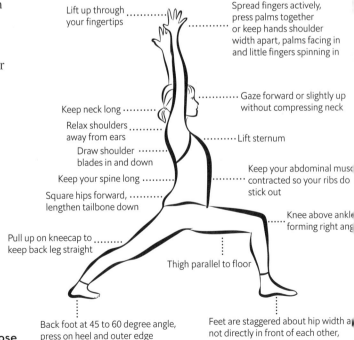

Lift up through your fingertips

Spread fingers actively, press palms together or keep hands shoulder width apart, palms facing in and little fingers spinning in

Gaze forward or slightly up without compressing neck

Keep neck long

Relax shoulders away from ears

Lift sternum

Draw shoulder blades in and down

Keep your spine long

Keep your abdominal musc[le] contracted so your ribs do[n't] stick out

Square hips forward, lengthen tailbone down

Knee above ankle forming right ang[le]

Pull up on kneecap to keep back leg straight

Thigh parallel to floor

Back foot at 45 to 60 degree angle, press on heel and outer edge

Feet are staggered about hip width a[part] not directly in front of each other, so hips can square forward

Figure 7.33   Warrior I Pose

Warrior II Pose (Virabhadrasana II)

Warrior II Pose is a strong, focused pose where you feel yourself fully expand from fingertip to fingertip. You build strength in your shoulders, legs, and groin in Warrior II. The pose stimulates and strengthens your abdominal muscles and relieves backaches.

1. Stand in Mountain Pose. Step your feet to about 3½ to 4 feet apart. Keep your hands at your hips.

2. Turn your back foot outward to about 60 to 90 degrees. Your front heel should be in line with the inner arch of your back foot.

3. Bend into your front knee so that it is above your ankle and your front thigh is parallel to the ground. Your front knee should be at a right angle and aimed toward the side of your little toe of your front foot. Keep your back leg straight. Your hips should be facing the long side of the mat.

4. Raise your arms so that they are straight and parallel to the ground, with your palms facing down and your fingers actively spread. Reach out in both directions evenly, so that your shoulders are directly centered above your hips, and you are neither leaning forward or backward.

5. Look forward over the fingers of your front hand. Draw your shoulder blades in and down, and relax your shoulders away from your ears. Breathe for 5 breaths. To come out of the pose, inhale and straighten both legs. Switch the position of your feet, and do the other side for 5 breaths.

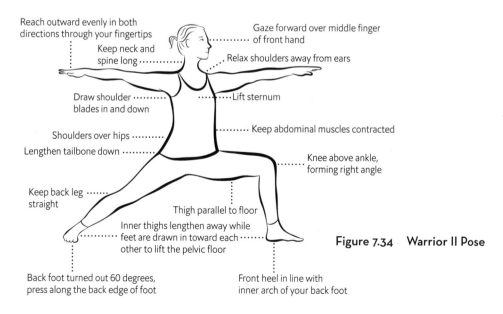

Reach outward evenly in both directions through your fingertips

Keep neck and spine long

Gaze forward over middle finger of front hand

Relax shoulders away from ears

Draw shoulder blades in and down

Lift sternum

Keep abdominal muscles contracted

Shoulders over hips

Lengthen tailbone down

Knee above ankle, forming right angle

Keep back leg straight

Thigh parallel to floor

Inner thighs lengthen away while feet are drawn in toward each other to lift the pelvic floor

Figure 7.34   Warrior II Pose

Back foot turned out 60 degrees, press along the back edge of foot

Front heel in line with inner arch of your back foot

Reverse Warrior Pose (Viparita Virabhadrasana)

Reverse Warrior Pose is technically a variation of Warrior II Pose that stretches your side body and chest. The pose can be used in transition between standing poses to create fluidity, such as between Warrior II and Extended Side Angle.

1. From Warrior II Pose, bring the palm of your back hand to your back thigh.
2. Flip your front hand so your front palm faces the sky. Inhale and sweep your extended front arm up and toward the sky. Continue to reach your front arm upward and back, with your front palm facing behind you.
3. Keep your front knee bent at a right angle. As you exhale, bend deeper into your front knee.
4. Lift your sternum toward the sky as you continue to reach upward with your raised arm. Breathe for 3 breaths as you feel a long stretch from the tips of your extended arm to your side torso. Return to Warrior II Pose, and switch feet to do the other side.

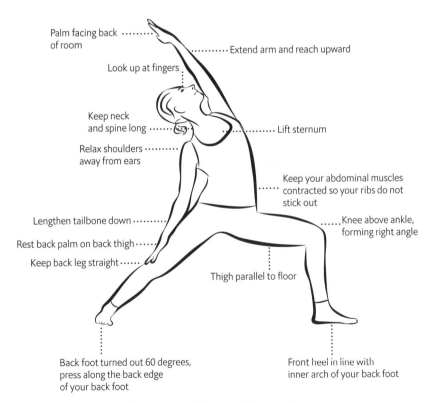

Palm facing back of room

Extend arm and reach upward

Look up at fingers

Keep neck and spine long

Lift sternum

Relax shoulders away from ears

Keep your abdominal muscles contracted so your ribs do not stick out

Lengthen tailbone down

Knee above ankle, forming right angle

Rest back palm on back thigh

Keep back leg straight

Thigh parallel to floor

Back foot turned out 60 degrees, press along the back edge of your back foot

Front heel in line with inner arch of your back foot

Figure 7.35   Reverse Warrior Pose

Low Lunge Pose (Anjaneyasana)

Low Lunge Pose, or Low Crescent Lunge, is calming and stabilizing, allowing you to stay close to the earth. The pose is used to prepare the body for the balance and strength needed in High Lunge. Low Lunge is also part of the Moon Salutation series, a soft and grounding sequence.

1. Start from Downward Facing Dog Pose, and step your right foot forward between your hands. Keep your hands shoulder width apart on the ground or on blocks flanking your front foot.

2. Keep your back knee lifted but not locked, and straighten your back leg. Your front knee should be above your ankle. Look forward without compressing your neck. This pose is a Low Lunge variation called Runner's Lunge. Runner's Lunge is often used to move into Pyramid Pose or as a modification of Low Lunge if you have knee injuries. If you find yourself rounding your back in an effort to reach the ground, place your palms or fingertips onto blocks on each side of your front foot. The purpose is not to touch the ground but to lengthen your spine. Use the support of the blocks to reach your chest forward and keep your torso long.

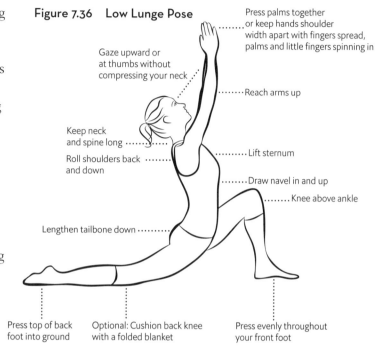

Figure 7.36   Low Lunge Pose

Gaze upward or at thumbs without compressing your neck

Press palms together or keep hands shoulder width apart with fingers spread, palms and little fingers spinning in

Reach arms up

Keep neck and spine long

Roll shoulders back and down

Lift sternum

Draw navel in and up

Knee above ankle

Lengthen tailbone down

Press top of back foot into ground

Optional: Cushion back knee with a folded blanket

Press evenly throughout your front foot

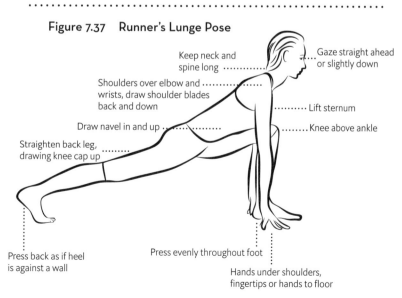

Figure 7.37   Runner's Lunge Pose

Keep neck and spine long

Gaze straight ahead or slightly down

Shoulders over elbow and wrists, draw shoulder blades back and down

Lift sternum

Draw navel in and up

Knee above ankle

Straighten back leg, drawing knee cap up

Press back as if heel is against a wall

Press evenly throughout foot

Hands under shoulders, fingertips or hands to floor

3. Lower your back knee to the ground, or onto a blanket for additional cushioning of your knee. Untuck your back toes. Your front knee should be above your ankle.

4. Inhale and place your hands on your knees or onto blocks next to your front foot. Lengthen your tailbone down.

5. Once you feel stable in your legs, raise your arms so that your fingertips reach toward the sky, palms facing in toward each other, little fingers rotating inward. You can also clasp your hands to form Releasing Mudra (page 225) or hook your thumbs together and spread the rest of your fingers wide like a flying bird. If you have shoulder injuries, place your hands directly under your shoulders onto blocks instead.

6. Lift your sternum to create a slight backbend. Contract your abdominal muscles, navel to spine, so that your ribs don't poke forward. Stay for 5 breaths. On each inhalation, lift yours arms a little higher toward the sky. With each exhalation, bend deeper and forward into your hips, but continue to draw your tailbone down. Do not push yourself so far that you are leaning forward. Your shoulders should be over your hips.

7. When you're ready to come out, lower your hands to your hips and then on each side of your front foot. Lift your back knee to Runner's Lunge, and step your back foot to meet the front foot to fold into Standing Forward Bend or return to Downward Facing Dog Pose. Repeat on the other side, and hold for the same amount of time.

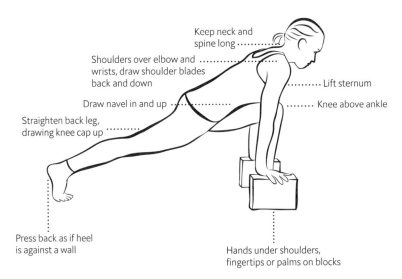

Keep neck and spine long ·········

Shoulders over elbow and ············ wrists, draw shoulder blades back and down

·········· Lift sternum

Draw navel in and up ···········

········ Knee above ankle

Straighten back leg, drawing knee cap up ·········

Press back as if heel is against a wall

Hands under shoulders, fingertips or palms on blocks

Figure 7.38   Runner's Lunge Pose modification with blocks

High Lunge (Alanasana)

High Lunge, or High Crescent Lunge, stretches in both directions toward the earth and sky. You must ground firmly into the legs to get balance and also lift upward with the arms. High Lunge improves balance and leg strength and simultaneously stretches your neck and shoulders. Prepare for High Lunge by first doing Low Lunge.

1. Start in Downward Facing Dog Pose. Step your right foot forward between your hands. Bend your front knee so that it is above your ankle, forming a right angle.

2. Root down in both legs, firming and straightening your back leg. Keep your back toes tucked. Your legs should be staggered on two separate tracks about hip width apart. Widen your stance for more stability.

3. Once you feel strong in your legs, inhale and lift your torso so that it is perpendicular to the ground. Exhale and place your hands on your hips, and bend deeper into your front knee to make sure it is at a right angle.

4. Lengthen your tailbone down and keep your abdominal muscles contracted, drawing your navel to your spine.

5. Inhale to sweep your arms to the sky. Press your palms together or spread your fingers wide, keeping arms shoulder width apart and face palms in, with little fingers rotating in.

6. Reach back with your back heel so that your back leg is straight. Stay for 5 breaths. Exhale to lower your torso to your front thigh and place your hands to frame the front foot in Runner's Lunge. Step back to Downward Facing Dog, and repeat on the other side.

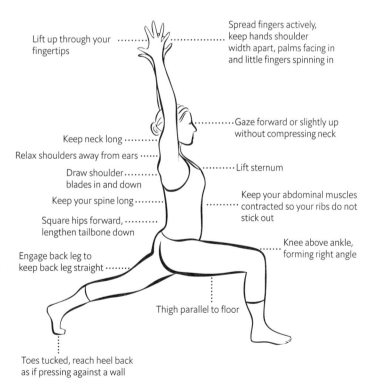

Lift up through your fingertips

Spread fingers actively, keep hands shoulder width apart, palms facing in and little fingers spinning in

Gaze forward or slightly up without compressing neck

Keep neck long

Relax shoulders away from ears

Draw shoulder blades in and down

Lift sternum

Keep your spine long

Keep your abdominal muscles contracted so your ribs do not stick out

Square hips forward, lengthen tailbone down

Knee above ankle, forming right angle

Engage back leg to keep back leg straight

Thigh parallel to floor

Toes tucked, reach heel back as if pressing against a wall

Figure 7.39   High Lunge Pose

Extended Side Angle Pose (Utthita Parsvakonasana)

Extended Side Angle Pose gives you a nice side stretch and helps you expand your sense of self by reaching either forward or lifting yourself upward. The pose also strengthens your legs and knees.

1. Start in Mountain Pose, and step your feet to 3½ to 4 feet apart. Turn out your back foot by about 60 to 90 degrees. Line your front heel with the arch of your back foot.

2. Inhale and raise both arms out to your sides, palms facing down, fingers spread wide.

3. Exhale and bend your front knee to a right angle, so that it is directly above your ankle, and your front thigh is parallel to the ground as much as possible without straining.

4. Reach your back arm toward the sky, perpendicular to the ground. Spread your fingers and continue to reach up actively. You can stay here or for a deeper side stretch, continue to reach your top arm forward and over your ear, with the palm facing the ground. Feel a long stretch from the outer edge of your back foot to the fingertips of your raised hand. Relax your shoulders away from your ears.

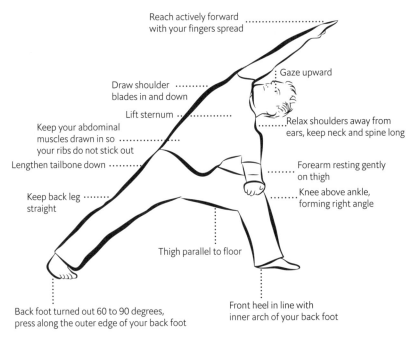

Reach actively forward with your fingers spread

Gaze upward

Draw shoulder blades in and down

Lift sternum

Keep your abdominal muscles drawn in so your ribs do not stick out

Relax shoulders away from ears, keep neck and spine long

Lengthen tailbone down

Forearm resting gently on thigh

Knee above ankle, forming right angle

Keep back leg straight

Thigh parallel to floor

Back foot turned out 60 to 90 degrees, press along the outer edge of your back foot

Front heel in line with inner arch of your back foot

Figure 7.40   Extended Side Angle Pose (Supported)

5. Continue to extend your torso over your front thigh, bending from the hip joint. Press into the outer edge of your back foot to keep your back leg straight and strong.

6. For Supported Extended Side Angle, bend and rest your front arm onto your front thigh gently, but do not put all your weight into this arm. Supported Extended Side Angle is a good first version of the pose.

When you are more warmed up, try practicing deeper variations by pressing your front hand onto a block or on the ground outside your front foot.

7. Turn your head to look up toward the thumb of your lifted hand. If you have neck injuries, do not turn your head to look up. Keep your head neutral and look ahead instead or down at the ground. Breathe for 5 breaths, continuing to use the top hand to lift you up so that you are not compressing your sides. Inhale to lift your torso and straighten both legs. Switch to do the other side.

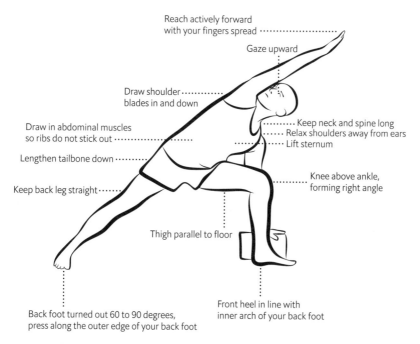

Reach actively forward with your fingers spread

Gaze upward

Draw shoulder blades in and down

Draw in abdominal muscles so ribs do not stick out

Lengthen tailbone down

Keep back leg straight

Keep neck and spine long
Relax shoulders away from ears
Lift sternum

Knee above ankle, forming right angle

Thigh parallel to floor

Back foot turned out 60 to 90 degrees, press along the outer edge of your back foot

Front heel in line with inner arch of your back foot

Figure 7.41 Extended Side Angle modification with block

Extended Triangle Pose (Utthita Trikonasana)

Extended Triangle Pose stretches your legs, shoulders, chest, and back and tones your arms and legs.

1. Start in Mountain Pose, and step your feet to 3½ to 4 feet apart with your right foot in front, left foot in the back. Turn your back foot out about 60 to 90 degrees. Line your front heel with the arch of your back foot.

2. Inhale and raise both arms out to your sides, palms facing down, fingers spread wide.

3. Exhale and reach forward with your right hand, palm down. Bring your torso toward the right and bend at your hip joint over your right leg, drawing your right hip joint back to create length on your right side. Rotate your torso to the left to keep your torso long on both sides.

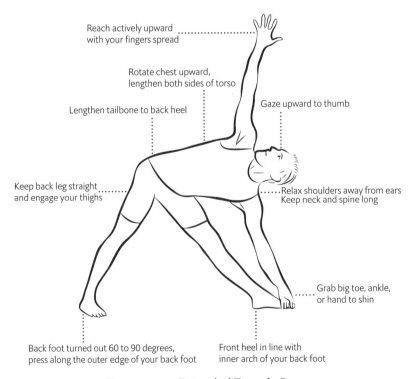

Reach actively upward with your fingers spread

Rotate chest upward, lengthen both sides of torso

Lengthen tailbone to back heel

Gaze upward to thumb

Keep back leg straight and engage your thighs

Relax shoulders away from ears
Keep neck and spine long

Grab big toe, ankle, or hand to shin

Back foot turned out 60 to 90 degrees, press along the outer edge of your back foot

Front heel in line with inner arch of your back foot

Figure 7.42   Extended Triangle Pose

4. Press into the outer edge of the back foot. Lengthen your tailbone toward your back heel. Draw in your abdominal muscles so that your ribs do not stick out.

5. Rest your right hand on your shin, ankle, or on a block or the ground on the outside or inside of your front foot. If you can reach the big toe of your front foot comfortably, grab it with your index and middle finger.

6. Stretch your left arm to the sky, perpendicular to the ground, and spread your fingers actively. Turn your head to look up at the thumb of your raised hand, or keep your head neutral. Stay for 5 breaths. Inhale to rise as you press on the back heel. Switch feet to repeat on the other side.

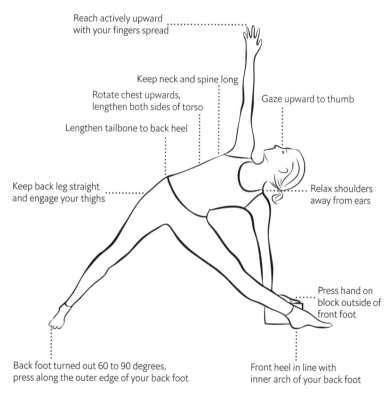

Reach actively upward with your fingers spread

Keep neck and spine long

Rotate chest upwards, lengthen both sides of torso

Gaze upward to thumb

Lengthen tailbone to back heel

Keep back leg straight and engage your thighs

Relax shoulders away from ears

Press hand on block outside of front foot

Back foot turned out 60 to 90 degrees, press along the outer edge of your back foot

Front heel in line with inner arch of your back foot

Figure 7.43   Extended Triangle Pose modification with block

Twisting Poses

It's important not to push yourself too far in twisting poses just to achieve a certain shape. To protect your spine and neck muscles, the twist should come from your center—from the lower half of your torso—your core and deep abdominal muscles. Avoid rounding your back or pulling yourself forward with your hands or twisting from your shoulders. Do not use your hands to tug or twist yourself rigorously as this can cause unsafe strain. Deep twisting poses should be avoided altogether during pregnancy.

Table 7.8   Twisting Poses

English Name	Sanskrit Name	Gaze	Modifications	Cautions & Contraindications
Revolved Fierce (Chair) Pose	Parivrtta Utkatasana	Beginner: Downward or to the side in the direction of the twist Experienced: Upward	• Hand onto block in front of feet • For deeper twist, arms spread and lower hand on ground or block outside of foot	Back or abdominal injury, pregnancy
Revolved Lunge Pose	Parivrtta Anjaneyasana	Beginner: Downward or to the side in the direction of the twist Experienced: Upward	• Back knee on ground • Hand onto block or ground inside or outside front foot • For deeper twist, spread arms or bind hands under thigh	Back or abdominal injury, pregnancy
Revolved Triangle Pose	Parivrtta Trikonasana	Beginner: Downward or to the side in the direction of the twist Experienced: Thumb of raised hand	• Hand on block inside or outside front foot • Keep one hand on hip instead of raised	Back or abdominal injury, pregnancy
Seated Spinal Twist	Ardha Matsyendrasana	Side in the direction of the twist or away from twist	• Lower leg extended • Arm hugging knee	Back or abdominal injury, pregnancy

Revolved Fierce Pose (Parivrtta Utkatasana)

Revolved Fierce Pose strengthens your quadriceps, knees, and gluteus muscles.

1. Start in Fierce Pose with your hands pressed together in front of your chest.

2. Inhale to lengthen your spine and lift higher through the top of your head.

3. Exhale to twist your left elbow over your right thigh. Widen your collarbone and continue to press your hands together at your chest. Twist from your abdominal core rather than using your elbow as leverage.

4. Press into your heels, and stay for 5 breaths. Make sure your knees are not going past your toes. Keep your weight in your heels and check to make sure your knees are even and in line with each other. It's common for the knee that you're twisting away from to stick out in front of the other. If so, draw your left thighbone gently back to get your knees even.

5. Exhale back to center to return to Fierce Pose, and fold forward into Standing Forward Bend to rest for 5 breaths. Repeat on the other side.

For a gentler twist, separate your hips shoulder width apart and place a block on its tallest side in front of your feet. Place one palm on the block and press down as your lift your other hand toward the sky. Look up at your raised hand, or, if you have neck injuries, keep your head neutral.

For a deeper twist, press your bottom hand on the ground outside your foot and reach up toward the sky with your other hand, spreading the collarbone and arms wide.

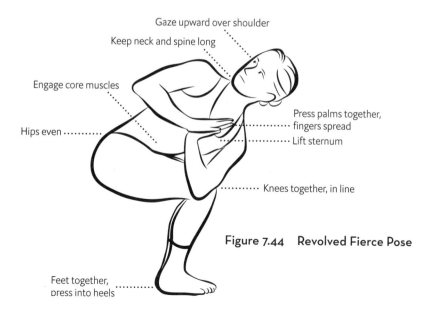

Gaze upward over shoulder
Keep neck and spine long
Engage core muscles
Hips even
Press palms together, fingers spread
Lift sternum
Knees together, in line
Feet together, press into heels

Figure 7.44   Revolved Fierce Pose

Revolved Lunge (Parivrtta Anjaneyasana)

Revolved Lunge is a twisting balance pose that stretches your psoas muscles and hips and strengthens your core, quadriceps, and gluteus muscles. The psoas muscles are major stabilizers of the lower back, so sufferers of lumbar back pain have to exercise extra caution in performing twists around these muscles.

1. Start in High Lunge with your back heel lifted. Bring your palms together in front of the center of your chest.

2. Inhale as you press your back heel back, as if against a wall (you can also do this against a wall for more support). Exhale and twist toward your front thigh, bringing your torso close to your thigh. If possible, hook the elbow of your lower arm over your front thigh.

   You can also bring your back knee down to provide more stability and feel more grounded. This can often help you achieve a safer, better twist from your core muscles.

3. Press your palms together and on each exhalation, twist a little deeper, with your chest rotating in the direction of the sky. Gaze upward past your shoulder or to the side. If you are a beginner or have a neck injury, keep your head neutral or look downward.

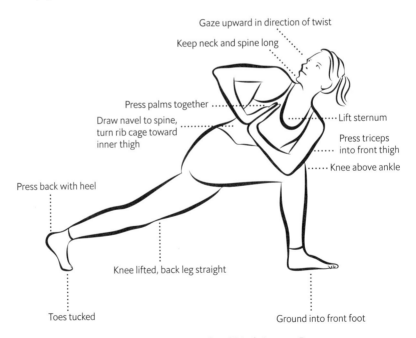

Gaze upward in direction of twist

Keep neck and spine long

Press palms together

Draw navel to spine, turn rib cage toward inner thigh

Lift sternum

Press triceps into front thigh

Knee above ankle

Press back with heel

Knee lifted, back leg straight

Toes tucked

Ground into front foot

Figure 7.45   Revolved High Lunge Pose

4. For a deeper twist, you can release your lower hand to the ground outside your front foot and lift your other hand toward the sky.

5. Stay here for 5 breaths. Release your twist by returning to center and placing both hands on the ground to frame your front foot in Low Lunge. Step back to Downward Facing Dog, and switch to the other side.

Before doing the full version of volved Lunge, it is a good idea to rm up the body and start with a s intense twist.

1. Start in Low Lunge with your right foot in front. You can keep your back left knee up or down, toes tucked. Inhale to lengthen your spine from head to toe.

2. Place your left hand to the inside of your front foot on the ground or onto a block. Exhale to twist gently toward your front thigh. Lift your right hand toward the sky.

3. Stay for 5 breaths, twisting a little deeper with each exhalation.

4. Exhale and release your twist. Bring your hands to the ground to frame your front foot in Low Lunge, then switch sides.

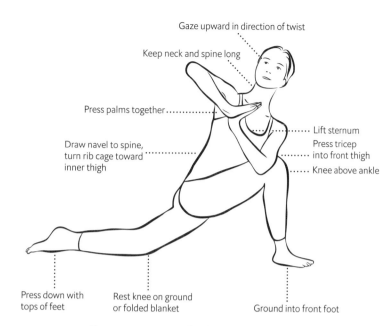

Gaze upward in direction of twist
Keep neck and spine long
Press palms together
Draw navel to spine, turn rib cage toward inner thigh
Lift sternum
Press tricep into front thigh
Knee above ankle
Press down with tops of feet
Rest knee on ground or folded blanket
Ground into front foot

Figure 7.46   Revolved Low Lunge Pose

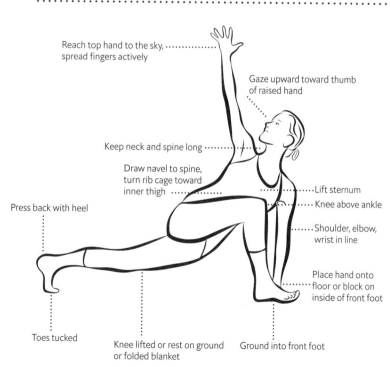

Reach top hand to the sky, spread fingers actively
Gaze upward toward thumb of raised hand
Keep neck and spine long
Draw navel to spine, turn rib cage toward inner thigh
Press back with heel
Lift sternum
Knee above ankle
Shoulder, elbow, wrist in line
Place hand onto floor or block on inside of front foot
Toes tucked
Knee lifted or rest on ground or folded blanket
Ground into front foot

Figure 7.47   Revolved Lunge modification

Revolved Triangle Pose (Parivrtta Trikonasana)

Revolved Triangle is a good pose for detoxification of "negative energy," providing a deep twist in your core muscles. Take caution especially if you have any back issues—be gentle and twist from your center rather than pulling yourself into a twist with your hands. Do not go past what feels right for your body, and use modifications with a block if more comfortable.

1. Start in Mountain Pose. Step your right foot back, so that your feet are 3½ to 4 feet apart. Point your left foot forward and turn your right foot about 45 degrees away from your midline. Put your hands on your hips. Your hips should face the right side of the mat.

   You have three options for your feet, depending on the level of difficulty that you prefer:

   Level 1. Keep your feet hip width apart.

   Level 2. Line your front heel with your back heel.

   Level 3. Line your front heel with the arch of your back foot.

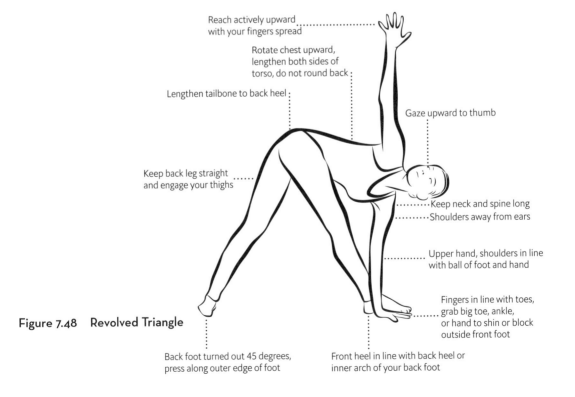

Reach actively upward with your fingers spread

Rotate chest upward, lengthen both sides of torso, do not round back

Lengthen tailbone to back heel

Gaze upward to thumb

Keep back leg straight and engage your thighs

Keep neck and spine long
Shoulders away from ears

Upper hand, shoulders in line with ball of foot and hand

Fingers in line with toes, grab big toe, ankle, or hand to shin or block outside front foot

Figure 7.48   Revolved Triangle

Back foot turned out 45 degrees, press along outer edge of foot

Front heel in line with back heel or inner arch of your back foot

2. Keep your left hand on your hip. Inhale to raise your right hand toward the sky and lengthen your spine.

3. Exhale to hinge at your hips as you reach your right hand toward the front of the mat.

Place your right hand on your front shin, a block on the inside or outside of the front foot, or grab the big toe of your front foot. Do not reach any farther if you start to round your back.

4. Inhale to continue to lengthen your back, keeping it flat and parallel to the ground. Exhale to rotate toward the left. Beginners or those with neck injuries can keep the head neutral and look straight ahead or downward.

5. Your left hand can stay at your hip. For a deeper twist, reach your left hand toward the sky and turn your head to gaze at the thumb of your raised hand.

6. Stay for 5 breaths. To exit the pose, turn back to the center, bring your hands back to your hips, and inhale to root into your feet as you lift your torso up, keeping a flat back. Step back to Mountain Pose, then breathe and switch sides.

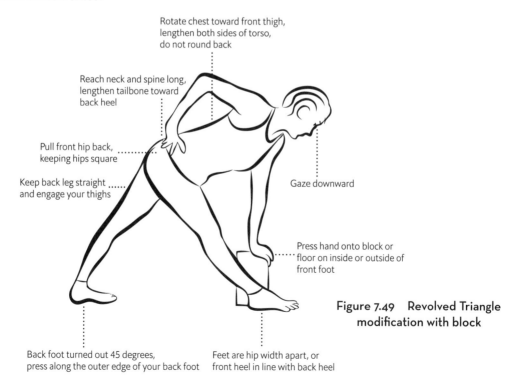

Rotate chest toward front thigh, lengthen both sides of torso, do not round back

Reach neck and spine long, lengthen tailbone toward back heel

Pull front hip back, keeping hips square

Keep back leg straight and engage your thighs

Gaze downward

Press hand onto block or floor on inside or outside of front foot

Figure 7.49 Revolved Triangle modification with block

Back foot turned out 45 degrees, press along the outer edge of your back foot

Feet are hip width apart, or front heel in line with back heel

Seated Spinal Twist (Ardha Matsyendrasana)

Seated Spinal Twist gently wrings out tension in your back and makes your spine more flexible. Use this pose to cool down and stretch your hip muscles.

1. Sit with your legs straight out in front of you. Bend your knees and slide your left foot under your right leg. Place your right foot on the ground over your left leg, to the outside of your left thigh, so that your right knee points to the sky. Keep both sitting bones evenly on the ground.

2. Place your right hand on the ground behind your buttocks to support the length of your back. Press down on your right hand to straighten your spine and sit taller.

3. Inhale to lift your left arm toward the sky. Exhale and twist toward the inside of your right thigh. The crook of your left arm can wrap over your right knee, hugging your right thigh in toward your chest. For a deeper twist, hook your right elbow to the outside of your left thigh, keeping your left arm bent and actively spreading your fingers.

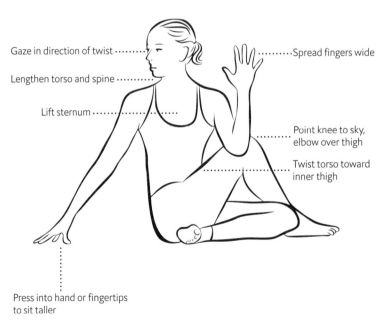

Gaze in direction of twist

Lengthen torso and spine

Lift sternum

Spread fingers wide

Point knee to sky, elbow over thigh

Twist torso toward inner thigh

Press into hand or fingertips to sit taller

Figure 7.50   Seated Spinal Twist

4. Gaze over your right shoulder in the direction of the twist. Or, if you have neck injuries, keep your head neutral and look straight ahead. Stay for 5 breaths. Exhale to release the twist. Switch your legs, and repeat on the other side.

If you have knee injuries or want a gentler twist, keep your bottom leg straight with your foot flexed, crossing your right foot over your left thigh.

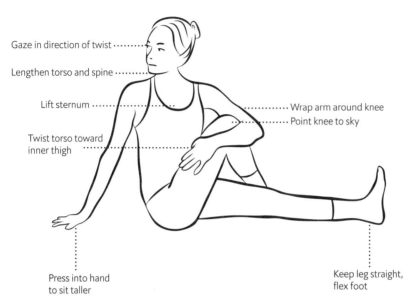

Gaze in direction of twist

Lengthen torso and spine

Lift sternum

Wrap arm around knee

Point knee to sky

Twist torso toward inner thigh

Press into hand to sit taller

Keep leg straight, flex foot

Figure 7.51   Seated Spinal Twist modification with lower leg straight

Balancing Poses

Balancing poses give you the opportunity to find your center of gravity, enhance focus and concentration, strengthen muscles, and improve coordination and balance. You might discover that one side of your body feels different from the other in these poses. Balancing poses also help us let go of a perfectionistic attitude. Even if you feel wobbly or shaky at first, let yourself enjoy the fluidity of your form. If you fall out of the pose, don't judge yourself and just try again if it feels right. The lesson of yoga is in the ability to let go of self-criticism and judgment and to try again. There is no perfect pose—even in the stillness of balancing poses, things are always changing. Our ability to ride the waves—or shakiness—is what builds our resilience.

Table 7.9 Balance Poses

English Name	Sanskrit Name	Gaze	Modifications	Cautions & Contraindications
Warrior III Pose	Virabhadrasana III	Downward	• Hands supported on blocks • Arms alongside torso • Hands clasped at lower back • Hands reaching to touch a wall	Hip or ankle injury
Half Moon Pose	Ardha Chandrasana	Beginner: Neck neutral Experienced: Upward at thumb of raised hand	• Lower hand on block 6 inches in front and outside of front little toe	Hip, groin, or ankle injury
Tree Pose	Vrksasana	Straight ahead	• Arms at chest or up • Big toe on ground as kickstand • Sole of foot to inside of standing leg's calf, or inner or upper thigh	Ankle injury
Eagle Pose	Garudasana	Straight ahead	• Big toe on ground outside ankle of standing foot as support • Hands on opposite shoulders	Elbow or knee injury
Side Plank Pose	Vasisthasana	Straight ahead	• One knee down • Cross leg and place foot on ground • Soles of feet against wall	Hand, wrist, elbow, or ankle injury

Warrior III Pose (Virabhadrasana III)

Warrior III makes your body focused and strong like an arrow. In this pose, you build balance and coordination and strengthen your back, legs, arms, shoulders, and core muscles. Warrior III has a component of a slight backbend as well, giving you an extra lift and stretch in your chest and shoulders.

1. Start in High Lunge Pose. Your front knee should be bent, and the toes of your back foot tucked under. Place both hands at your hips to make sure that your hips are facing forward. You can keep your hands at your hips or use other variations. You can bring your hands together in front of your chest in Salutation Seal Mudra (page 223). For a shoulder stretch, clasp your hands behind your lower back.

2. Press evenly into your front foot as you shift your weight gradually to the front foot. Draw your navel toward your spine and contract your core muscles. Inhale to lift your back foot as you lean your torso toward your front thigh.

3. Exhale to slowly extend both legs, without locking the knee of your standing leg. Press into big toe mound and heel of your standing foot. Your back leg reaches backward behind you. Lift your back leg higher so that it is parallel to the ground. Flex your foot and point the toes of back foot downward so that your hips are even, and one is not higher than the

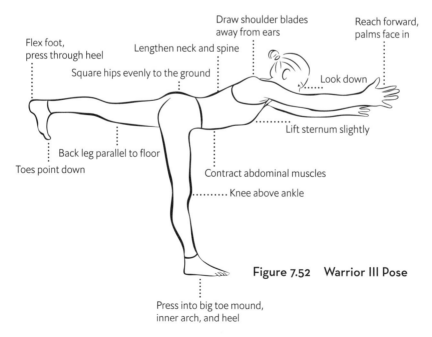

Flex foot, press through heel

Lengthen neck and spine

Draw shoulder blades away from ears

Reach forward, palms face in

Square hips evenly to the ground

Look down

Back leg parallel to floor

Toes point down

Lift sternum slightly

Contract abdominal muscles

Knee above ankle

Figure 7.52 Warrior III Pose

Press into big toe mound, inner arch, and heel

other. Press back with your back foot, as if you were actively pushing your heel against a wall.

4. If you feel stable here, reach forward with both hands so that your arms are in line with your head and neck and parallel to the ground. Turn your palms toward each other and draw your shoulder blades away from your ears. Lift your sternum and reach actively forward with your hands.

   If your hands are clasped behind your back, lift your hands away from your lower back and lift your sternum for a slight backbend.

   Another arm variation is extending your arms backward alongside your torso, parallel to the ground. Point your thumbs outward away from your body.

5. Gaze downward. Stay for 5 breaths if comfortable. Exhale to step back to High Lunge or draw your back leg in toward your standing leg to place both feet together for Mountain Pose.

Supported Warrior III uses blocks to increase stability in this balancing pose. Place two blocks, one directly below each shoulder. Place your hands on these blocks so that your shoulder, elbow, and wrist are perpendicular to the ground. Press on the blocks as you continue to lift your sternum so that your torso and back leg are parallel to the ground.

Another option is to use the wall. Stand about an arm's length away from the wall. As you shift forward for Warrior III, reach toward the wall with your hands, using your fingertips against the wall as support.

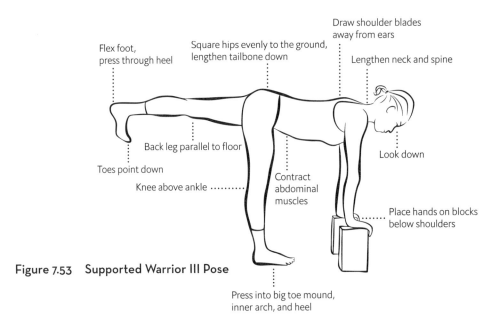

Draw shoulder blades away from ears

Flex foot, press through heel

Square hips evenly to the ground, lengthen tailbone down

Lengthen neck and spine

Back leg parallel to floor

Look down

Toes point down

Knee above ankle

Contract abdominal muscles

Place hands on blocks below shoulders

Figure 7.53   Supported Warrior III Pose

Press into big toe mound, inner arch, and heel

Half Moon Pose (Ardha Chandrasana)

If you want to take flight, try Half Moon Pose. The balance pose feels like flying, expands your chest and shoulders, and strengthens your legs and hips.

1. Start in Warrior II Pose with your arms extended, right foot forward. Make sure that your hips are facing the long edge of the mat. For the Half Moon with block variation, place a block 6 inches in front of and 6 inches outside the little toe of your front foot. Place your left hand onto your hip.

2. Inhale and shift your weight into your front leg. Ground firmly throughout the inner arch, outer edge, ball, toes, and heel of your front foot. Keep your front knee bent.

3. Exhale and shift slowly forward as you lift your back leg and start to extend your standing leg, without locking it.

4. Extend your right arm toward the ground or the block that you had set up. Your hand should be in line with your shoulder, and adjust the block as necessary. Tent your fingertips so that they touch lightly onto the ground or a block.

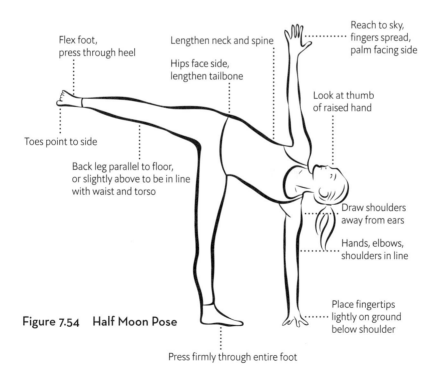

Flex foot, press through heel

Lengthen neck and spine

Hips face side, lengthen tailbone

Reach to sky, fingers spread, palm facing side

Look at thumb of raised hand

Toes point to side

Back leg parallel to floor, or slightly above to be in line with waist and torso

Draw shoulders away from ears

Hands, elbows, shoulders in line

Place fingertips lightly on ground below shoulder

Figure 7.54   Half Moon Pose

Press firmly through entire foot

5. Raise your back leg farther so that it becomes parallel to the ground, or slightly above, to keep in line with your waist and torso. Flex your back foot actively, as if you are pressing against the wall with your heel. Point your toes to the left side of the mat, so your hips face the side of the mat.

6. Keep your neck and spine long, reaching toward the front. You can choose to gaze toward the side. You can keep your left hand at your hip. Or, for a deeper pose, lift your left hand to reach toward the sky with your fingers spread actively. Gaze toward the thumb of your lifted hand.

7. Breathe for 5 counts. To exit the pose, look at your standing foot. Bring your left hand back to your hip and slowly lower your left foot and place next to your right foot. Fold forward in Standing Forward Bend. Switch to repeat on the other side.

For additional support, try doing Half Moon Pose against a wall. In Warrior II, line up the right side of your body (right thigh, shoulder, and hip) so that it is a few inches away from the wall. Move into Half Moon, with your torso, back, and hips supported by the wall behind you.

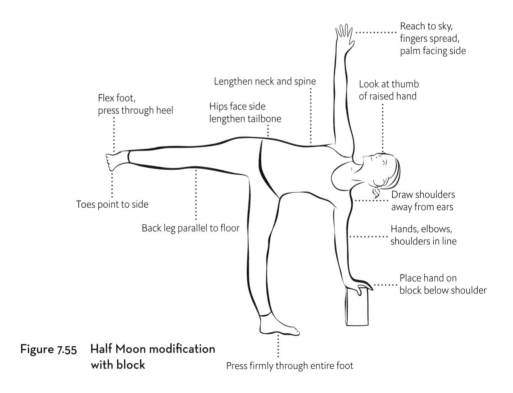

Reach to sky, fingers spread, palm facing side

Lengthen neck and spine

Look at thumb of raised hand

Flex foot, press through heel

Hips face side lengthen tailbone

Toes point to side

Draw shoulders away from ears

Back leg parallel to floor

Hands, elbows, shoulders in line

Place hand on block below shoulder

Figure 7.55 Half Moon modification with block

Press firmly through entire foot

Tree Pose (Vrksasana)

1. Stand in Mountain Pose with your feet hip width apart and firmly grounded in the "four corners" of your feet. Look forward and find a place straight ahead of you to focus your gaze.

2. Shift your weight to your right foot as you begin to lift your left foot. You have three options for your raised foot:

   Option A. Kickstand. Support yourself by using your foot as a kickstand. Place the sole of your left foot against your ankle so that your left toes are touching the ground and your left heel is pressed against your lower calf of the other leg.

   Option B. Inner calf. Press the sole of your left foot on the inside of the calf of your other leg, toes pointing downward.

   Option C. Inner thigh. Press the sole of your left foot on the inside of your mid or upper thigh and point your toes downward.

   Do not place the sole of your foot on your knee—this can be harmful on the joint.

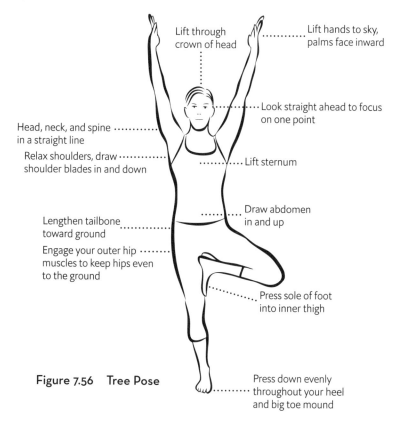

Lift through crown of head

Lift hands to sky, palms face inward

Look straight ahead to focus on one point

Head, neck, and spine in a straight line

Relax shoulders, draw shoulder blades in and down

Lift sternum

Draw abdomen in and up

Lengthen tailbone toward ground

Engage your outer hip muscles to keep hips even to the ground

Press sole of foot into inner thigh

Figure 7.56   Tree Pose

Press down evenly throughout your heel and big toe mound

3. Keep your hips even to the ground. Press on the big toe mound of your standing leg.

4. Press your hands together in front of your chest. You can stay with your hands in Salutation Seal Mudra (page 223) in front of your chest. Or, inhale and slowly raise your arms to the sky, palms facing inward. Continue to lift through the top of your head, and keep your spine long. Lift your sternum. Lifting your arms can often create neck tension, relax your shoulders away from your ears.

5. Take 5 breaths. You may feel wobbly at first or need to step out of Tree Pose at times, but this is normal. Exhale and lower your hands, palms pressed in front of your chest. Release your hands alongside your body as you lower your left foot to return to Mountain Pose. Shake the body to loosen any tension and return to Mountain Pose to repeat on the other side.

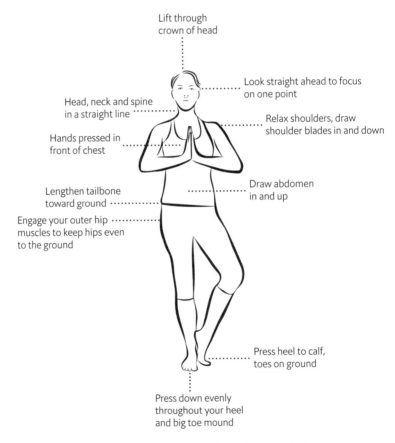

Lift through crown of head

Look straight ahead to focus on one point

Head, neck and spine in a straight line

Relax shoulders, draw shoulder blades in and down

Hands pressed in front of chest

Lengthen tailbone toward ground

Draw abdomen in and up

Engage your outer hip muscles to keep hips even to the ground

Press heel to calf, toes on ground

Press down evenly throughout your heel and big toe mound

Figure 7.57 Tree Pose with modified kickstand

Eagle Pose (Garudasana)

Feel regal in this pose named after the mythical "King of Birds" who burned bright with fire and light.

1. Stand in Mountain Pose with your feet hip width apart. Stand tall with your neck and spine long, and lift through the crown of your head. Look straight ahead and find a point to fix your gaze.

2. Contract your abdominal muscles and shift your weight onto your right foot. Gently bend both knees. Inhale and lift your left foot off the ground. Cross your left knee over your right thigh. For more support, place your left big toe onto the ground outside your right ankle, acting like a kick-stand. Or, if comfortable, continue to wrap your left toes behind the lower calf of your standing leg and ankle.

3. Press evenly throughout the sole of your foot on the ground. Keep your neck and spine long and do not round your back. Continue to contract your abdominal muscles.

4. Inhale and raise your arms parallel to the ground, wrap your left elbow under your right arm. Your right elbow rests in the crook of your left elbow. Bend both elbows, and lift your elbows away from your chest

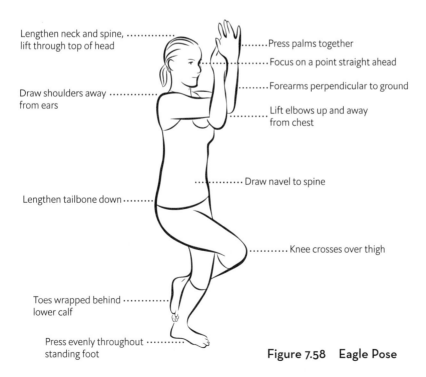

Lengthen neck and spine, lift through top of head

Press palms together

Focus on a point straight ahead

Forearms perpendicular to ground

Draw shoulders away from ears

Lift elbows up and away from chest

Draw navel to spine

Lengthen tailbone down

Knee crosses over thigh

Toes wrapped behind lower calf

Press evenly throughout standing foot

Figure 7.58   Eagle Pose

so that your forearms are perpendicular to the ground. If comfortable, continue wrap your forearms around each other so that your palms press together.

If you have shoulder or elbow discomfort or find that you are rounding your back, try a different arm variation. Place your left hand on your right shoulder and wrap your right hand to your left shoulder, giving yourself a hug. In either arm variation, draw your shoulder blades down and shoulders away from your ears.

5. Stay for 5 breaths. With each exhalation, gently reach your elbows forward and sit a little deeper. Exhale and unwind your arms and legs, returning to Mountain Pose. Repeat on the other side.

Side Plank Pose (Vasisthasana)

Side Plank strengthens your balance and strengthens your arms, wrists, and legs. Beginners may have a hard time staying in this pose so try the variations first.

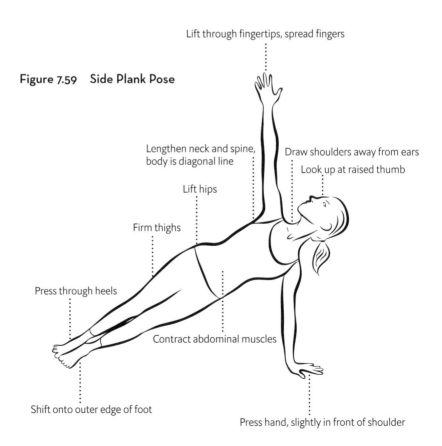

Lift through fingertips, spread fingers

Figure 7.59   Side Plank Pose

Lengthen neck and spine, body is diagonal line

Draw shoulders away from ears

Look up at raised thumb

Lift hips

Firm thighs

Press through heels

Contract abdominal muscles

Shift onto outer edge of foot

Press hand, slightly in front of shoulder

1. Start in Downward Facing Dog. Shift onto outer edge of your right foot. Turn your torso toward the left, shifting weight onto your right hand and outer right foot and right hand. Your right arm should be extended with your right hand slightly in front of your shoulder. Bring your left hand to your left hip.

2. Depending on the level of support you want in this pose, you have different options for your legs.

   Option A. Knee down variation. Bring your right knee down to the ground below your hip. Press your shin to the ground with your knee at a 90-degree angle and right thigh perpendicular to the ground. Extend your left leg straight, and press your left foot on the floor. Press along the outer edge of your left foot to stabilize your lower body. You can stay here or lift your back leg toward the sky so that it is parallel to the floor.

   Option B. Foot down variation. Keep your right leg straight and press into the outer edge of your right foot to keep your side body long. Cross your left leg in front of your right knee. Place your left foot onto the ground firmly so that your shin is perpendicular to the ground. Press into your left foot and outer edge of your right foot to continue to lengthen through the right side of your body.

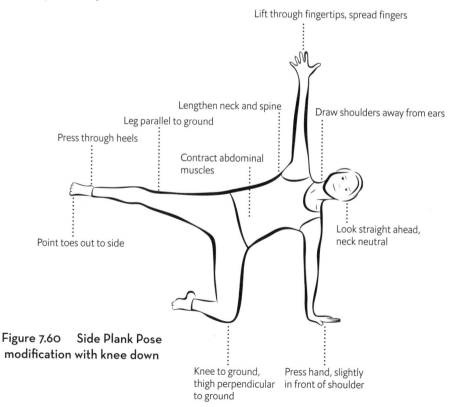

Lift through fingertips, spread fingers

Lengthen neck and spine

Leg parallel to ground

Draw shoulders away from ears

Press through heels

Contract abdominal muscles

Point toes out to side

Look straight ahead, neck neutral

Figure 7.60 Side Plank Pose modification with knee down

Knee to ground, thigh perpendicular to ground

Press hand, slightly in front of shoulder

Option C. Wall variation. Practice Side Plank Pose against the wall for additional support of your heels. Start in Downward Facing Dog with your heels pressing against the wall. Then, when you move onto the outer edge of your right foot, press the sole of your foot against the wall. Stack your left foot on top of your right foot, pressing the soles of both feet against the wall. Press through the heels of both feet in Side Plank.

Option D. Shift onto the outer edge of your right foot. Stack your left foot onto your right foot. Keep both feet flexed. Press through both heels as if you are in Mountain Pose.

3. If you feel stable here, raise your left hand toward the sky, spreading your fingers, palm facing away from you.

4. Your entire body from heels to top of head should be in one long, straight diagonal line. Keep your head in neutral position to look straight ahead or turn to look upward at the thumb of your raised hand.

5. Stay for 5 breaths or until ready to exit the pose. Bring your left hand down to the ground and turn your torso back toward the ground. Bring your knees down and rest in Child's Pose. Reverse sides and repeat on the other side.

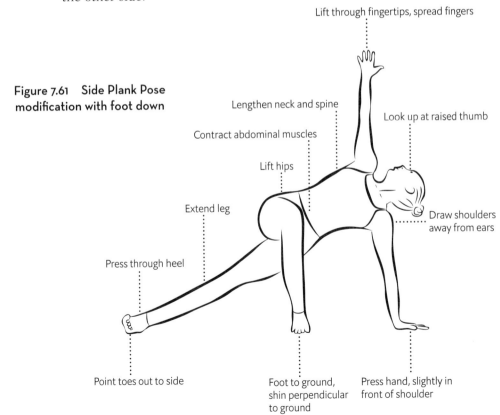

Figure 7.61 Side Plank Pose modification with foot down

Lift through fingertips, spread fingers

Lengthen neck and spine

Look up at raised thumb

Contract abdominal muscles

Lift hips

Draw shoulders away from ears

Extend leg

Press through heel

Point toes out to side

Foot to ground, shin perpendicular to ground

Press hand, slightly in front of shoulder

Backbend Poses

Backbend poses can feel radiant and expansive. But if done with too much intensity without warming up the body first, you can crunch your neck or overarch your lower back, causing strain or pain. So, it's important to prepare for these poses and go easy. In general, you should start with more gentle backbends and gradually progress to more strenuous backbends only when your body has warmed up. For the majority of us, our thoracic spine in our upper torso is naturally stiffer than our lower back. So, it's common (and harmful) for us to overarch and strain the lower back or neck to compensate for the stiff thoracic spine so as to achieve a backbend shape. Be careful not to crank your neck back too far in these poses either, as this can cause compression of your neck. Take caution in prone backbends if you are pregnant, since it places pressure on your abdominal area, and avoid them during your second and third trimester.

Table 7.10   Backbend Poses

English Name	Sanskrit Name	Gaze	Modifications	Cautions & Contraindications
Crocodile Pose	Makarasana	Eyes closed	• Hands to opposite elbows to prop torso up • Rest chin in palms and elbows on floor • Hands to opposite shoulder blades and rest head in crook of elbows	Back, neck, or abdominal injury; pregnancy
Cobra Pose	Bhujangasana	Tip of nose Do not compress neck.	Bend elbows and keep low to the ground for gentler version	Back, neck, or abdominal injury; carpal tunnel syndrome; pregnancy
Upward Facing Dog Pose	Urdhva Mukha Svanasana	Tip of nose Do not compress neck.	Hands onto blocks	Back, neck, or abdominal injury; spinal stenosis

(continued)

Table 7.10 Backbend Poses (*continued*)

English Name	Sanskrit Name	Gaze	Modifications	Cautions & Contraindications
Locust Pose	*Salabhasana*	Tip of nose Do not compress neck.	• Lift thighs and chest with rolled blankets under each • Keep legs grounded • Hands under shoulders off or on the ground • For deeper backbend, hands clasped at lower back, lift away from tailbone	Back, neck, or abdominal injury; pregnancy
Bow Pose	*Dhanurasana*	Tip of nose Do not compress neck.	• Support thighs with blanket underneath • Half Bow variation	Back, neck, or abdominal injury; pregnancy
Camel Pose	*Ustrasana*	Forward or up	• Hands at back of pelvis • Hands on heels • Toes turned under to lift heels • Against a wall • Blanket under knees or ankles	Back, neck, or abdominal injury; pregnancy
Reverse Tabletop Pose	*Ardha Purvottanasana*	Eyes closed or up	For deeper version, try Reverse Plank: keep legs straight and extended, soles of feet on the ground	Neck injury
Fish Pose	*Matsyasana*	Third Eye	Two blocks or rolled blanket under shoulders	Back or neck injury
Bridge Pose	*Setu Bandha Sarvangasana*	Eyes closed or up	Supported Bridge with block	Neck injury

Crocodile Pose (Makarasana)

If you're looking for some stress relief, Crocodile Pose is a calming pose that releases tension, improves headaches, fatigue, and insomnia.

1. Lie on your abdomen with your feet untucked. Cross your forearms under your head, palms facing down, and rest your forehead on your hands. Close your eyes. You have other options for your hands as well:

    Option A. Cross your arms with your hands on opposite shoulders and rest your head in the crook of your elbows.

    Option B. Cross your arms with your elbows below your shoulders to prop up your torso and let your head relax downward.

    Option C. Rest your elbows on the ground shoulder width apart and bring the base of your palms together. Place your chin in your palms.

2. Space your legs hip width apart. Relax and feel your entire body grounded on the floor.

3. Inhale fully and exhale to relax any tension in your body. Let your body relax deeper into the ground. Breathe for 5 counts.

4. To exit, bring your hands underneath your shoulders and press up into Tabletop or up and back into Child's Pose.

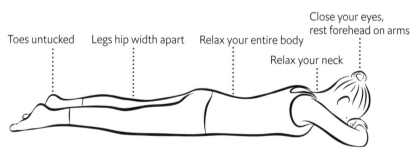

Toes untucked   Legs hip width apart   Relax your entire body   Relax your neck   Close your eyes, rest forehead on arms

Figure 7.62   Crocodile Pose

Cobra Pose (Bhujangasana)

Cobra Pose expands your chest and stretches your front torso. It can be part of Sun Salutation A series or done on its own. Start with gentle version. Keep your elbows bent and hugged in close to your torso. Once this is comfortable, work toward Cobra Pose by straightening your arms, but only as far as you can go while maintaining a connection to the ground with your pubic bone, thighs, and tops of your feet. Cobra can feel exhilarating, so there is a temptation to overdo it and strain the neck or lower spine.

1. Lie on your stomach. Your legs should point directly behind you with the tops of your feet on the ground. Your knees should be hip width apart.

2. Bring your hands on the ground underneath your shoulders, and spread your fingers wide. Draw your elbows close to your torso.

3. Inhale and press the tops of your feet into the floor, rooting your thighs and pubic bone into the ground. Press gently into your hands and use your back muscles to lift your chest away from the floor.

4. You can stay with your elbows bent, and hug them in toward your torso for a gentler version called Baby Cobra.

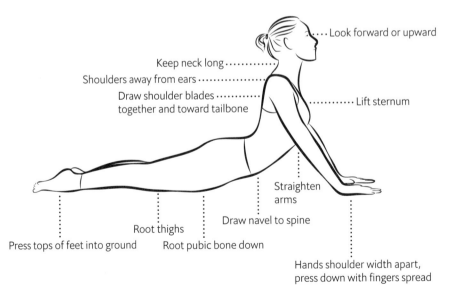

Figure 7.63   Cobra Pose

For a deeper backbend, continue to press on your hands and gradually extend your arms until fully straightened.

5. Draw your shoulders away from your eyes. Draw your shoulder blades together and toward your tailbone.

6. Lift your sternum. Contract your abdominal muscles so that your ribs don't jut forward. Keep your neck long and avoid throwing your head back, which compresses your neck.

7. Stay for 2–3 breaths. Exhale and gently release to the ground.

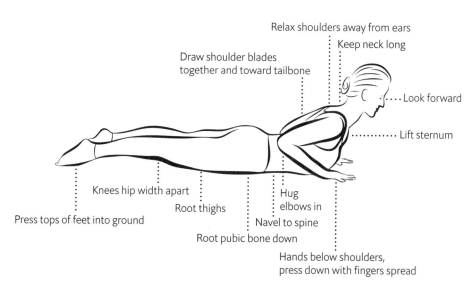

Figure 7.64   Baby Cobra Pose: gentler version of Cobra Pose

Upward Facing Dog Pose (Urdhva Mukha Svanasana)

Upward Facing Dog energizes your upper body and stretches your chest and abdomen. It is used in Sun Salutation series. Try this pose after you have warmed up your back already with Cobra Pose.

1. Lie on your stomach with the tops of your feet on the ground. Place your hands next to your rib cage with your elbows bent and your forearms nearly perpendicular to the floor.

2. Inhale and press into your palms. Straighten your arms and lift your torso, hips, and knees off the floor. Squeeze your elbows in toward your torso, so your elbow creases face forward. Roll your shoulders back, drawing your shoulder blades together and down toward your tailbone.

3. Draw your abdomen in toward your spine and press the tops of your feet into the ground. Lift your sternum forward and upward and widen your collarbones.

4. Lengthen through the back of your neck to prevent any compression. Lift through the top of your head. Look past the tip of your nose, which should be slightly upward.

5. Stay for 3 breaths. Exhale and release gently back to the ground.

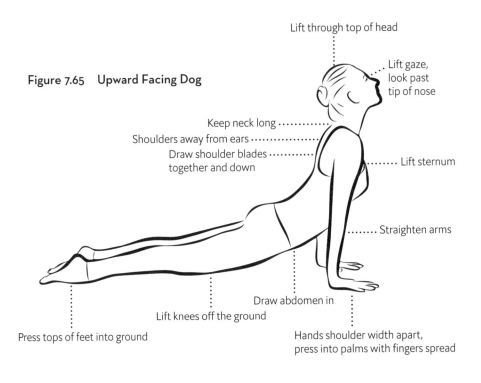

Lift through top of head

Lift gaze, look past tip of nose

Figure 7.65   Upward Facing Dog

Keep neck long

Shoulders away from ears

Draw shoulder blades together and down

Lift sternum

Straighten arms

Draw abdomen in

Lift knees off the ground

Press tops of feet into ground

Hands shoulder width apart, press into palms with fingers spread

Locust Pose (Salabhasana)

This prone pose is also a gentle backbend that stretches your chest and strengthens your back. Place a blanket under your hips and ribs for more padding.

1. Lie on your stomach with your arms alongside your torso, palms facing up. Rest your cheek or forehead against the ground. Keep your feet hip width apart.

2. Exhale and lift your chest away from the floor and lift your sternum. At the same time, lift your legs away from the ground. Reach through your heels to lengthen your legs. Your feet stay hip width apart. For more support, place a rolled blanket underneath your chest and your thighs to help provide lift in both areas.

3. Lift your arms away from the floor, and reach back actively with your fingers spread. Your fingers should point behind you. If this feels too intense on your lower back, try Option A or B. For a deeper backbend, try Option C.

   Option A. Keep your legs and tops of your feet on the ground and lift your chest only.

   Option B. Bring your hands underneath your shoulders, palms facing down. Lift your hands and chest off the ground at the same time, and spread your fingers wide. This should feel easier on your neck and shoulders.

   Option C. For a deeper stretch, interlace your fingers behind your back. Lift away from the base of your back when you inhale and lift your chest and legs.

4. Draw your shoulders away from your ears and draw your shoulder blades together and down. Look forward or past the tip of your nose as long as you keep your neck long and extended. Avoid bending your neck too far back, which can cause compression in your vertebrae.

5. Stay for 5 breaths. Release your chest and legs back down to the ground. Let your hands relax alongside your torso, palms facing up. Rock your hips gently from side to side or bend your knees and gently sweep your shins from left to right, like windshield wipers, behind you to loosen your lower back.

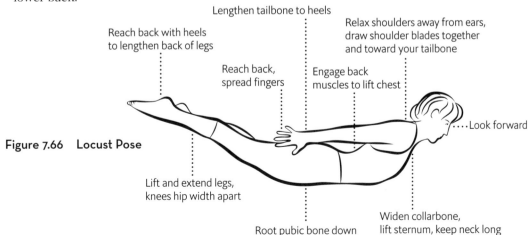

Lengthen tailbone to heels

Relax shoulders away from ears, draw shoulder blades together and toward your tailbone

Reach back with heels to lengthen back of legs

Reach back, spread fingers

Engage back muscles to lift chest

Look forward

Figure 7.66   Locust Pose

Lift and extend legs, knees hip width apart

Root pubic bone down

Widen collarbone, lift sternum, keep neck long

Bow Pose (Dhanurasana)

Bow Pose is a more intense backbend than Locust Pose and expands the chest, strengthens your back, and improves your pose. Place a blanket under your torso and pelvis for more padding.

1. Lie on your stomach with your arms by your side, palms facing up. Bend both knees so that your feet are closer to your bottom. Your knees should be hip width apart throughout the pose.

2. Inhale and draw your shoulder blades together. Lift your arms up, reach behind you, and grab the outside of your ankles with your hands. If it is difficult to reach your ankles, do not force the pose and do Locust Pose instead.

3. Contract your abdominal muscles and press your heels away from your bottom, which will lift your chest and thighs higher off the ground.

4. Lift through the top of your head, and keep your neck and spine long. Look straight ahead, but do not compress the back of your neck. Relax your shoulders away from your neck.

5. Stay for 5 breaths and let go of your ankles, relaxing your arms and legs back to the ground. To loosen your lower back, rock your hips gently from side to side or bend your knees and gently sweep your feet from right to left, like windshield wipers, behind you.

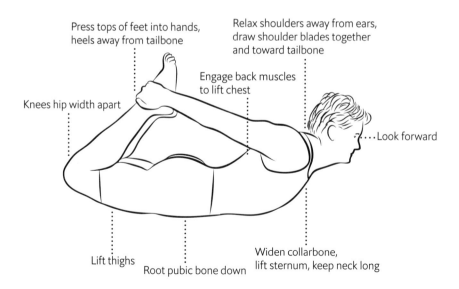

Figure 7.67   Bow Pose

If it is difficult to reach both ankles at the same time, but you are able to reach one at a time comfortably, try Half Bow Pose instead.

1. Lie on your stomach with your arms by your side, palms facing up. Bend both knees so that your feet are closer to your bottom.
2. Reach toward your right foot with your right hand and grab the outside of your right ankle.
3. Reach your left hand forward, palm facing the ground.
4. Inhale to lift your chest and both shoulders away from the floor, pressing your right heel away. Raise your left arm parallel to the floor and reach actively forward with your fingertips.
5. Stay for 5 breaths. Release your leg, chest, and arms to the ground. Switch sides.

Camel Pose (Ustrasana)

Camel Pose stretches your neck, chest, and abdomen. You should take caution in this pose to protect your neck and lower back, since the pose can cause neck strain or lower back compression if done improperly. Do not push yourself past what is comfortable in this pose.

The point of the pose is not to touch your heels, but to lift and expand your chest toward the sky. So, if you reach for your heels and find that your hips are behind your knees, then you are likely also losing the lift in the chest. If you have never done Camel Pose before, you can check whether you should attempt to reach your heels by doing Camel Pose facing a wall. Press your hips and thighs against the wall. When you reach back toward your heels or blocks outside your feet, do not let your hip points and thighs leave the wall. If you cannot reach your heels and keep your hip points against the wall, then keep your hands at the back of your pelvis instead.

1. Kneel on the floor with your knees hip width apart and your hips over your knees so that your thighs are perpendicular to the floor. For extra padding, use a folded blanket under your knees and ankles.
2. Press into the ground with the tops of your feet.
3. Contract your lower abdomen to draw your tailbone down. Your front hip points should be pointing upward. If this is difficult to feel, kneel in front of a wall so that the front of your thighs are touching the wall and keep your hip points pressed against the wall.

4. Place your hands on the back of your pelvis, so that the base of your palms are above your buttocks. You can either point your fingers up along your back or down, depending on what is comfortable for your wrists. Gently press your hands so that they spread your pelvis down and your tailbone lengthens.

5. Inhale and roll your shoulders back. Draw your shoulder blades together to expand your chest and lift your sternum.

6. Lean slightly into your hands but focus on lifting your hip points and chest toward the sky. Keep your head lifted and your hips over your knees. If you are doing Camel Pose against a wall, lean back only as far as possible without letting your hip points leave the wall. You can stay here for 5 breaths and keep your gaze forward.

7. If you are comfortable enough to do a deeper backbend, very gently and slightly twist to the right to place your right hand on the heel of your

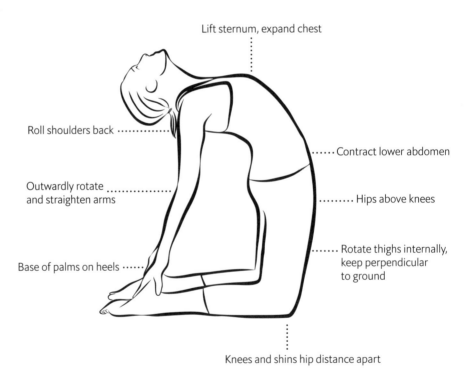

Figure 7.68 Camel Pose

right foot. Once this is stable, return back to center and gently twist to the left to place your left hand on the heel of your left foot. If you cannot reach your heels, lift your heels by turning your toes under. Or place blocks at the highest height outside each heel. Straighten and externally rotate your arms so that your elbow creases face forward.

8. Press the base of your palms against your heels. Press your thighs forward to keep them perpendicular to the ground. Your neck should be continuous with the curve of your spine so that it is not compressed. Do not throw your head back because this can cause neck strain.

9. Stay in this pose for 5 breaths. To exit, return your hands to the back of the pelvis. When you come up, lead with your chest and not your head, as this can cause neck strain. Inhale as you contract your abdominal muscles to lift your chest over your knees.

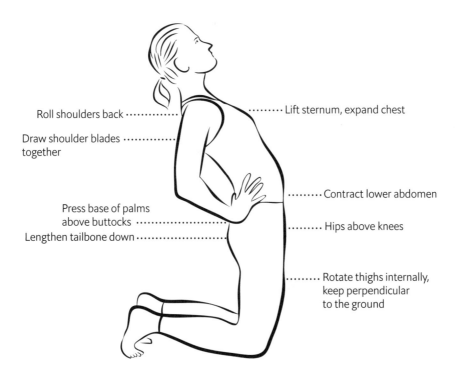

Roll shoulders back

Draw shoulder blades together

Lift sternum, expand chest

Contract lower abdomen

Press base of palms above buttocks

Hips above knees

Lengthen tailbone down

Rotate thighs internally, keep perpendicular to the ground

Figure 7.69   Gentle Camel Pose

Reverse Tabletop Pose (Ardha Purvottanasana)

Reverse Tabletop is also known as Half Upward Plank Pose. The pose stretches the front of your body and strengthens your core. The pose can be paired with energy releasing breaths, such as Lion's Breath (page 96).

1. Start seated with your legs extended in front of you. Bend your knees and place your feet hip distance apart and about 1½ to 2 feet in front of your hips.

2. Place your hands below your shoulders. Spread your fingers and point them forward.

3. Inhale and lift your hips up to the sky. Continue lifting until your hips are even with your shoulders and knees. Lift until the front of your body is parallel to the ground and your knees are directly above your ankles.

4. Gently move your head so that it is in line with the rest of your torso, but do not let your neck fall back too far, which can cause neck strain. Gaze up at the sky. Exhale and release a Lion's Breath. Stay for 3 breaths. Exhale and lower to the ground.

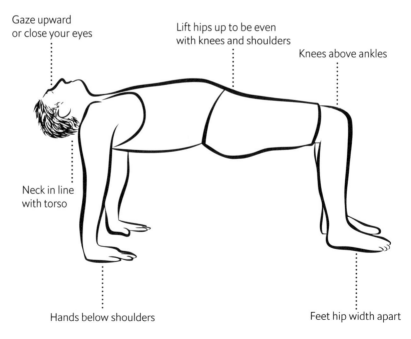

Gaze upward or close your eyes

Lift hips up to be even with knees and shoulders

Knees above ankles

Neck in line with torso

Hands below shoulders

Feet hip width apart

Figure 7.70   Reverse Tabletop

Fish Pose (Matsyasana)

Fish Pose stretches the muscles between your rib cage that help you breathe better and also relaxes your throat muscles.

1. Lie on your back. Keep your feet on the floor with your knees bent.

2. Inhale and gently lift your pelvis a few inches off the floor. Slide your hands, palms down, underneath your hips, and then rest your hips on your hands.

3. Bring your forearms and elbows close to your torso. Inhale and press down on your forearms and elbows to lift your head and upper torso off the ground. Draw your shoulder blades together and toward your tailbone as you expand your chest and lift your sternum toward the sky.

4. Your hand can gently rest on the ground or on a block, but do not place weight on your head. The muscles of your back and chest are lifting your torso, so there should be no pressure on your head and neck.

5. Your legs can be in three different variations:
   Option A. Keep your knees bent and soles of the feet on the ground.
   Option B. Extend your legs on the ground, and feet flexed. Press through your heels.
   Option C. Cross your legs as in Easy Pose.

   If you have any lower back discomfort, return to Option A.

6. Close your eyes and focus on the point between your forehead, your Third Eye. Stay for 5 breaths. Exhale and release your torso and head to the ground. Draw your knees into your chest, and rock side to side to loosen any tension in your lower back. Circle your knees clockwise a few times and then counterclockwise to massage your lower back.

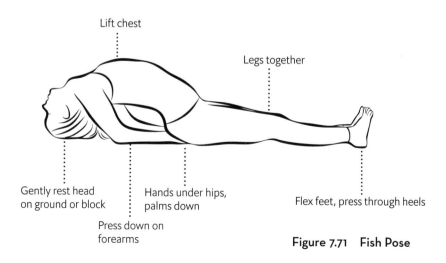

Lift chest

Legs together

Gently rest head on ground or block

Hands under hips, palms down

Flex feet, press through heels

Press down on forearms

Figure 7.71 Fish Pose

1. Set up two blocks so that one will be lengthwise to support the spine of the upper torso. If this does not feel good on your spine, you can also place the block horizontally so that the block will be underneath and support both shoulder blades.

2. Place the second block above the other about a foot apart. The second block will support the head, so it can be either at its tallest or medium height, depending on what is comfortable for your neck. Try both heights to see what is most comfortable.

3. Lie gently back onto the blocks, positioning the first block between your shoulder blades. The second block will go under your head.

4. Let your arms relax to your sides, palms facing the sky. Adjust the blocks as needed so that there is no neck or back discomfort. Stay for 5 breaths. Exit slowly by gently rolling off the blocks to one side, using your hands to support you.

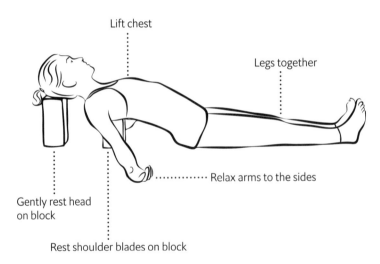

Figure 7.72   Supported Fish Pose

Bridge Pose (Setu Bandha Sarvangasana)

Bridge Pose is a calming pose that can be used to wrap up your practice. The pose stretches the chest and hips and strengthens your back. You can place a folded blanket under your neck and shoulders to protect your neck.

1. Lie on your back. Bend your knees and place your feet flat on the ground as close to your sitting bones as possible. Your heels should be below your knees and hip width apart. Your feet and thighs should be parallel to each other. Place your arms alongside your torso, palms down, fingers pointing to the front of the mat.

2. Contract your abdominal muscles and flatten your lower back to seal the space between your lower back and the ground. This will tilt your pelvis slightly toward you.

3. Exhale and press into the inner edges of your feet and your arms. Lift your hips to the sky, keeping the pelvic tilt. Keep lifting your hips and reach forward with your thighs until your thighs are nearly parallel to the floor.

4. Lengthen your tailbone toward your knees. Keep your knees directly above your ankles.

5. Roll your shoulders under and broaden your shoulder blades. One option is to clasp your hands together underneath your pelvis. Press down on your forearms and shoulder blades. You should not feel pressure on your neck in this pose.

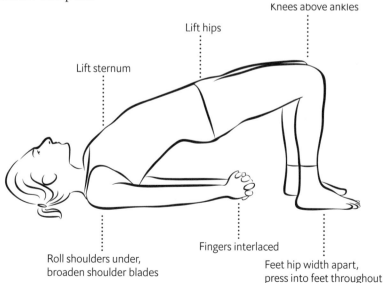

Knees above ankles

Lift hips

Lift sternum

Roll shoulders under, broaden shoulder blades

Fingers interlaced

Feet hip width apart, press into feet throughout

Figure 7.73   Bridge Pose

6. Stay for 5 breaths and exit slowly by releasing your hips gently to the ground. Hug your knees into your chest, and rock side to side to loosen any tension in your back. Circle your knees clockwise a few times and then counterclockwise to massage your lower back.

For a restorative version of Bridge, try Supported Bridge Pose.

1. Lie on your back and bring your knees close to your tailbone with your feet flat on the ground hip width apart.
2. Lift your hips to a comfortable height. Place a block underneath your sacrum. You can place it on the lowest, medium, or tallest height, depending on how it feels on your back and chest.
3. Rest your arms alongside your body. With your hands palms down, reach forward with your fingertips. Exhale and relax your body onto the block.

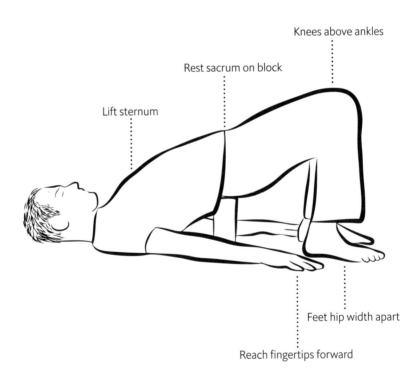

Figure 7.74   Supported Bridge Pose

Hip Opener Poses

The psoas is a deep muscle connecting your spine to your legs and is critical for stabilization of your abdominal core and being able to lift your legs as you walk. The psoas originates from the sides of your lumbar and thoracic spine, runs through your pelvis and attaches to the thigh (femur) bones in your legs. The deep muscle is also closely connected to breathing since it is attached to the diaphragm through connective tissue and ligaments of the diaphragm. It is important to breathe intentionally in hip opener poses to relax tension in these muscles.

Table 7.11   Hip Opener Poses

English Name	Sanskrit Name	Gaze	Modifications	Cautions & Contraindications
Yogi Squat (Garland Pose)	Malasana	Forward or upward	Block underneath sacrum	Hip, groin, or knee injury
Goddess Pose	Utkata Konasana	Forward	Chi breath	Shoulder, hip, groin, or knee injury
Bound Angle Pose	Baddha Konasana	Down	Blocks under knees	Hip, groin, or knee injury
Reclining Bound Angle Pose	Supta Baddha Konasana	Eyes closed, Third Eye	Blocks under knees	Hip, groin, knee, or lower back injury
Lizard Pose	Utthan Pristhasana	Forward or downward	Forearms or hands on blocks	Hip or groin injury
Reclining Pigeon Pose (Figure Four Pose)	Supta Kapotasana	Tip of nose	• Reclining Pigeon with supporting foot propped against a wall • Seated Reclining Pigeon	Hip or groin injury
Half Pigeon Pose (One-Legged Pigeon, Sleeping Pigeon)	Eka Pada Rajakapotasana	Eyes closed	Blocks underneath back thigh or pelvis, Reclining Pigeon reclined or seated	Hip, groin, or knee injury

Yogi Squat (Malasana)

Yogi Squat, or Garland Pose, is grounding and calming. The squatting position releases digestive issues and relaxes muscles that allow your body to eliminate waste more easily.

1. Start in Mountain Pose with your feet wider than hip distance apart, heels in, toes out.

2. Bend your knees until your hips are a few inches off the floor, keeping your back straight and lift through the top of your head. If this is uncomfortable, sit on a block for support or add a folded blanket under your heels to lift them.

3. Press your palms together in front of your chest. Bring your elbows inside your knees one at a time. Press your upper arms against your inner thighs and press your thighs back in return.

4. Lift your sternum and relax your shoulders away from your ears.

5. Stay for 5 breaths. To exit, sit down onto the ground or gently release your hands in front of you to the ground and return to standing.

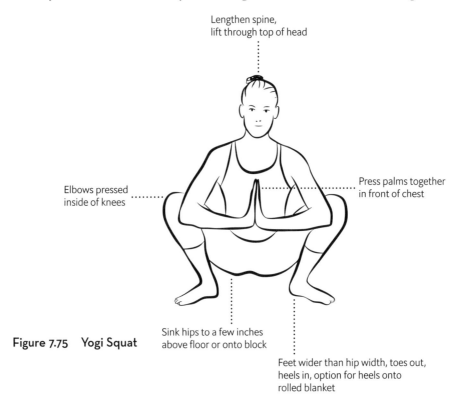

Lengthen spine, lift through top of head

Elbows pressed inside of knees

Press palms together in front of chest

Sink hips to a few inches above floor or onto block

Feet wider than hip width, toes out, heels in, option for heels onto rolled blanket

Figure 7.75 Yogi Squat

Goddess Pose (Utkata Konasana)

Goddess Pose represents a healing and revitalizing feminine force. Pair Goddess Pose with breathing from the solar plexus to release energy from the center of your being, or *hara*, in Japanese martial arts.

1. Stand in Mountain Pose and then bring your feet about 2 to 3 feet apart, toes turned out about 45 degrees. Bend your knees so that your knees are in line with your ankles and your hips are the same height as your knees.

2. Raise your arms to shoulder height and bend your elbows so that your fingertips point to the sky. Spread your fingers actively. Lift your sternum and widen your collarbone. If this is painful for your shoulders, you can keep your palms pressed together in front of your chest.

3. Draw your tailbone down to the ground. Draw your shoulders away from your ears. Stay here for 5 breaths.

4. You also have two options to pair breath and movement in Goddess Pose.

    Option A. Release negative energy. Bend your elbows out to the side of the room so that your forearm is parallel to the ground and your palms are facing your chest. Inhale through your nose deeply, imagining being filled with vital energy at your solar plexus. Exhale through your mouth with a rapid whooshing sound as you turn and push your palms forward with force, as if you are pushing a heavy door open in front of you. Inhale as you draw your palms back in toward your solar plexus. Repeat this 5 times.

    Option B. Bring in positive energy. Bend your elbows at 90 degrees, palms facing your head, your forearms are perpendicular to the ground. Inhale through your nose to draw in energy. Exhale through your mouth with the forceful sound "ha" as you draw your fists down alongside your ribs. This draws energy into the center of your body.

5. To exit, step your feet together to stand in Mountain Pose.

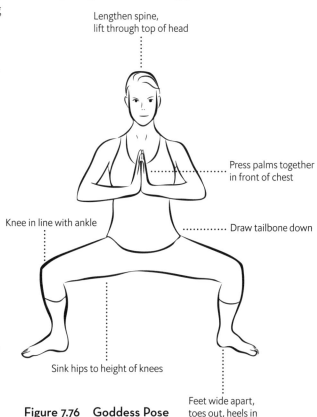

Lengthen spine, lift through top of head

Press palms together in front of chest

Knee in line with ankle

Draw tailbone down

Sink hips to height of knees

Feet wide apart, toes out, heels in

Figure 7.76   Goddess Pose

Bound Angle Pose (Baddha Konasana)

1. Sit on the ground with your legs straight out in front of you. If your hips and groin area are tight, then you can sit on a block or folded blanket.

2. Exhale and bend your knees, bringing your heels close to your pelvis. Then gently release your knees to the sides so that the soles of your feet press together. Root the outer edge of the feet on the ground.

3. Grasp the big toe of each foot with your first and second finger and thumb of each hand. If you can't reach your toes, gently wrap each hand around the same-side ankle or shin.

4. Sit tall and lift through the crown of your head. Your pelvis should be neutral so that you are neither rounding nor arching your lower back. Relax your shoulders away from your ears and draw your shoulder blades together gently and down. Lift your sternum and relax your thighs.

5. *Do not press or force your knees down.* Stay in this pose for 5 breaths. To exit, use your hands to lift your knees away from the ground and extend your legs out in front of you.

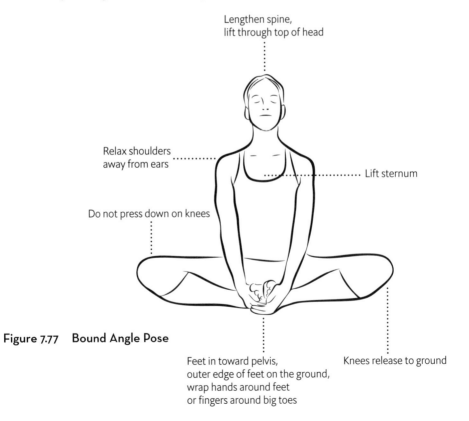

Lengthen spine, lift through top of head

Relax shoulders away from ears

Lift sternum

Do not press down on knees

Figure 7.77 Bound Angle Pose

Feet in toward pelvis, outer edge of feet on the ground, wrap hands around feet or fingers around big toes

Knees release to ground

Reclining Bound Angle Pose (Supta Baddha Konasana)

Reclining Bound Angle Pose is a restorative pose to relax your hips and legs. The pose is also useful to practice breath awareness.

1. Lie back on the ground. Place your feet flat on the ground close to your tailbone. Press your lower back down to seal the space between your lower back and the ground. This will cause your pelvis to tilt slightly toward you. Keep this tilt in order to prevent the lower back from arching in this pose.

2. Exhale and gradually allow your knees to open and move toward the ground. Try to keep your feet as close to your groin as comfortable. If it becomes uncomfortable on your back, knees, or groin, then support your knees with a folded blanket, cushion, or block to reduce any groin strain. Bring the soles of your feet together and let the outer edges of your feet rest on the ground.

3. *Do not force your knees toward the ground.* Relax your shoulders away from your ears and release your arms to the sides so that they are about 45 degrees away from your torso, palms facing the sky.

4. Stay here for 5 breaths. You can practice breath awareness in this pose. To exit, use your hands to guide your knees gently back together. Hug your knees to your chest. Circle your knees clockwise a few times and then counterclockwise, to loosen and massage your lower back.

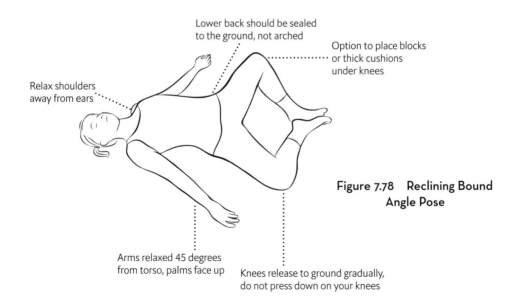

Lower back should be sealed to the ground, not arched

Option to place blocks or thick cushions under knees

Relax shoulders away from ears

Arms relaxed 45 degrees from torso, palms face up

Knees release to ground gradually, do not press down on your knees

Figure 7.78   Reclining Bound Angle Pose

Lizard Pose (Utthan Pristhasana)

Lizard Pose stretches your hips and prepares your body for deeper hip opener poses, such as Half Pigeon.

1. Start in Downward Facing Dog. Step your right foot forward between your hands. Gently heel-toe your front foot to outside of your right hand, so that your foot is slightly outside your right shoulder.

2. Both of your hands should be on the inside of your right foot. You can stay here with your arms straight and your back knee extended or rest your back knee on the ground or a folded blanket for a more restorative pose. Stay here for 5 breaths.

3. For a deeper pose, begin to walk your hands slightly forward and lower your torso. Sink your hips deeper forward as you place your forearms on the ground or onto blocks.

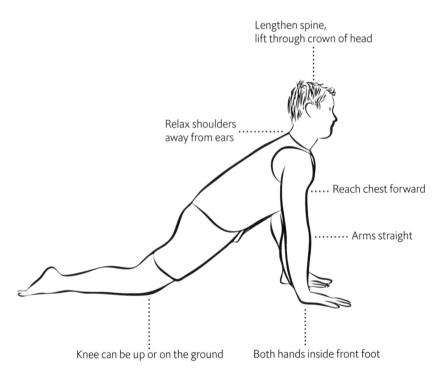

Lengthen spine,
lift through crown of head

Relax shoulders
away from ears

Reach chest forward

Arms straight

Knee can be up or on the ground

Both hands inside front foot

Figure 7.79   Lizard Pose

4. Continue to reach your chest forward to lengthen your spine. Draw your shoulder blades together and toward your tailbone, and do not round your back. You have the option to keep your back knee on the ground or, for a more challenging and active pose, lift your back knee and straighten your back leg.

5. Stay for 5 breaths. Look forward as you reach your chest forward. Or gaze downward if your neck has any discomfort. To exit, press into your hands to step back to Downward Facing Dog. Repeat on the other side.

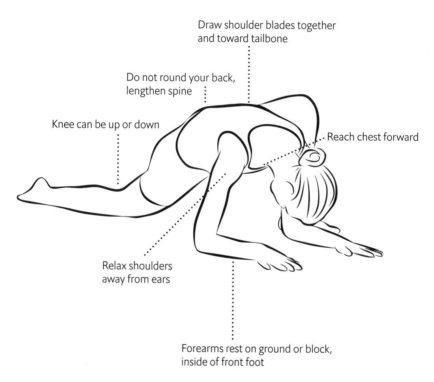

Draw shoulder blades together and toward tailbone

Do not round your back, lengthen spine

Knee can be up or down

Reach chest forward

Relax shoulders away from ears

Forearms rest on ground or block, inside of front foot

Figure 7.80 Lizard Pose: deeper stretch with forearms down

Reclining Pigeon, or Figure Four, Pose (Supta Kapotasana)

1. Lie on your back. Bend your knees with the soles of your feet flat on the ground.

2. Cross your left ankle over your right knee, so that your left ankle is pointed to the side. Keep your left foot flexed to protect your knee.

3. Reach your hands behind your right thigh to hug your right thigh toward your chest. If it feels comfortable, for a more intense stretch, lift your right foot off the floor and hug your right thigh closer in toward your chest. Keep your sacrum rooted into the ground. Optional: Tuck your chin in gently toward your chest so that your neck rests comfortably on the ground.

4. Stay for 5 breaths. Release your left foot to the ground and switch sides.

Other variations include Reclining Pigeon against the wall. Prop the foot of your supporting leg against a wall. Adjust the intensity of the stretch by moving the supporting foot up or down the wall to increase or decrease the hip stretch.

You can also do Reclining Pigeon Pose while seated with the sole of the foot of the supporting leg flat on the ground. Increase the intensity of the hip stretch by gently bringing the supporting leg in closer to your hips or walk the foot farther away to lessen the stretch.

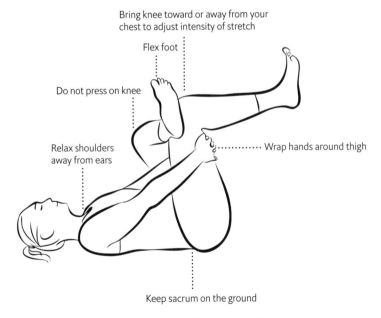

Bring knee toward or away from your chest to adjust intensity of stretch

Flex foot

Do not press on knee

Relax shoulders away from ears

Wrap hands around thigh

Keep sacrum on the ground

Figure 7.81 Reclining Pigeon or Figure Four Pose on your back

Half Pigeon Pose (Eka Pada Rajakapotasana)

Half Pigeon is an intense stretch for your hip flexors, groin muscles, and glutes that settles your mind and calms your body. Use Half Pigeon only after you have warmed up your body with hip openers, such as Lizard or Reclining Pigeon. Given the intensity of the stretch from gravity, do not do Half Pigeon if it feels uncomfortable. There are many other options with a similar stretch that are less intense, such as Lizard or Reclining Pigeon. It is important to modify this pose to support the body so that it is as comfortable as possible. If you are able to get into Half Pigeon comfortably, but find that your hips cannot reach the ground, add blocks underneath your sitting bone under your front hip. Support your body to ensure that your hips are even.

1. Start in Tabletop Pose. Bring your right knee behind your right wrist. Keep your right thigh parallel to the side of the mat and gradually inch your right foot forward until it is in front of your left hip. Your right knee can stay at a 45-degree angle. For a deeper stretch, continue to move

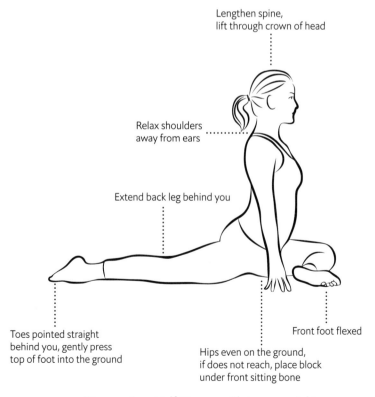

Lengthen spine, lift through crown of head

Relax shoulders away from ears

Extend back leg behind you

Toes pointed straight behind you, gently press top of foot into the ground

Hips even on the ground, if does not reach, place block under front sitting bone

Front foot flexed

Figure 7.82   Half Pigeon with torso upright

your right foot away from your left knee until your right shin is parallel to the top of the mat. Flex your right foot, toes in toward your shin.

2. Curl your left toes under so that the top of the foot is on the ground. Slide your left leg toward the back of the mat until your hips are lowered on the ground. If your hips cannot reach the ground, place a block or folded blanket under the sitting bone on either side. Make sure your hips are squared forward and even to the ground. Check to make sure your left leg and toes are pointed straight behind you.

3. Place your hands alongside your hips, and straighten your arms. Lengthen your spine and lift through the crown of your head. Stay here for 2 to 3 breaths.

4. If it feels comfortable, start to walk your arms forward to a 45-degree angle to the ground. Press down gently with your front shin and top of your back foot. Stay here for 2 to 3 breaths.

5. For a deeper pose (Sleeping Half Pigeon Pose), continue to walk your arms forward until your forearms touch the ground. You can stay here and keep your head lifted, gazing forward with your neck neutral. Or cross your arms, and relax your forehead on your arms. If your forehead does not reach the ground, place your forehead on a block or folded blanket to keep your neck neutral. Stay for 5 breaths. If this feels too intense, bring your torso upright again with your arms straight, hands next to your hips.

6. To exit, walk your arms back toward your hips. Press both palms on the ground to lift your hips gently and step back to Downward Facing Dog. Repeat on the other side. You may notice that your left and right sides are different, which reminds you to accept yourself as you are.

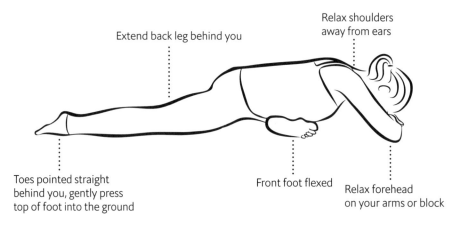

Extend back leg behind you

Relax shoulders away from ears

Toes pointed straight behind you, gently press top of foot into the ground

Front foot flexed

Relax forehead on your arms or block

Figure 7.83   Sleeping Half Pigeon

Cool-Down Poses

These poses calm your body and mind. Use them toward the end of your practice or when you need to feel more grounded.

Table 7.12　Cool-Down Poses

English Name	Sanskrit Name	Gaze	Modifications	Cautions & Contraindications
Reclining Hand to Big Toe Pose	Supta Padangusthasana	Toes	• Strap around arch or ball of foot • Extended foot pressed against wall • Fingers grab big toe of raised foot	Back injuries
Staff Pose	Dandasana	Tip of nose	Folded blanket or block under hips	Lower back injury. If you cannot do at least 90 degrees between leg and torso in Reclining Hand to Big Toe, sit on a block.
Seated Forward Bend	Paschimottanasana	Toes	Seated on block, strap around feet	Neck or lower back injury. If you cannot do at least 90 degrees in Reclining Hand to Big Toe, use block and strap.
Seated Head to Knee Forward Bend	Janu Sirsasana	Toes	Seated on block, strap around foot	Knee or lower back injury. If you cannot do at least 90 degrees in Reclining Hand to Big Toe, use block and strap.
Knee to Chest Pose	Apanasana	Eyes closed, forward	Calves resting on chair	Knee or abdominal injury, pregnancy
Happy Baby Pose	Ananda Balasana	Eyes closed, forward	Hands at outer edge of feet or big toes	Knee or ankle injury, pregnancy
Reclining Spinal Twist	Supta Matsyendrasana	Over extended arm	Eagle legs for deeper twist	Knee or lower back injury, pregnancy
Supported Shoulder Stand	Salamba Sarvangasana	Eyes closed	Block underneath sacrum	Neck injury, pregnancy, headache, glaucoma, high blood pressure
Legs up the Wall Pose	Viparita Karani	Eyes closed	Calves resting on chair seat	Back injuries, headache, glaucoma, high blood pressure
Corpse Pose	Savasana	Eyes closed	Side-lying on left with blanket between knees, inclined with head on propped bolster	Back injury, second and third trimester of pregnancy (try side-lying option)

Reclining Hand to Big Toe Pose (Supta Padangusthasana)

Reclining Hand to Big Toe Pose helps you gradually increase the flexibility of your hamstrings without hurting your lower back. We recommend using a strap in this pose. If you have a lot of flexibility, you have the option to wrap your fingers around your big toe if you are able to reach your foot while keeping both legs straight.

This pose is very useful to help you determine how much you can safely fold forward in forward bends. If you are able to lift your raised leg in Reclining Hand to Big Toe to 90 degrees in this pose, then that means that you are able to sit upright in Staff Pose safely without hurting your lower back. If you are able to bring your raised leg closer to your head past 90 degrees, then you should be able to safely do Seated Forward Bend and Seated Head to Knee Forward Bend with some folding forward. However, if you cannot bring your raised leg to 90 degrees in this pose, then you should sit up on a block and use a strap in Staff Pose. This also means that you should avoid folding forward in Seated Forward Bend and Seated Head to Knee Forward Bend. Folding forward in such forward bends without bending your knees or using a block and strap under these conditions can lead to rounding your back and lower back strain or injury.

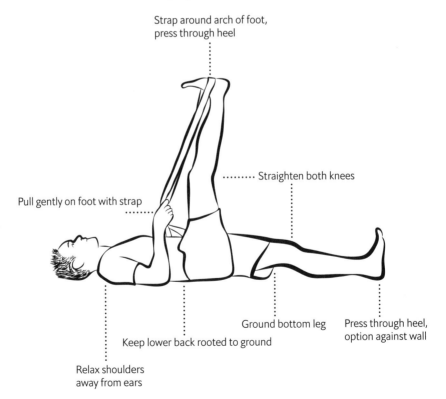

Figure 7.84   Reclining Hand to Big Toe Pose

1. Lie on your back with your legs extended. If your head is not comfortable on the ground, place a folded towel under your head to support your head and neck.

2. Draw your left knee in toward your chest. Keep your right knee extended and press your right thigh down to the floor actively. Flex your right foot, pressing through the heel. If it is difficult to activate your right leg muscles, use a wall and press your right heel against the wall.

3. Wrap a strap around the arch of your left foot and hold the ends of the strap in both hands. Inhale and slowly straighten your left knee, pressing your left heel toward the sky. Release any tension in your front torso and shoulders. Broaden your shoulder blades and widen your collarbones.

4. For a deeper stretch, wrap the ends of the strap around your hands and use the strap to help pull in your foot gently toward your head. You should feel a more intense stretch along the back of your leg, but do not be forceful. Your lower leg should remain on the floor.

5. Exhale to release your raised leg to the floor gently using the support of the strap. Reverse to repeat on the other side.

Staff Pose (Dandasana)

Staff Pose is a simple and foundational pose that prepares you for seated poses, grounds your body, and improves your poses. Before doing Staff Pose, first assess your hamstring flexibility in Reclining Hand to Big Toe Pose with a strap. If you are able to bring your legs to 90 degrees comfortably on both sides in Reclining Hand to Big Toe Pose, then you should be able to sit upright in Staff Pose comfortably. If not, then ease Staff Pose by placing a block or folded blanket underneath your hips to reduce the risk of straining your lower back. You can also use this pose to do all three muscle locks, or *bandhas*: abdominal, chin, and pelvic floor (Chapter 8).

1. Sit on the floor with your legs together and straight out in front of you. Flex your feet and press through the heels. If it is difficult to activate your leg muscles, then press both your heels into a wall.

2. Place your hands on the ground beside your hips, palms down, and press down to sit up tall. You can also place blocks under your hands if it is difficult to reach the floor.

3. Lift your sternum up and widen your collarbone. Lift through the top of your head to lengthen your spine. Stay for 5 breaths.

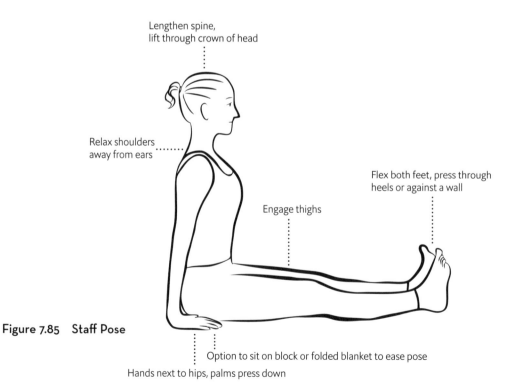

Lengthen spine,
lift through crown of head

Relax shoulders
away from ears

Flex both feet, press through
heels or against a wall

Engage thighs

Figure 7.85 Staff Pose

Option to sit on block or folded blanket to ease pose

Hands next to hips, palms press down

Seated Forward Bend (Paschimottanasana)

Seated Forward Bend is calming and improves fatigue and digestion. Check the flexibility of your hamstrings before doing this pose. If you are able to bend your raised leg comfortably on both sides so that your raised leg is past 90 degrees toward your head in Reclining Hand to Big Toe Pose, then you can bend forward in Seated Forward Bend. If not, sit on a block or folded blanket and use a strap around the arches of your feet instead of bending forward.

1. Start from Staff Pose. Sit on the ground with your feet extended straight in front of you. You can place a block or folded blanket under your sitting bones. Flex your feet and press through your heels actively. If it helps you keep your leg muscles active, press your heels against a wall.

2. Inhale and lift your sternum toward the sky. Raise your hands toward the sky to lengthen the sides of your body. Keep your torso long and lean forward, hinging at your hips, not your waist. It is important to focus on maintaining length in your spine and not focus on making a certain forward shape, which can lead to rounding your back, causing lower back strain and injuries.

3. Gaze forward at your feet. Stay for 5 breaths. With each inhalation, lengthen your torso. With each exhalation, release gently into your forward bend. To exit, return to sit upright and release your hands next to your hips.

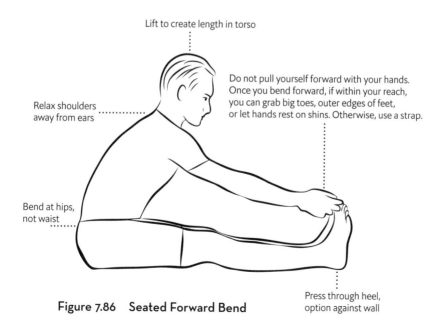

Lift to create length in torso

Do not pull yourself forward with your hands. Once you bend forward, if within your reach, you can grab big toes, outer edges of feet, or let hands rest on shins. Otherwise, use a strap.

Relax shoulders away from ears

Bend at hips, not waist

Press through heel, option against wall

Figure 7.86   Seated Forward Bend

This pose is not about reaching your toes. Do **not** pull yourself forward with your hands to try to reach your toes and do not pull on the strap, either. Allow your hands to rest on your shins or outside of your feet—wherever your hands comfortable land once you have bent at your hips. If you are using a strap, loop a strap behind the arches of your feet and hold onto the ends with your hands with your elbows straight. Do not pull yourself forward with the strap. *Focus on creating length in your back and front torso instead.*

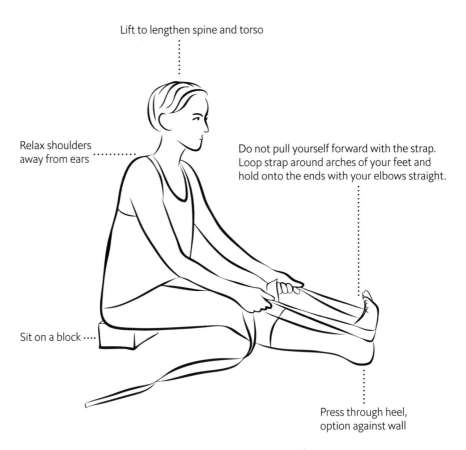

Lift to lengthen spine and torso

Relax shoulders away from ears

Do not pull yourself forward with the strap. Loop strap around arches of your feet and hold onto the ends with your elbows straight.

Sit on a block

Press through heel, option against wall

Figure 7.87   Forward Bend modification: seated on block with strap

Seated Head to Knee Forward Bend (Janu Sirsasana)

Seated Head to Knee Forward Bend is calming and helps relieve anxiety and stress.

1. Start in Staff Pose with your legs extended straight in front of you. Bend your right knee and place the sole of your foot on the inside of your left thigh. Your right knee should be comfortably on the ground. If not, place a folded blanket under the right knee.

2. Place your right hand on your inner right groin and your left hand on the ground next. Press gently into your hands to swivel your torso toward your left thigh so that your navel lines up with the middle of your left thigh. Your hips, chest, and navel should now be square with your left leg.

3. Use a strap to loop around the arch of your left foot and hold onto the ends with your hands. Sit tall to lengthen your spine and torso and ground down into your sitting bones. Keep the foot of your extended leg flexed.

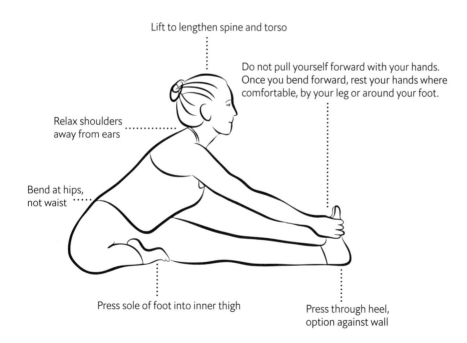

Lift to lengthen spine and torso

Do not pull yourself forward with your hands. Once you bend forward, rest your hands where comfortable, by your leg or around your foot.

Relax shoulders away from ears

Bend at hips, not waist

Press sole of foot into inner thigh

Press through heel, option against wall

Figure 7.88   Seated Head to Knee Pose

4. If you were able to bend your leg in toward your head comfortably in Reclining Hand to Big Toe Pose on both sides past 90 degrees, then you can try a deeper stretch. Inhale to reach both hands toward the sky, lengthening your side body and torso. Exhale and bend gently forward at your hips. Rest your hands where they land, whether it is your shins or foot.

    The purpose of the pose is to lengthen your spine and torso—not to create a forward bending shape. *Do not round your back or pull yourself forward with your hands, which can cause lower back strain or injury.*

5. Stay for 5 breaths. Inhale and lift your torso upright and switch legs to repeat on the other side.

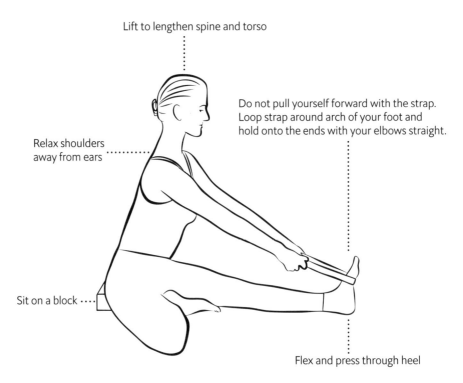

Lift to lengthen spine and torso

Do not pull yourself forward with the strap. Loop strap around arch of your foot and hold onto the ends with your elbows straight.

Relax shoulders away from ears

Sit on a block

Flex and press through heel

Figure 7.89   Head to Knee Pose modification: seated on block with strap

Knee to Chest Pose (Apanasana)

This simple pose is reassuring and quiets the mind and body. The meaning of its Sanskrit name is "downward flowing life force." The pose is useful to release tension in your lower back between poses.

1. Lie on your back. Draw your knees to your chest and hug your knees with your hands. You can interlace your fingers or place one hand on top of the other.
2. Release your lower back into the mat. Draw your shoulder blades together and toward your tailbone. You can rock side or side or gently circle your knees clockwise and then counterclockwise.
3. Gently bring your chin slightly toward your chest to relax your neck.
4. Stay for 5 breaths. To exit, exhale and extend your arms and legs to the ground.

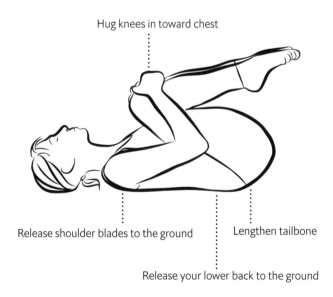

Hug knees in toward chest

Release shoulder blades to the ground · Lengthen tailbone

Release your lower back to the ground

Figure 7.90   Knee to Chest Pose

Happy Baby Pose (Ananda Balasana)

Happy Baby Pose is a calming hip opener that relieves stress and anxiety. Try this pose at the end of your practice.

1. Lie on your back and draw both knees in toward your chest.
2. Grab onto the outside edges of your feet with your forearms in front of your shins. You also have the option to hold the inside arches of your feet, ankles, or shins. Flex your feet and push up into your hands.
3. Bring your knees slightly wider than your shoulders. Bring your ankles above your knees, if possible, so that your shins are perpendicular to the floor. Spread your lower back on the ground.
4. Stay for 5 breaths. To exit, release your feet and draw your knees back into your chest, then roll onto your side.

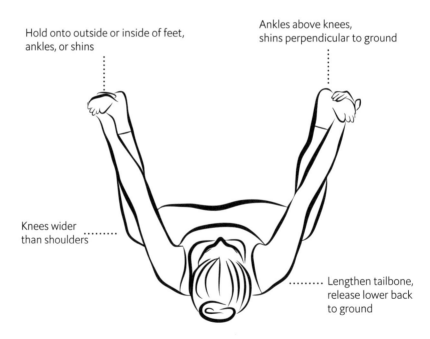

Hold onto outside or inside of feet, ankles, or shins

Ankles above knees, shins perpendicular to ground

Knees wider than shoulders

Lengthen tailbone, release lower back to ground

Figure 7.91   Happy Baby Pose

Reclining Spinal Twist (Supta Matsyendrasana)

Reclining Spinal Twist is good for fighting fatigue and promoting digestion. The pose gently warms up your spine and can relieve pain in your lower back and hips.

1. Lie on your back. Exhale and press your lower back to the ground. Bend your left knee in toward your chest.

2. Exhale and open your arms out to both sides, palms down, arms in line with your shoulders. Cross your left knee over your right leg, keeping both shoulders rooted on the ground. Keep your right leg extended straight in front of you.

3. You can use your right hand to gently relax on your left knee. Turn your head to the left to look over your left hand. Make sure that your left shoulder remains close on the ground. Stay for 5 breaths.

4. To get out of the pose, press both hands into the ground and contract your abdominal muscles to inhale and lift your left knee back to center. Reverse legs and switch to twist to the other side.

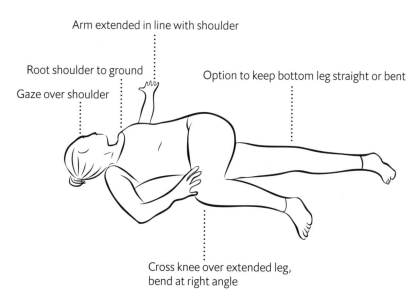

Arm extended in line with shoulder

Root shoulder to ground

Gaze over shoulder

Option to keep bottom leg straight or bent

Cross knee over extended leg, bend at right angle

Figure 7.92   Reclining Spinal Twist

For a deeper twist, try the Two Knee version.

1. Lie on your back. Exhale and press your lower back into the ground. Bend your knees and lift your feet off the ground, keeping your abdominal muscles contracted. Bring your knees together.

2. Exhale and open your arms out to both sides, palms down, so that your arms are in line with your shoulders.

3. Inhale and bring your heels a little higher than your knees. Exhale and gently lower your knees to your right. Your knees should be at the same line of your hips and at about a 90-degree angle.

4. Slowly turn your head toward the left to gaze over your left hand. Your left shoulder should be rooted to the ground. Stay for 5 breaths.

5. To get out of the pose, press both hands into the ground and contract your abdominal muscles to inhale and lift your knees back to center. You can also use your hands to help guide your knees back to center if this is more comfortable. Switch sides and repeat.

Supported Shoulder Stand (Salamba Sarvangasana)

Shoulder stand is a type of yoga pose called an inversion, or a pose that raises your chest above your head. Inversions are typically done at the end of your practice. Since Shoulder Stand can put too much pressure on your head and neck, especially without guidance from a teacher, here is a gentler modification of Shoulder Stand.

1. Keep a block within reach. Lie down on your back with your knees bent and feet flat on the ground. Inhale and lift your hips to place a block on its lowest height underneath your sacrum.

2. Once you feel stable on the block, raise one leg at a time up toward the sky. Extend both legs straight to the sky, feet flexed.

3. Relax your arms alongside your torso or overhead, palms up. Stay for 5 to 10 breaths.

After doing an inversion like Supported Shoulder Stand, balance your body with a counterpose, such as Fish Pose or Child's Pose.

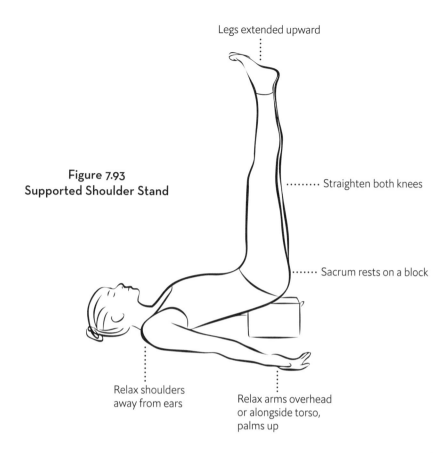

**Figure 7.93
Supported Shoulder Stand**

Legs extended upward

········ Straighten both knees

······· Sacrum rests on a block

Relax shoulders
away from ears

Relax arms overhead
or alongside torso,
palms up

Legs up the Wall Pose (Viparita Karani)

If you've been sitting at a desk or standing on your feet all day, then Legs up the Wall Pose is great to recirculate your blood and wind down at the end of the day. This pose is useful for headaches, stress, and insomnia. You can use a folded blanket or cushion at the base of the wall to support your hips if it feels more comfortable. You can end your practice in this pose.

1. Sit next to the wall with one side against the wall, your knees bent, and feet flat on the ground. Lie on your back and gently pivot your body to bring the back of your legs against the wall.

2. Get your sitting bones as close to the wall as possible and relax your head, neck, and back on the ground. If comfortable, your body should form a 90-degree angle.

3. If you are uncomfortable, try adding additional padding under your lower back. Press your feet on the wall to lift your hips slightly and slide a cushion or folded blanket to give your lower back support.

4. Relax your arms either above your head or alongside your torso about 45 degrees away, palms up. Relax your shoulders away from your ears and draw your shoulder blades together and toward your tailbone. Stay for 5 to 10 breaths.

5. To exit, press your feet on the wall to lift your hips and remove any prop under your back. Bend your knees toward your chest and roll gently to one side.

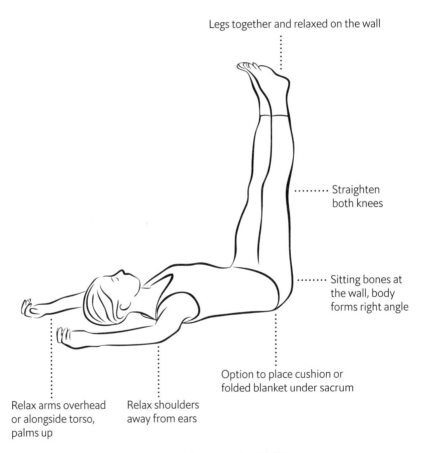

Legs together and relaxed on the wall

Straighten both knees

Sitting bones at the wall, body forms right angle

Option to place cushion or folded blanket under sacrum

Relax arms overhead or alongside torso, palms up

Relax shoulders away from ears

Figure 7.94 **Legs up the Wall Pose**

Corpse Pose (Savasana)

Corpse Pose is a calming final resting pose that can release tension and relieve stress and insomnia.

1. Lie on your back. It is important that your body be neutral in this pose to prevent any back discomfort. Bend your knees and keep your feet on the floor hip distance apart. Lift your pelvis off the floor and slide your tailbone away and rest your pelvis back on the ground. Extend your legs so that your knees are hip width apart and let your knees open gently outward. If you feel discomfort in your lower back in this pose, make sure that you are neither arching nor rounding your lower back.

2. Rest your arms alongside your torso about 45 degrees away, palms facing the sky. Relax your shoulders away from your ears.

3. Lengthen the back of your neck by gently moving your chin toward your chest. You can also support your neck with a folded blanket.

4. Close your eyes and relax for 10 to 20 breaths. To exit the pose, bring your knees to your chest and rock side to side or in circles in both directions. Roll to one side. Exhale and gently use your hands to press your torso upright. Your head will be the last to come up.

If you are in the third trimester of pregnancy, or lying on your back is uncomfortable, elevate your head and chest on a bolster or cushion, or try Side-Lying Corpse Pose (page 296). Lie back and rest on your left side with a pillow between your legs. Your right knee is slightly in front of your left leg. Place another cushion between your arms for added support.

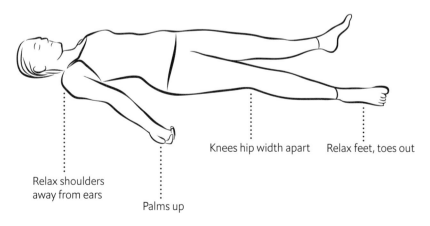

Relax shoulders away from ears

Palms up

Knees hip width apart   Relax feet, toes out

Figure 7.95   Corpse Pose

CHAPTER 8

Deepen Your Practice: Muscle Locks (*Bandhas*) and Hand Expressions (*Mudras*)

To perform every action artfully is yoga.

SWAMI KRIPALU

Mudras are symbolic hand gestures or bodily postures that communicate a specific meaning.[1] Mudras, which means "seals" in Sanskrit, are postures in the hatha yoga tradition that direct and concentrate energy in the body. One type of mudra is hand expressions, or *hasta mudras*, which convey specific spiritual meanings and can often be seen in ancient renderings of Buddha.

Mudras can also involve other parts of the body. Muscle "locks," or *bandhas*, are considered a type of mudra, or sealing posture. These muscle locks are focused, deep muscular contractions of the body. When these muscle locks are activated, you can build stronger, more stable yoga poses and improve yoga breathing, too.

Both muscle locks and hand mudras are important elements that deepen your yoga practice and prepare your mind for meditation. Once you are familiar with the basics of yoga postures, breathing, and meditation, you can add these two elements to your practice. Integrate muscle locks and hand mudras to intensify your focus, keep your body active in the pose, and build more awareness during breathing exercises, postures, and meditation.

Many styles of yoga view muscle locks as essential for yoga postures. Muscle locks are intended to seal and concentrate energy, or *prana*, in the body. The term *bandhas* means to lock, hold, bind, or tighten. In scientific terms, muscle locks are intentional muscle contractions of specific muscles in your body.

Muscle Locks (*Bandhas*)

There are three types of muscle locks used in yoga, and the combination of all three makes up the fourth muscle lock. Muscle locks stabilize your postures, focus your breathing, and calm your mind for meditation.

> We recommend that you learn muscle locks with the guidance from an experienced yoga teacher to ensure safety. These locks should not be practiced if you are pregnant or if you have medical conditions, injuries, or recent surgeries in the focused area of the muscle lock. These exercises should never be painful—do not force your body to do something that doesn't feel right. As with all other parts of yoga, start with listening to your body and being aware and compassionate toward your body and mind.

Table 8.1   Muscle Locks (*Bandhas*)

Muscle Lock	Sanskrit Name	Anatomical Location	Chakra	Use with
Root Lock	*Mula Bandha*	Perineum, pelvic floor contraction	First (Root) Chakra, Second (Sacral) Chakra	Inhalation retention, and Mountain, High Plank, Downward Dog, Warrior II Poses
Upward Abdominal Lock	*Uddiyana Bandha*	Abdominal and trunk core muscles, behind navel	Third (Solar Plexus) Chakra	Exhalation, exhalation retention, Breath of Fire, Bellows Breath, standing poses (Mountain, Goddess)
Chin Lock	*Jalandhara Bandha*	Chin, neck flexion	Fifth (Throat) Chakra	Inhalation retention, seated poses, forward bends
Great Lock	*Maha Bandha*	Combination of throat, abdomen, pelvic floor	First, Second, Third, Fifth Chakra	Seated poses, seated forward bends
Tongue Lock	*Jiva or Kechari Bandha*	Tongue, soft palate of mouth	Lalana, Talu, Kala (Roof of Mouth) Chakra	Victorious Breath, Chin Lock, meditation

Root Lock (*Mula Bandha*)

In the *Hatha Yoga Pradipika*, a classic Sanskrit text on hatha yoga written in the fifteenth century, Svatmarama says that practicing Root Lock attains "total perfection." While in yoga we do not seek perfection, this does highlight the importance of the Root Lock, which is the primary *bandha* in many yoga traditions. It is named for the first or most basic chakra, the "Root Chakra." Root Lock is a muscle contraction of your pelvic floor, the deep layers of muscle fibers and tissues of your pelvis. The most superficial layer is what contracts your anal sphincter. There are deeper sets of pelvic floor muscle layers above the superficial layer; one is like a hammock running side to side between your sitting bones, and an even deeper layer of pelvic floor muscles, the pelvic diaphragm, runs front to back between your pubic bone and tailbone. These muscles of Root Lock are also connected to lower fibers of deep abdominal layers. When you engage Root Lock, you lift these layers of the pelvic floor inward and upward, which stabilizes and calms your body and concentrates energy in your pelvic region. Root Lock stimulates pelvic nerves in the root chakra, the lowest chakra along the spine. Root Lock is a contraction of the deeper layers of pelvic floor muscles and does not require contracting the superficial layer.

How do you find and activate the muscles used in Root Lock? For some, it may be easier first to find the pelvic floor muscles used to stop and start the flow of urine, the same muscles used in Kegel exercises. Then, try finding your pelvic floor muscles in Yogi Squat. Squat with your heels in, toes out, and your torso leaning in between your legs, but keep your spine upright. Press your hands together at heart center. As you inhale, draw the muscles in and up, gently bringing together parts of your pelvic floor as if they were two halves sliding together like an elevator door. Imagine gently drawing up energy from the earth and into your pelvic floor. Exhale and release and relax these muscles, without letting your pelvic floor collapse completely.

In scientific terms, Root Lock is similar to Kegel exercises, or pelvic floor contractions. Surprisingly, perhaps, Kegel exercises have been shown to improve lung function and increase the amount of air your lungs can hold as well as increase the volume of breath that you can exhale.[2] Pelvic floor contraction has also been shown to activate your "core," the deep abdominal and lumbosacral muscles around your spine when walking, which means better support and protection for your lower spine. Together, these studies suggest that using Root Lock helps you breathe better and be physically safer in yoga poses, breathing exercises, and meditation.

Some yoga styles encourage keeping Root Lock active throughout the entire yoga practice, which we do not recommend since continuous contraction of your pelvic floor can be overly stressful and straining for most people. It is important not to overdo Root Lock or Kegel exercises since overuse and repeated overcontraction can overly tighten the muscle. As always, it's important to listen to your body and get a sense of whether and when it feels good to activate Root Lock.

Root Lock Exercise 1: Root Lock with Rhythmic Breathing

Once you have identified your pelvic floor muscles, try doing pelvic floor contraction along with breath retention in rhythmic breathing. Inhale slowly through your nose for 5 counts. Pause to retain your breath for 5 counts and simultaneously gently contract your pelvic floor muscles inward and upward. Imagine subtly pulling energy up from the pelvic floor like the tide of the ocean. Let go of Root Lock and exhale for 5 counts. Inhale deeply for 5 counts. Engage Root Lock again when you pause for breath retention for 5 counts. And release with exhalation for 5 counts. Continue this pattern for 10 cycles of breath, using Root Lock during breath retention and releasing with exhalation.

Root Lock Exercise 2: Root Lock with High Plank Pose

Root Lock can be added to a wide variety of standing yoga poses like Mountain, Yogi Squat, Warrior II, and seated forward bends. In general, you can activate Root Lock on inhalation during a pose, and release it during exhalation upon transition to another pose. In this exercise, add Root Lock to High Plank Pose. Find a small wall space and place your mat perpendicular to the wall, so that the small edge of the mat is along the wall. Come to Tabletop Pose on your hands and knees, facing away from the wall. Do a gentle warm-up of 5 cycles of alternating Cat and Cow Pose. When you feel ready, press back to Downward Facing Dog so that your heels press against the baseboard of the wall. Take 5 deep Victorious Breath cycles. Inhale and shift forward to High Plank Pose or modified High Plank Pose with your knees supported on the ground. Keep reaching your heels toward the wall so that they touch and press against the baseboard of the wall. Add Root Lock by contracting your pelvic floor muscles and hold it with Victorious Breath for 5 full breath cycle counts. Then, release Root Lock and move back to Downward Facing Dog for 5 counts. Continue alternating between the two poses for 5 sets. When you are finished with your last High Plank, release Root Lock and relax into Child's Pose for 10 counts.

During this exercise, you should feel a long line of energy in High Plank from your pelvis to your inner thighs and reaching to the bottom of your heels. Your pelvic muscles have to be active to lift your spine so that our middle doesn't buckle upward or downward. If it is difficult to find Root Lock in High Plank, place a yoga block so that its narrow width is held between your inner thighs. Press on the yoga foam block in High Plank actively and contract your pelvic floor muscles.

Chin Lock (*Jalandhara Bandha*)

Chin Lock is a position where your neck is drawn inward and downward toward your chest, with your sternum lifted upward. Chin Lock releases the tension at the back of your neck at the suboccipital region, at the base of your head and top of your neck. In the yoga tradition, Chin Lock lets energy, or *prana*, flow downward in the body.

Anatomically, the maneuver presses on your carotid sinus and carotid bodies, areas of your carotid arteries, which run through your neck on both sides. These areas contain chemical and pressure receptors that regulate your blood pressure, heart rate, and breathing rate. These same receptors get turned on, when you have a higher level of carbon dioxide in the body, and send messages to the rest of your body to increase your heart rate and quicken your breath to get rid of the excess carbon dioxide. As the carbon dioxide level increases, there is a subjective sense of air hunger. Chin Lock presses on these receptors in the neck arteries, preventing them from speeding up your heart rate and breath as your carbon dioxide levels rise. You will feel less breathless, so you are able to keep your breath and heart rate slow and steady. This stops you from hyperventilating and getting lightheaded during yoga breathing. In some yoga traditions, Chin Lock is used during all yoga breathing to prevent lightheadedness. Since it can be difficult to learn Chin Lock and yoga breathing at the same time without supervision, we recommend adding Chin Lock later, once you become more familiar with yoga breathing techniques.

As with other muscle locks, Chin Lock is best learned with supervision from a yoga teacher. If you have any neck or joint issues or such medical conditions as osteoporosis, be very cautious, as sudden and severe neck flexion can lead to injuries. It is important not to force your chin into a position that exceeds your natural flexibility. Do not perform Chin Lock if you have cardiac issues, including past heart attacks, stroke, arrhythmias, or carotid sinus issues. Stimulating the carotid sinuses in these medical conditions by overflexing the neck can be medically dangerous. If you have had fainting episodes or cardiovascular issues, talk to your doctor first before trying Chin Lock.

Some yoga styles add Chin Lock during breath retention at the end of the inhalation or exhalation. Don't try to hold this lock for the entirety of your breath cycle as a beginner. Also, remember to go easy, since many demonstrations of Chin Lock overdo the flexion. It doesn't take a lot of flexion to instantly and noticeably reduce breathlessness. It should feel easy and natural.

Basic Chin Lock Exercise

As a beginner, try Chin Lock at the end of inhalation during retention and release Chin Lock upon exhalation. Do Chin Lock while seated in Easy Pose or Hero Pose. Take 5 deep Victorious Breaths to relax your body. After you feel relaxed, inhale for 5 counts, retain your breath. Draw your shoulder blades toward each other, and lift the top of your sternum toward your chin. Now, softly relax your chin inward so that your chin lowers toward your raised sternum. Do not force your chin toward your sternum or vice versa. They do not need to touch. The underside of your chin where you chin meets your throat should be drawn upward, toward the top of your head. Lengthen the back of your neck, and relax your shoulders. Keep your chest lifted as your retain your breath for 5 counts. Release the lock by returning your head to neutral position and exhale for 5 counts. Relax your shoulders and chest. Repeat this pattern of inhalation, retention with Chin Lock, and release with exhalation. You can add Chin Lock during breath retention after inhalation or exhalation in breathing exercises, such as rhythmic breathing.

If you feel any pain or neck strain during Chin Lock, stop immediately and gently return your head to neutral position, with your head level and eyes looking straight ahead. Beginners can try holding a rolled kitchen towel between their neck and chin while keeping their sternum lifted. Once again, in Chin Lock, a little flexion is usually enough.

Chin Lock can be performed in seated poses, forward bends, and Bridge Pose. Chin Lock is also useful in Shoulder Stand Pose, but we do not recommend trying this without supervision from an experienced yoga teacher, given the higher risk for neck and shoulder injuries from significant body weight on your neck and shoulders in this inversion.

Upward Abdominal Lock (*Uddiyana Bandha*)

The Upward Abdominal lock is a deep abdominal muscle contraction that is done after exhalation on an empty stomach and should never be done after inhalation. Upward Abdominal Lock contracts the deep abdominal muscles inward and upward and toward the back, so that your diaphragm rises and the belly is scooped in. Do not practice this muscle lock if you are pregnant or have abdominal medical conditions, such as a hernia.

Biomechanical and exercise studies have found that you need these trunk muscles to be active to keep your spine stable. Upward Abdominal Lock engages many layers of your abdominal muscles, including deep core muscles, which are the trunk muscles surrounding and supporting your lower back and spine. When you use Upward Abdominal Lock, you are able to better protect your spine and lower back.

Abdominal hollowing, a maneuver that is nearly identical to Upward Abdominal Lock, has been used in physical therapy and rehabilitation as a way to activate the transverse abdominal muscles, protect the lower back, and treat lower back pain. Scientists have studied the use of abdominal hollowing during exercise and found that it better protects the lower, or lumbosacral, spine. Researchers used electrodes to measure trunk muscle activation during walking and found that when people did an abdominal hollowing, many more core trunk muscles were active, which protects and stabilizes the spine.[3] Abdominal hollowing activated local trunk muscles responsible for stabilizing your lumbar spine of your lower back, including the multifidus, transverse abdominus, and internal oblique abdominals. These same muscles were not activated when people didn't use abdominal hollowing. Another similar study on stair-climbing found that protective core muscles were active with abdominal hollowing, but inactive if you did not do the maneuver.[4]

Basic Upward Abdominal Lock Exercise

You can try Upward Abdominal Lock from a standing position or lying down, but it's easier for most people to learn standing up. Stand with your feet hip width apart. Rest your hands on your thighs and gently round your torso so that your back is curved as in Cat Pose. Inhale deeply, and exhale fully and forcefully through your nose. After you exhale completely, contract and draw your abdominal muscles in and up. Add Chin Lock gently, and hold for 5 counts while retaining your breath. Release Chin and Upward Abdominal Lock by relaxing your head, neck, and abdomen. Inhale and exhale gently, and return to normal breathing.

It's important to remember that you don't need to do Upward Abdominal Lock forcefully to get its benefits. A slight contraction of your abdominal muscles in poses can be protective of the spine, such as in standing poses, such as Mountain Pose or Warrior I or II Poses. If you engage Upward Abdominal Lock too suddenly, forcefully, or unevenly, you can hurt your back. We recommend working with an experienced yoga teacher to do this muscle lock safely if you're unfamiliar with it.

Great Lock (*Maha Bandha*)

Great Lock is the combination of all three muscle locks at once. It should be learned only under supervision from a trained yoga teacher. You should try this only when you are comfortable with all three muscle locks separately. You can do Great Lock while seated or in such poses as Seated Forward Bend. Sit in a comfortable pose. Exhale completely and contract your pelvic floor muscles to activate Root Lock. Now, draw your abdominal muscles in and up for Upward Abdominal Lock. Keep your spine erect and tall, lift your sternum gently, and press your chin toward your throat for Chin Lock. Remember not to force your chin to touch your sternum. After a few seconds, release your entire body and all three muscle locks. Return your chin to neutral position and inhale naturally. You can resume normal breathing or continue to seated meditation. Great Lock can help you transition more quickly and smoothly to meditation.

You can also use a combination of locks during your breathing practice. In the Ashtanga tradition, Victorious Breath is done with both Root Lock and Upward Abdominal Lock, in which the pelvic floor and abdominal muscles are drawn inward and upward during inhalation.

Tongue Lock (*Jiva or Kechari Bandha*)

In ancient yoga texts, Tongue Lock is thought to catch and purify nectar from a minor chakra (*Bindu*) at the back of the head as energy flows past the roof of the mouth and downward to the fifth (throat) chakra. Tongue Lock is said to activate a minor chakra called *Lalana*, also known as *Talu* or *Kala*, which located at the roof of the mouth. Tongue Lock is useful as a point of focus during meditation and helps you extend breath retention during breathing techniques. Physically, the muscle contraction of the tongue should lower saliva production, reduce the need to swallow, and relieve tension and pain in the neck and jaw area. When you do Tongue Lock, imagine that you are forming a pot or reservoir to store positive energy and concentration.

Basic Tongue Lock Exercise

Sit in a comfortable seated pose, such as Easy or Hero Pose, with your spine erect. Inhale deeply through your nose for 5 counts to prepare for Victorious Breath. Pause your breath for breath retention. Stick out your tongue to lengthen your tongue. Keep this length as you curl your tongue and press the tip of your tongue as far back as possible to the roof of your mouth. Imagine saying the letter *N* silently. Close your mouth, continue to press your tongue against the roof of your mouth for 5 counts of breath retention. Imagine that you are collecting positive energy with your tongue at the back of your throat. Exhale for 5 counts through your nose, keeping Tongue Lock in place. Imagine purifying any negative energy as your exhale. Air should pass through the back of your throat to make the sound of the ocean. Relax your tongue after full exhalation. Repeat this pattern for 5 cycles of breath. You can skip the step of sticking out your tongue after the first few cycles.

You can use Tongue Lock during breathing exercises, such as rhythmic breathing and Victorious Breath, or hold it during meditation.

Hand Mudras

Take a minute to notice how you are sitting or standing. Now, pay attention to what your hands and fingers are doing. Are your hands touching or separated? Are they relaxed or tense? Are your hands clenched or loose? Hands express and convey your inner state or mood, intentionally or not. The mind-body connection posits that our mind influences how we hold our body, and the position of our body can affect our mind. This goes for the position of your hands as well, which can direct and affect your energy, focus, or mood.

Hand mudras are expressions of your hands and fingers that direct the flow of energy in the body. Just like breath, hand mudras can focus your mind and enhance mental and physical awareness. These mudras are found throughout ancient Hindu and Buddhist art, scriptures, and texts. The term *mudra* means a mark, gesture, or sealing posture. Mudras in the South Asian culture appear in spiritual practices of Hinduism, Buddhism, and Taoism, Indian classical dance, and Camatic music, a major type of classical music originating in southern India.[5] In Buddhism, mudras represent and stand for specific events and teachings from the Buddha's life.

There are dozens of hand mudras with a variety of different spiritual and symbolic meanings. Hand mudras in yoga can provide comfort, focus, and serenity. You can think of them as doing yoga with your hands. Mudras are accessible to people of all ranges of physical mobility. Some people do mudras for as long as forty-five minutes a day. Use hand mudras during yoga poses to concentrate and guide your attention, or do them in combination with breathing in order to connect the mind with the body, enhance focus, and prepare for meditation. When first learning hand mudras, it is easiest to try them in a comfortable seated pose, but you can also do them lying down, standing, walking, or while doing balancing yoga poses, such as Tree Pose or Dancer.

An important part of practicing mudras is listening to your body and mind. A big surprise about mudras is that they are both fun and effortless. First, figure out how you're feeling and what your intention is for your mudra practice. Does your mind feel scattered; are you looking for more focus? Are you feeling exhausted and want to feel more restored? Choose the variation based on how you want to influence your mind and body, and find out how it affects you. As with any other technique in yoga, explore what feels right for you. Practicing mudras encourages certain states of mind and also paves the way for meditation.

The two broad categories are separate hand mudras (*asamyukta-hasta*) and combined hand mudras (*samyukta-hasta*). In the Hindu tradition, each finger of the hand is associated with a natural element, an energy center (*chakra*) and symbolic characteristics of such energy centers:

Thumb: fire (*agni*), solar plexus chakra, wisdom, ego, self-esteem
Index finger: air (*vayu*), heart chakra, compassion
Middle finger: space/ether (*akash*), throat chakra, trust, creativity
Ring finger: earth (*prithvi*), root chakra, stability, self-confidence
Little finger: water (*jal/apas*), sacral chakra, joy, cravings

In the Buddhist tradition, each finger of the hand is also associated with a natural element:[6]

Thumb: water
Index finger: space
Middle finger: earth
Ring finger: fire
Little finger: air

When two fingers touch in a mudra, this symbolizes union of the different elements. In Buddhism, the right hand typifies male qualities (yang), such as power and action, and the left hand represents feminine qualities (yin), including knowledge and wisdom.

There are dozens of mudras, and we have included a sampling here along with their symbolic meanings.

Individual Hand Mudras

Mudras of Wisdom (Jnana Mudra) *and Consciousness* (Chin Mudra)

The most commonly practiced mudra in yoga is *Jnana Mudra* and *Chin Mudra*, which are the same hand positions but facing different directions. (*Chin* here is Sanskrit, not the body part.) Touch the tip of your index finger to your thumb and keep your other fingers actively extended and spread. When your palm and fingers are pointed to the sky, it is called *Jnana Mudra*, the mudra of wisdom and knowledge. When your palm and fingers face the earth, it is called *Chin Mudra*, the mudra of consciousness or teaching.

Both mudras represent the union of your individual self with the outside world. The index finger symbolizes inspiration and energy from the outside world, while the thumb represents energy from your inner self or ego, or intuition. (In some texts, the symbolism of the index finger and thumb are reversed.) By connecting these two fingers in the circle of this mudra, you bring the universe and the individual self together. This union symbolizes knowledge, balance, peace, and harmony.

Table 8.2 Hand Expressions (*Hasta Mudras*)

Mudra	Mudra Sanskrit Name	Symbolic Meaning or Purpose
Wisdom Mudra	*Jhana or Gyan*	Union of individual and universe, knowledge, letting-go of ego
Consciousness Mudra	*Chin*	Union of individual and universe, consciousness, teaching
Life Mudra	*Pran*	Vitality, nourishment
Energy Mudra	*Apan*	Patience, focus, detoxification
Beak Mudra	*Mukula*	Focused energy, relaxation
Meditation Mudra	*Dhyana*	Meditation, contemplation
Salutation Seal Mudra	*Anjali*	Gratitude, reflection, harmony, peace, balance, repose
Heart Embrace Mudra	*SvaBhava*	Compassion, grounding
Connected Mind Mudra	*Hakini*	Recharge mental energy, access memory
Refreshing Mudra	*Ushas*	Energizing, wakefulness, morning, creativity
Overcoming Mudra	*Ganesha*	Resilience, courage, determination, perseverance
Releasing Mudra	*Ksepana*	Detoxification, letting go, stress relief
Heart Lotus Mudra	*Hridaya Padma*	Compassion, gratitude, renewal, growth
Lotus Mudra	*Padma*	Compassion, love, openness, transformation
Love Mudra	*Anahata Chakra*	Love, courage, compassion
Enlightenment Mudra	*Uttarabodhi*	Energizing, strength, union
Confidence Mudra	*Vajrapradama*	Strength, confidence, trust

You can use Wisdom or Consciousness Mudra with both hands in seated poses, such as Easy or Hero Pose. Rest your hands on your knees or thighs. How do you choose between *Jhana* or *Chin Mudra*? If you are seeking more energy or insight, turn your palms upward (*Jhana*) as if to "catch" the energy that comes from above. If you are looking for a more calming and grounding effect, face your palms downward (*Chin*) to the earth, for stability. You can also use Wisdom and Consciousness Mudras in balance poses, such as Tree Pose.

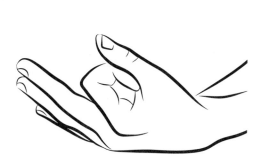

Figure 8.1 Wisdom Mudra

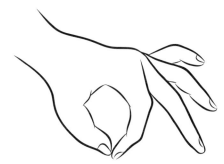

Figure 8.2 Consciousness Mudra

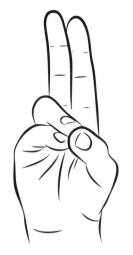

**Figure 8.3
Life Mudra**

Life (Prana) Mudra

Life Mudra represents vitality and assertiveness. Use this mudra in both hands when you are in seated postures. Press the tips of your thumb, ring finger, and little finger together. Extend your index and middle fingers so that they're straight. Use this mudra to help clear your mind and improve your sense of feeling empowered and strong.

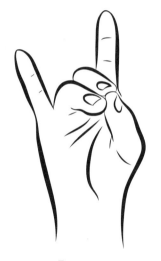

**Figure 8.4
Energy Mudra**

Energy (Apan) Mudra

Energy Mudra represents patience, balance, and detoxification. Bend your middle and ring fingers of both hands in toward your palms so that their tips can touch your thumb tips. Extend your index and little fingers so that they are straight and active. Place both hands in your lap in Energy Mudra, palms facing upward. Combine this mudra with ratio breathing or Victorious Breath. Imagine filling yourself with positive energy or positive thoughts as you inhale, and exhale negative energy or negative thoughts as you exhale. Focus on being patient with yourself even if you are experiencing negative or distracting thoughts.

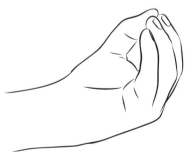

Figure 8.5   Beak Mudra

Beak (Mukula) Mudra

Beak Mudra is a simple mudra that symbolizes focused energy, self-healing, and relaxation. Bring all your fingers together to touch, creating a cupped shape with your hands. You can place this mudra on a part of your body that needs healing. Imagine that healing energy is flowing to the tips of your fingers. As you breathe slowly and smoothly, imagine watering that part of your body with the healing energy of this mudra.

Combined Hand Mudras

Meditation (Dhyana) Mudra

The Buddha is commonly depicted seated with hands in his lap in this mudra. This mudra is useful for calming and centering during meditation. Practice meditation mudra in your lap or at your navel center by forming a bowl with your hands, with your palms facing up. Your fingers are extended and touching each other, with one set of fingers resting on the others and your thumbs are touching. Hold this mudra during meditation or breathing techniques. The right hand usually rests on top of the left hand. Remember to switch so that the other set of fingers are resting on top. This change in position might feel funny at first because most people have a more natural way that they hold their hands out of habit. Breaking the usual habit will help make you more aware of your body. This mudra represents the calmness that meditation brings the mind.

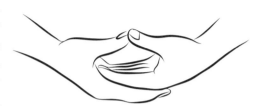

Figure 8.6   Meditation Mudra

Salutation Seal (Anjali) Mudra

Salutation Seal Mudra represents reflection, inner harmony, peace, and balance. This mudra, known as Prayer Mudra, is also used spiritually as a sign of reverence or gratitude or as gesture of respect. Sit in Easy or Hero Pose or stand in Mountain Pose. Bring your palms and fingers together in front of your heart and let your thumbs rest on your sternum gently. Press your fingers and palms together evenly and firmly, making sure that your dominant hand does not push harder and releasing it slightly if the dominant hand is creating imbalance. Use this mudra with meditation or ratio breathing. You can also use it in such postures as Tree Pose or Twisting Fierce Pose or modification of such poses as Fierce Pose if you have a shoulder injury.

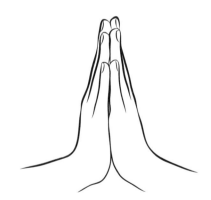

Figure 8.7   Salutation Seal Mudra

Heart Embrace (SvaBhava) Mudra

Heart Embrace Mudra is a warming, restorative mudra that recovers your sense of calm when you are feeling vulnerable or exhausted. Cross your hands over your chest, placing one hand on top of the other. Let yourself enjoy the feeling of comfort. Let your thumbs touch and the fingers spread like wings across your heart. Relax your neck and shoulders, letting your elbows relax. If you are winding down a hectic day, try using heart embrace mudra in a supine position, such as Corpse Pose, and combine it with simple breath awareness or even ratio breathing.

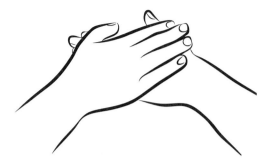

Figure 8.8   Heart Embrace Mudra

Connected Mind (Hakini) Mudra

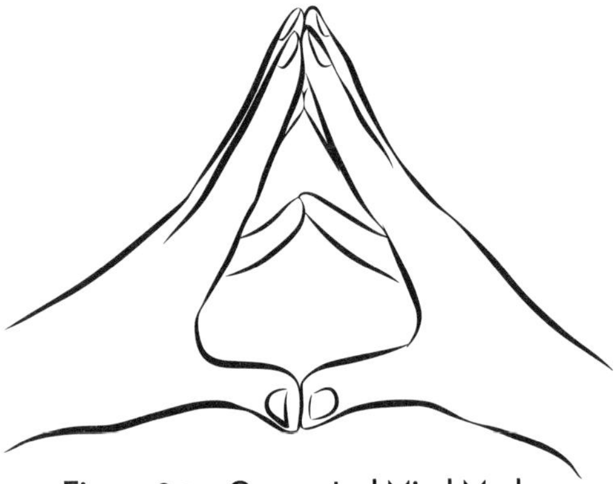

Connected Mind Mudra is useful when you are feeling disorganized, flighty, or scattered. This calming mudra allows you to feel whole and connected. Hold your elbows out at your sides and bring your palms to face each other and press your fingertips firmly together, forming a tent. Keep your fingers active so that you can begin to feel heat building up at your fingertips. Continue to breathe deeply as your actively form this mudra with your hands.

Figure 8.9   Connected Mind Mudra

Refreshing (Ushas) Mudra

Refreshing Mudra is said to stimulate your sacral chakra, the second chakra, which is associated with creativity and sexuality and the element water. The mudra is useful in the morning to stimulate energy and promote wakefulness and alertness. Interlace your fingers at your chest, drawing your elbows wide, or at your abdomen. You can do Refreshing Mudra while lying supine or when in a seated pose.

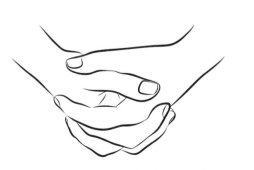

Figure 8.10   Refreshing Mudra

Overcoming (Ganesha) Mudra

Overcoming Mudra represents endurance, perseverance, and resilience. When you are feeling that you need to pick yourself up after being blue or down, use this mudra to cultivate determination. In a seated position, bring your left hand to your chest and face the palm outward. Bend the fingers in toward the palm. Grasp the left hand with your right hand, your right palm facing your chest. Fill yourself with the feeling of courage. Draw your elbows wide, and keep your hands at your sternum. Combine Overcoming Mudra with Victorious Breath to feel strong and courageous.

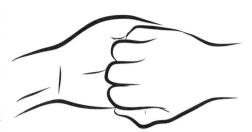

Figure 8.11   Overcoming Mudra

Releasing (Ksepana) Mudra

Releasing Mudra is a gesture that represents letting go and pouring out negative energy. Use this mudra to relieve stress and let go of things that have been difficult to let go. Bring your palms together and interlace your middle, ring, and little fingers. Extend your index fingers so that their tips are touching, like an arrow. Cross your thumbs over each other. Remember to try interlacing your fingers the opposite way (the way that doesn't feel natural) so as to break habits. Use this mudra in such poses as Warrior I, High Crescent Lunge, Low Lunge, or Mountain Pose. With each exhalation, imagine releasing negative energy through your index fingers, like shooting arrows.

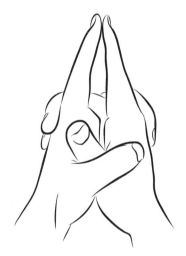

Figure 8.12   Releasing Mudra

Heart Lotus (Hridaya Padma) Mudra

Heart Lotus Mudra represents compassion, gratitude, and healing renewal. The mudra also represents inner self and growth. Your fingertips actively press each other, with your palms curved outward, forming a small space, cupped between your hands. Hold the mudra at your chest. Imagine that your hands create the shape of a lotus bud, filled with hope, compassion, rejuvenation, and growth. You can also try holding Heart Lotus at the location of your Third Eye chakra of your forehead and look through the opening of the space between your hands.

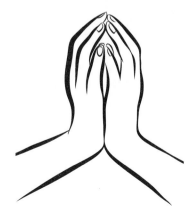

Figure 8.13   Heart Lotus Mudra

Lotus (Padma) *Mudra*

The lotus blossom represents an open and compassionate heart. The lotus flower also symbolizes transformation since it blossoms on the surface of water in spite of its dark muddy roots. The Lotus Mudra signifies light and beauty in the midst of darkness. Do Lotus Mudra in seated postures, such as Easy or Hero Pose. Bring the bases of your palms together and imagine a strong root to the lotus plant. Press your thumb tips and fingertips of your little fingers together so that they are firmly connected but not tight. Imagine yourself rooted and blossoming as you extend and separate your fingers so that they blossom like petals of a flower. As you hold Lotus Mudra, focus on the feeling of openness and connectedness with others. You can combine Lotus Mudra with Loving Kindness (*metta*) meditation.

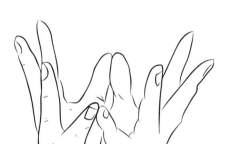

Figure 8.14   Lotus Mudra

Love (Anahata Chakra) *Mudra*

Press your index fingers together and move your thumbs away from the index fingers, and press the thumb tips together. Curve your middle and fourth fingers toward each other, interlocking them to form the shape of a heart, with the thumbs at the bottom of the heart. Raise your little fingers and press their tips together. Imagine using your index and little fingers to send out compassion and to radiate love and care.

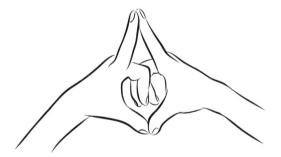

Figure 8.15   Love Mudra

Enlightenment (Uttarabodhi) Mudra

The Enlightenment Mudra is useful when you're feeling like you need some inspiration and hope. The Enlightenment Mudra represents interconnectedness and union. The power of the mudra has been compared to a "lightning rod" used for instilling inspiration and cultivating strength.[7] Interlock the middle, ring, and little fingers and press your index fingertips together. Your palms should be separated. Pull the thumbs away from the index fingers and toward you, keeping the thumb tips pressing against each other. Hold this mudra at your chest when you are in a seated position. Focus on feelings of interconnectedness and union. You can practice Enlightenment Mudra in Warrior I Pose and Warrior III Pose.

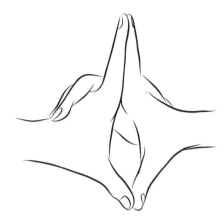

Figure 8.16   Enlightenment Mudra

Confidence (Vajrapradama) Mudra

The Confidence Mudra builds inner strength, trust and confidence. The Sanskrit term for this mudra (*vajrapradama*) means "thunderbolt." It's useful to get rid of doubt, insecurity, or feelings of hopelessness. Use this mudra to build confidence and trust in yourself. Interlace and cross your fingers in front of your chest to form a strong net with your hands. Draw your elbows out wide. Spread your thumbs wide toward the ceiling. Focus on feeling strong and solid. Close your eyes and imagine the brightness and power of a thunderbolt dissipating any sense of self-doubt or mistrust.

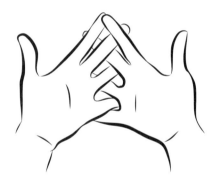

Figure 8.17   Confidence Mudra

✦

Muscles locks and hand mudras are both ways to cultivate a state of mind and build a stronger mind-body connection. Explore how they feel and use them as tools to deepen your breathing, postures, and meditation practice. Don't get so perfectionistic about form that you forget to enjoy the feelings these shapes of the body and hands cultivate.

CHAPTER 9

Learn How to Meditate (Dhyana)

Yoga is the practice of quieting the fluctuations of the mind.

PATANJALI, *YOGA SUTRAS*

Take a moment and find a comfortable seat. Close your eyes. Slowly scan from the top of your head and notice how each part of your body feels. Are you clenching your jaw? Do your neck and shoulders feel tight or hunched from a long day at your desk? Continue to scan downward to your chest, torso, and lower back. How do they feel? Now, pay attention to your hips, legs, and feet. Do you notice any tension, tightness, or pain in your body? When you've reached the bottom of your feet, open your eyes.

You've just done a short meditation.

What do you think of when you hear the word *meditation*? Do you imagine having to sit in a dark room trying to empty your mind? For a lot of people, meditation can bring up concerns about being bored or restless. But there are many techniques of meditation. For some styles, you don't have to stay still. You can meditate while you are walking to work or waiting in line at the grocery store. You can meditate while sitting comfortably in a quiet, relaxed space in your home. You may be surprised to discover that the experience can be as simple as breathing and can produce incredibly centering and relaxing results. Our goal is to help you find a way to meditate that works for you, and then we'll show you how to build meditation into your daily life.

What Is Meditation?

Meditation is an ancient practice with roots in the contemplative practices of many religions across the world, including Buddhism. Meditation has become popularized in the secular world as a form of mental exercise—a practical tool for stress reduction, clarity of mind, and overall wellness. With regular practice, meditation gives you more mental flexibility and calmness so you can feel less bothered by mental chatter and more focused.

Pema Chödrön, a Tibetan Buddhist meditation teacher, describes meditation as "a compassionate openness and the ability to be with oneself and one's situation through all kinds of experiences."[1] She compares the meditative space to a sky that is "spacious, vast enough to accommodate anything that arises." Jon Kabat-Zinn, founder of the popular form of meditation called Mindfulness-Based Stress Reduction, describes meditation as "the intentional self-regulation of attention from moment to moment."[2]

Why Meditate?

The original purpose of poses and movement in yoga was to prepare your mind and body for meditation. Meditation can offer so many benefits. The ancient roots of meditation place meditation within a greater context of spiritual practices and ethical teachings.[3] Meditation can be part of a greater spiritual practice, but it can also be secular. Meditating regularly leads to many personal changes, including mental and physical health benefits that are backed by science.[4]

Here are the many areas in which meditation can be transformative. Notice the overlap with the many benefits of yoga outlined in Chapter 3.

Broaden your capacity to observe. Meditation has been shown to improve your ability to be more aware of both inner and outer experiences. It helps you be more self-aware and be able to be attuned to outer experiences, including how other people are feeling. Over time, meditation can make you more empathic.

Know and describe what you're feeling or thinking. Meditation puts you in touch with your feelings and thoughts, so that you can better understand and articulate your inner experiences. This helps you not only be able to have more insight into what you're going through but also be better able to share and communicate with others. Meditation can help you connect in your relationships.

Act with awareness based on what is happening now. Meditation stops you from going on autopilot. It might at first seem like an "escapist" type of practice, but actually it helps you sit with what is happening right *now*. Meditation brings your attention to the present moment, as opposed to being burdened by what has happened in the past or anxieties about the future. You are still fully able to act from experiences and be motivated by future goals, but, by being in the present moment, you can avoid feeling weighed down by baggage or being paralyzed with the fear of moving forward. Like drawing a bow, you must first pull backward to shoot the bow farthest and with true conviction.

Be less judgmental and critical of yourself and others. Meditation develops more empathy and compassion for yourself and nurtures compassion toward others. It encourages you to take on a nonjudgmental attitude—to rid yourself of the nagging voice in your head that can be so critical of yourself and others. You're also more equipped to catch yourself when you're judging and criticizing.

Feel more centered. Meditation helps temper your reactions so that you don't have to react immediately or get carried away with any particular feeling or situation. When you meditate, you are practicing letting thoughts and feeling come and go, rise and fall, without having to react, get rid of, or change them. This leads to being able to steady the way that you process emotions. You end up having more time to respond and feel less urgency to react. It puts on the emotional brakes so that you get more space between your thoughts and feelings and your actions.

Reduce stress and anxiety. Meditation has been shown to reduce stress and improve overall well-being.[5] It has been used in several health-care programs to reduce stress and has been shown to decrease anxiety in people with generalized anxiety disorder.[6]

Be in touch with your "gut" intuition. Meditation helps you be in touch with your own intuition. One study shows that meditation may even help you connect with your unconscious and have an earlier awareness of your intentions. In a 1980s experiment, psychologist Benjamin Libet, who asked participants who were hooked up to brain electrodes, to press a button whenever they wanted, and report the time on the clock when they consciously became aware of their intention to press the button. Libet's experiment showed that brain activity in areas in charge of moving the finger occurred hundreds of milliseconds *before* people reported that they decided to press the button. In a 2016 study, researchers tried a variation of the same experiment (without the brain electrodes) with longtime meditators who had at least three years of meditation experience, comparing them to people who didn't meditate. Meditators were a lot faster at realizing their intention to move their finger. Researchers concluded that meditation gives you earlier and better access to your unconscious.[7]

Build your ability to adapt or deal with difficult situations with more flexibility. Meditation builds your mental resilience and gives you a balanced, relaxed, yet actively attentive mind. Your mind becomes like an ocean. It still has movement and rocky waves, but each individual ripple has less overall impact in the expansive ocean of your mind. Meditation helps you become more flexible and adaptive to what is happening now. Science has also backed this up, showing that meditation enhances cognitive flexibility.[8]

Sharpen your attention and memory. Meditation improves several measures of attention[9] in adults and children. It has improved school behavior, academic performance, and attention in school-age children and teens.[10] Researchers continue to study whether meditation could also help children with attention deficit/hyperactivity disorder (ADHD). Short meditations can start building the capacity to learn to pay attention and sit still.

Have you ever noticed how you are more forgetful when you're stressed? Stress actually leads to more cell death and less growth of neurons in your hippocampus, an area critical for memory. Meditation counteracts the negative effects of stress on memory and promotes more activity and growth in the hippocampus and other areas associated with memory.

Improve your mood. Meditation isn't always a path to feeling better about something or happier, but it has been shown to boost your mood generally. Loving kindness meditations have been shown to spur people into an "upward spiral" of positive emotions[11] and enhance the feeling of being social connected.[12]

Get better sleep. Meditation has been shown to improve sleep quality and be effective in treating chronic insomnia.[13] It also boosts your body's nighttime level of melatonin, a natural hormone that regulates our sleep-wake cycle and is used to treat insomnia and jetlag.[14]

Boost your immune system and protect your body from the harmful physical effects of chronic stress and aging. There is much emerging research on meditation being able to boost your immune system.[15] One fascinating study found that meditators produced more antibodies, the fighter cells of the immune system, when they got a flu (influenza) vaccine compared to people who did not meditate and got the same vaccine.[16]

Meditation also lowers stress hormones and decreases inflammation in the body. Chronic stress is a contributor to many physical illnesses, including many illnesses related to inflammation, including diabetes and cardiovascular and auto-immune diseases. One small study found that by adding meditation to walking on a treadmill, people with type 2 diabetes were better able to control their blood sugar and lower stress hormone cortisol levels doing just regular walking.[17]

Help heal anxiety, depression, trauma, and addictions. There is growing evidence that meditation can play an important role in the clinical treatment of psychiatric disorders including anxiety and depression.[18] Adding meditation and mindfulness to exercise has been shown to reduce the symptoms of depression. Another study found that adding meditation before jogging reduced depression symptoms by 40 percent in only eight weeks.

Meditation is a promising tool to help ease suffering related to trauma, including anxiety, depression, or post-traumatic stress disorder (PTSD). It has helped reduce trauma symptoms in veterans with PTSD[19] and women survivors of violence.[20]

Meditation can help pave the road toward recovery as well. Smokers who practiced mindfulness had less craving activity found on brain imaging when they were shown a picture of someone lighting a cigarette, demonstrating the powerful protective effect that meditation can provide for those in recovery.[21] It heightens awareness of triggers and also reduces stress and the need to react immediately, and both increased awareness and delayed impulsiveness promote sobriety.[22]

What's the Science Behind Meditation?

Science in the last few decades has advanced our understanding of how meditation changes the body and mind by examining the power of meditation at the neurobiological, hormonal, anatomical, and functional level. Researchers define meditation as a complex mental process that changes our emotional control, memory, sensory perception, hormones, and nervous system. Meditation trains our mind to be focused and relaxed at the same time, which balances our nervous system and lowers our blood pressure, heart rate, and breathing rate, but just enough so we're still awake and focused. Meditation cushions the way our body reacts to stress over time, leading to lower stress hormone levels and less inflammation overall in the body.[23]

Meditation also acts by harnessing the proven power of the mind—and brain—to grow and change through experience, even in adulthood, through a process called neuroplasticity, or cortical plasticity. Neuroplasticity is the concept that the pathways and structures in our brain can be transformed through experience.

When you meditate regularly, you are "working out" your mind and making areas that manage attention, emotional regulation, motivation, and body awareness "stronger." Long-term meditation has been shown to have lasting changes to brain activity as measured by electroencephalogram (EEG), or brain wave, patterns in areas related to positive emotions and attention. We also see this effect with functional brain imaging, which tracks brain activity in real time by measuring blood flow. Meditators have enhanced activity in large areas of the prefrontal cortex of their brain. The prefrontal cortex is the area of the brain in charge of making good decisions, having appropriate social manners, and expressing your personality. It's in charge of weighing the consequences of actions, keeping you focused on goals, and helping you imagine how other people are feeling. In other words, it's a really important part of the brain that makes us human and connected with others. Meditation also increases activity and growth in the other areas in the brain in charge of processing and regulating emotions.

One of the most fascinating findings suggests that meditation has the power to change the structure of your brain. A Harvard study using brain imaging found that people who were experienced meditators had more gray matter in specific brain areas related to attention, body awareness, and sensory processing compared to expected sizes for people at their age.[24] Experienced meditators also had more gray matter in the frontal cortex. The natural aging process causes the brain to shrink over time and the outer layer, or cortex, thins with age. In the prefrontal cortex, fifty-year-old experienced meditators had the brain volume you would expect in a twenty-five-year-old, suggesting meditation could help buffer the effects of age on the mind.

A second Harvard study found that as few as eight weeks of mindfulness meditation helped grow areas of the brain involved in thinking about the self, emotional regulation, learning, memory, attention, empathy, and compassion.[25] In contrast, areas of the brain involved in anxiety, fear, stress, and emotional reactivity got smaller. Who wouldn't want such benefits?

How Do I Get Started?

The key to meditation is regular practice. With practice, it becomes easier and evolves. Meditation is like a mental muscle. The more you practice, the more you are able to do it more smoothly and easily. Studies have shown that experienced meditation activates fewer parts of the brain compared to people new to meditation, corroborating the idea that meditation becomes easier with practice and requires less mental effort.

Think of trying meditation as an experiment, because, for a lot of people, meditation is really tricky and challenging. That's normal, because we are much more used to distractions or a frantic pace of life. We suggest starting with as little as one minute a day for the first few days—or even week. And once you get used to a minute, you can build on that and try a little longer, say, 3 to 5 minutes. Pretty soon, you'll notice that you're meditating for 10 to 15 minutes with less effort than it took you for the first minute of meditation when you first started! So, relax, build gradually, and don't worry if it doesn't seem to "work" at first. We're interested in your creating a habit and figuring out what works for you gradually, rather than to try to sit for 30 minutes for the first time and then give up because it's an awful, uncomfortable experience. Don't be discouraged early on if you feel like you're not reaping all the benefits of meditation at first—it takes at least a month or so to start to notice some changes. Even though we encourage you to try a little at a time and increase it gradually, meditation shouldn't be so uncomfortable that you feel more overwhelmed or unraveled than when you started.

Remember, our motto is—don't do it if it doesn't feel right for you.

Here are some of our tips for getting started with your meditation practice. In our 8-week program, you will try out eight different types of meditations to see what works for you.

Pick a regular time of day to meditate. You can choose a regular time, such as in the morning, at noon, or at nighttime before bed. Schedule anywhere between 5 and 30 minutes a day to practice meditation and add it to a routine that you already have. Protect this time by putting away distracting devices.

Find a comfortable posture. For most of these meditations, except active ones, such as walking meditation, you do them in a comfortable seated position. You can sit in Easy or Hero Pose with an optional block underneath your tailbone, or on a chair with your feet flat on the floor. Make sure that your shoulders are relaxed away from your ears and your spine is tall.

We find it helpful to check in with six areas of your body before you get started with the meditation: your seat and spine, legs, shoulders and chest, hands, face, and eyes.

1. *Seat and spine.* Root your tailbone into the ground or chair so that your spine and can feel long and tall. You should feel solid and stable in your foundation.

2. *Legs.* Depending on your posture, your legs can be crossed or folded underneath you. Your knees should not be higher than your hips in Easy or Hero Pose, so add blocks under your seat to correct this.

3. *Shoulders and chest.* Check your shoulders to make sure they are relaxed away from your ears. Broaden your chest so that you feel expansive and wide.

4. *Hands.* Choose a mudra for your hands and rest them comfortably in your lap or on your knees.

5. *Face.* Relax the muscles of your face and make sure you're not grimacing or clenching your jaw. Let your face be serene.

6. *Eyes.* Relax your eyes to prevent any eye strain and let your gaze be soft and gentle.

Find or create a comfortable space. Create a comfortable, private space that you can use regularly. Close your office door, retreat to a bedroom, even a bathroom stall, if you have no privacy at work. Some people even meditate on buses or subways.

Remember your intention. Remind yourself why you would like to meditate.

Be easy on yourself. Remember that your experience of meditation will change day to day and will feel different, so don't judge yourself if it feels harder on some days than others. The fundamental principle of meditation is making friends with yourself without harboring any judgment or criticism. It's not a competition and there is no "perfect" or "right" way to meditate.

What If I'm Too Busy to Meditate?

It's very common to feel that you're too busy to schedule a time to meditate. That's why we recommend finding a regular time to meditate, building it into your morning or bedtime routine for as few as one to five minutes a day. Regular meditation actually gives you *more* time in the day. How? Meditation improves your concentration and attention so that you can work more efficiently throughout the day. It also helps you learn how to respond to stress more calmly, so that you can feel not so rushed and can be more effective in difficult situations.

Is Meditation for Everyone?

Meditation has a lot of proven physical and mental health benefits, but not everyone enjoys the experience of it. Even though it can be extremely relaxing and calming, meditation isn't intended to be curative or to make you a happier person. Meditation and its heightened awareness can bring up difficult feelings, such as frustration or sadness. The awareness of these emotions means that meditation doesn't always feel good.

Meditation is generally safe and accessible. However, if you have a history of severe anxiety, panic disorder, trauma, dissociation, or psychosis, you should discuss meditation with your mental health professional first to make sure it's safe for you. There have been a few small studies and anecdotes reporting that meditation can worsen panic or anxiety symptoms for some people. We recommend carefully considering with your doctor whether meditation could be harmful. One 1992 study done by Dr. David Shapiro found that two out of twenty-seven long-term meditators with an average of four years of meditation training suffered from profoundly distressing symptoms during and after meditation, including worsening panic, anxiety, depression, or pain. But this area has not been well studied. In our clinical practice, certain types of meditation can be distressing to some, particularly during acute times of grief, depression, and trauma.

If you are feeling unsafe or experience such symptoms as dissociation, flashbacks, panic, or severe anxiety during meditation, then stop immediately. As with any other exercise in this book, stop when something feels distressing or painful.

Remember, our motto is—don't do it if it doesn't feel right for you.

Meditation Techniques

There are many techniques of meditation rooted in many different traditions—modern and ancient, secular and spiritual. The key in any of these techniques is to find the balance between a focused and relaxed state of mind. Many people think you have to try really hard and put in a lot of effort to concentrate. But training your mind is like dealing with an overly excited puppy; you don't want to be too restrictive and harsh, but can gently guide and direct it.

There are three general categories of meditation: focused attention, open monitoring, and natural presence. Focused attention is where you concentrate on something external, such as a candle flame; something physical, such as your breath; or an internal feeling, such as compassion or kindness. Open monitoring is when you merely observe passing feelings and thoughts or all the sounds and sights around you, but you don't focus on any passing thought, feeling, or object in particular. Natural or effortless presence, which is a more advanced technique, has no object to focus on. You allow your mind to just observe and exist in the moment, letting go of any passing thoughts or emotions. Some techniques combine different elements from these three categories.

People often think of meditation as sitting down to "empty your mind," "think of nothing," or "make your mind an empty canvas," but there are actually many styles of meditation that welcome and recognize the many thoughts and feelings that come and go through your mind. Many forms of meditation recognize that you will likely have distracting thoughts that come and go at any given point. But the key is not getting caught up or carried away by any particular thought; you acknowledge and try to let them go. This general form of meditation is called open monitoring.

Our 8-week program outlined in the next chapter incorporates a number of different meditation techniques.

Table 9.1   General Categories of Meditation

General Category of Meditation	Description	Good for
Focused Attention	Focused attention, or concentrative, meditation cultivates your attention to a single object, such as your breath, or an image, feeling, or sound.	Beginners, intermediate
Open Monitoring	Open monitoring uses open awareness, which expands your mind and welcomes thoughts and feelings. Develops awareness and nonreactivity.	Beginners, intermediate
Natural/Effortless/ Objectless Presence	Does not focus on anything in particular except being in the present moment. Trains the mind to not be attached to any particular thought, feeling, or object and to be in "pure presence" or "pure being." Also known as desirelessness.	Intermediate, advanced

Table 9.2 Forms of Meditation

Forms of Meditation	Description	Good for
Affirmations or Self-Affirmations	Psychological technique to focus thinking about core values; can be effectively used to increase changes to more positive behavior	Self-confidence, positive thinking
Atiyoga, or Dzogchen, Meditation	Meaning "great perfection," an advanced form of Buddhist meditation that encourages spontaneity and resting in a relaxed and natural state	Spiritually minded
Breathing Meditation	Meditation involving focusing on the breath; often an easy way to begin your meditation practice	Beginners; sleep, stress reduction, concentration, body awareness
Body Scan	Deeply relaxing form of mindfulness meditation that increases body awareness by bringing your focused attention to each part of your body in a gradual upward fashion from your toes to the top of your head	Beginners; deep relaxation, sleep, stress reduction, chronic pain
Chakra Meditation	Meditations based on balancing and healing the different chakra centers of the body. Each meditation focuses on a theme associated with specific chakra.	Balance energy, spiritually minded
Guided Imagery Meditation or Visualization	Technique using words, sounds, or images to guide the imagination and evoke a positive situation, sensation, or emotion	Deep relaxation, stress reduction, chronic pain
Guided Meditation	Broad term referring to a teacher or person guiding a person through meditation by using text, audio, or video with words, music, or sound	Beginners; people who prefer more verbal cues
Insight (Vipassana) Meditation	Traditional Buddhist mindfulness meditation that emphasizes awareness of the breath, noticing objects, labeling thoughts or feelings, and returning to a point of focus, such as the breath	Beginners; secular, awareness, nonreactivity
Kundalini Meditation	Variety of different meditations, including mantra and active breathing techniques	Spiritually minded, open-minded
Loving Kindness (*Metta*) or Compassion Meditation	Meditation that focuses on developing feelings of kindness and compassion toward oneself and then gradually extending this compassion toward others to increase empathy	Improve self esteem, less self-critical, sense of empathy
Mantra Meditation	Sounds, words, or phrases, spoken aloud or in the mind, as the object of concentration	Concentration
Mindful Walking	Form of mindfulness paired with movement, often in nature; walking meditation is walking paired with mantra, breath, or focused attention on body and natural environment	Beginners; restlessness, renewal, stress relief

(continued)

Table 9.2 Forms of Meditation (*continued*)

Forms of Meditation	Description	Good for
Mindfulness Meditation	Combination of open monitoring and focused attention that encourages observing internal thoughts and external sensations, including sights and sounds, without getting carried away with them	Beginners; secular, concentration, descriptive observation, nonjudgmental attitude, nonreactivity
Mindfulness-Based Stress Reduction	Structured 8-week mindfulness program developed by Jon Kabat-Zinn that teaches principles derived from Buddhism and yoga	Beginners; structured, secular, chronic pain, anxiety, stress, depression
Nada (Sound) Yoga	"Union through sound"; different sources of sound and vibration, including voice, mantras, and music	Relaxation, concentration, calming
Self Inquiry or "I Am" Meditation	Form of effortless presence meditation focusing the mind on the feeling of being and the question "Who am I?" turning the focus inward	Advanced; inner peace
Shikantaza	Form of objectless meditation or effortless presence associated with Soto Zen school in Japan founded by Dogen; the practice of "just sitting" requires staying alert without focusing on the breath or any sensations or thoughts	Advanced; focus on present moment
Taoist Meditation	Many different types of meditations within the Taoist tradition, including insight, breathing, and visualization	Those interested in nature and philosophy
Tonglen	Tibetan Buddhist "giving and taking" or "sending and receiving" meditation focused on deep connectedness with others and wish for all to be free from suffering; breathe in hot, heavy air, representing the suffering of others, and breathe out cool, light air, sending kindness toward oneself and others	Dealing with negativity, stress, nurturing love, compassion, social connectedness, spiritual growth
Transcendental Meditation ("TM")	Structured technique involving repetition of a mantra to achieve a state of thought-free awareness	Focus, relaxed mental state
Yoga Nidra	Peaceful practice that creates a state of deep relaxation similar to sleep in terms of its restorative properties, but without loss of consciousness	Stress relief, relaxation, trauma, insomnia
Zen (*Zazen*)	General term for seated meditation in the Zen Buddhist tradition and can be practiced in various forms, such as focused attention on the breath or Shikantaza objectless meditation	Awareness, nonreactivity, focused on present

Breath Meditation (Week 1)

Doing focused breathing exercises is an easy way to try focused awareness meditation. Three-Part Breath is a form of breath meditation that helps you feel more grounded. You can also do rhythmic breathing as a form of breath meditation.

Table 9.3   Breath Meditation

1.	Start in a comfortable position on your back, such as Reclining Bound Angle or Corpse Pose. Another option is to place your feet flat on the ground, hip distance apart, as if you are going into Bridge Pose. Let your spine and lower back release on the ground.
2.	Place your hands alongside your torso and let your shoulders relax away from your ears. You can also place one hand on your chest and the other on your abdomen, if you want to feel the rise and fall of your breath.
3.	Start to **tune into your breath.**
4.	Relax your mouth, let your face go soft, and sigh out all your breath with an open mouth.
5.	Inhale and exhale slowly through your nose and feel your belly, rib cage, and chest expand **on the inhalation and release like the gentle waves of the ocean on the exhalation.**
6.	Notice if you're clenching your jaw—it's very common to carry tension there. **Relax your jaw** and let it be open slightly. Rest your tongue gently behind your lower teeth. Imagine the roof of your mouth as an expansive dome. Feel your temples relax on both sides.
7.	Continue to breathe. If you get distracted by any thoughts, just let them come and go. **Gently bring your mind back to the sensation of your breath**, flowing in and out of your body.
8.	Count your breath from 1 to 10: *in-one, out-one, in-two, out-two,* and so on. If you get distracted, restart the count at 1. Don't struggle to keep track. If you feel restless or distracted, breathe louder, using your Victorious Breath. Let the sound of your breath fill the room and keep bringing your mind gently back to the sound of your breath. If you prefer to use an affirmation instead of counting, try saying to yourself with each breath, "I breathe in joy and peace, I breathe out suffering and negative energy."
9.	Stay on your breath for 5 to 15 minutes. If you're a beginner, try 1 to 3 minutes at first and work your way up to 5 minutes. Don't compete with yourself. Once 5 minutes feels comfortable, do 10 minutes.

Mindfulness Body and Sound Meditation (Week 2)

Mindfulness meditation is also known as nonreactive awareness. *Mindfulness* has been defined as "paying attention in a particular way: on purpose, in the present moment, and nonjudgmentally."[26]

Think of mindfulness meditation as a way of learning to stay on the sidewalk while you carefully watch traffic pass by. It gives you the chance to stay on the sidewalk, observing passing traffic and listening to the sounds on the street, without having to do or change anything. You may be tempted to jump in a car or try to stop traffic, but just gently draw yourself back onto the sidewalk.

Table 9.4 Mindfulness Body and Sound Meditation

1.	Start in a comfortable meditation position of your choice (standing, seated, or lying down).
2.	Notice how you are standing, lying, or sitting down. Where does your body make contact with the ground or the chair? What does it feel like? Notice the position of your head and neck, your arms, and your legs.
3.	Start to tune into the sensations in your body with **curiosity and interest.**
4.	Notice the sensations in your body. Do they feel warm or cool? Tingling or vibrating? Pulsing or steady? Soft and subtle, or loud and clear? Expanding or shrinking? Moving or still? Where do you feel tension?
5.	Continue to observe your body sensations for about 5 minutes.
6.	You may **notice thoughts coming and going.** Let them come and go like cars in traffic. You may observe them from afar, but don't get carried away or rush after any one in particular.
7.	Let go of body sensations.
8.	Now bring your attention to the sounds in the room. **Simply listen passively.** Do you hear traffic, birds, or other noises outside? Do you hear noises inside the room? Are they soft or loud? Sharp or dull? Long or short? Let your mind simply witness all the different sounds inside and outside the room. Observe the gap of silence in between sounds as well.
9.	Continue to listen to the sounds with curiosity and interest for 5 minutes.
10.	If you have a **particular sensation in your body or sound** that is pulling away your attention, then **allow yourself to focus on it.** Bring all your attention to that sensation or sound and notice all the dimensions of how it feels or sounds. Then allow it to evaporate.
11.	Let yourself relax your attention gradually and gently open your eyes.

Walking Meditation (Week 3)

You can do mindful walking indoors, in a mall, city, or nature, and even on a treadmill. It does not have to be for a long period of time, and can be as short as one to two minutes. You could even set your initial goal to try mindful walking for only ten steps.

Mindful walking or walking meditation relaxes the mind and is easy to add to your everyday routine. For a more nurturing experience, try walking in nature. The Japanese art of *shinrin-yoku* (forest bathing) uses a mindful walk through the forest to relax, absorb nature, and relieve stress. For mindful walking, don't rush yourself and walk at a pace where you can comfortably match an equal number of steps smoothly with your breath, creating an equal ratio of steps per inhalation and exhalation, such as inhaling for three steps and exhaling for three steps. Thích Nhất Hạnh, a Vietnamese Zen teacher, suggests visualizing yourself as a tiger walking slowly, and you will find that your steps become as majestic as the steps of a tiger.

Table 9.5 Walking Meditation

1.	Start walking at a steady and regular pace that is comfortable to you. You can be in nature or in the city, or even in the grocery store or in a mall—you can do this pretty much anywhere you can walk safely.
2.	Notice the feeling of your feet on the ground as you walk. **Spend a few minutes observing the sensations of your body as you walk.** Keep a relaxed pace.
3.	Next, figure out the natural pace of your steady breath based on your steps. Maybe your breath is naturally 3 steps in and 3 steps out, or 5 steps in and 5 steps out. Try to make the number of the inhalations and exhalations the same. Beginners, you may find that your inhalation and exhalation are not the same number of steps, but you can stay with that ratio if it is comfortable and work toward a more even inhalation and exhalation.
4.	Once you determine a smooth and steady number of steps per breath, you can **count and match your breath with your steps.** For example, inhale for 4 steps, and exhale for 4 steps, and so on, counting to yourself *in-two-three-four, out-two-three-four.*
5.	You can also use phrases instead of counting your steps. For example, **"Breathing in, I feel calm. Breathing out, I feel strong."**
6.	If you are out in nature or a place that feels peaceful, then you can stop to **observe the sights, sounds, and smells around you** as you continue to breathe steadily and smoothly.
7.	Continue with your walking meditation for as little as a few minutes or up to 30 minutes or longer.

Gazing Candle Meditation (Week 4)

Candle or gazing (*trataka*) meditation is a focused attention meditation that is useful to help your concentration and have a renewed sense of energy. If you don't have access to a candle, you can also use an online video of a candle flame or watch leaves fluttering in the wind or ocean waves at the shoreline. The key to this meditation is to have a point of focus with some interest where you can gaze steadily and softly. Alternatively, the point of focus could be internal, such as by closing your eyes and focusing on the point between your brows, the Third Eye. It's important not to stare too hard, to avoid straining your eyes. Your gaze should be soft and gentle.

Table 9.6   Gazing Candle Meditation

1.	Light a candle on a table in front of you about 3 to 4 feet away, so that you can sit upright and see the flame at eye level or slightly below.
2.	Sit upright in a comfortable posture so that your neck and shoulders are relaxed. You can use Easy or Hero Pose.
3.	Take 4 or 5 deep breaths to relax and **close your eyes as you tune into your breath.**
4.	Open your eyes and look at the flame. **Let your gaze be soft and focused.** Imagine that the flame is your anchor in the room.
5.	Continue to **observe the flame steadily** with as little blinking as possible but without straining your eyes.
6.	Observe the intensity, color, movement, and shape of the flame.
7.	Pick a point within the flame, and focus gently on it for 2 or 3 minutes. If your eyes become dry or start to water, close your eyes for a break for about 10 to 20 seconds.
8.	**Close your eyes and visualize the candle flame at the point between your brows,** your Third Eye. Let that image fill you with warmth, compassion, and renewed energy. With your eyes closed, look gently upward at that point between your brows for 2 to 3 minutes.
9.	**Relax your eyes** and open them again to gaze at the flame. Repeating this process as long as comfortable, between 5 and 15 minutes.
10.	It's normal to have distracting thoughts or feelings during this meditation—let them come and go. Draw your attention gently back to the flame and the rise and fall of your breath. You can also close your eyes and focus on your breath for a few minutes to center yourself.

Compassion or Loving Kindness (*Metta*) Meditation (Week 5)

The compassion, or *metta*, meditation trains your mind to be more compassionate toward yourself and others. The practice has been shown to increase optimism, positive emotions, and social connectedness. Loving kindness meditation improves the ability to empathize and read other people's emotions.[27] It is associated with changes in brain activity to viewing emotions in others and changes brain activity in areas of emotional processing.[28] A brain imaging study found that compassionate training increases altruistic behavior and increases brain activity in regions associated with social awareness and emotional regulation.[29]

Table 9.7 Compassion Meditation

1.	Start in a comfortable seated position.
2.	Close your eyes and **focus on the area of your heart in the center of your chest.** Imagine that the sun is shining into that space to fill it with light and warmth. As you visualize this, repeat these phrases in your mind. You can also modify them if your wish. *May I be free from suffering.* *May I be happy.* *May I be peaceful and at ease.* Continue repeating these phrases in your mind for about 3 minutes as you imagine the light and warmth expanding in your chest.
3.	Now, **think of someone whom you have loving and kind feelings toward,** a loved one or family member. Imagine sending that person warmth and light from your heart center. As you visualize this, repeat in your mind: *May you be free from suffering.* *May you be happy.* *May you be peaceful and at ease.* Continue repeating these phrases in your mind for 2 to 3 minutes as you imagine sending stronger and brighter light and warmth toward the person.
4.	Next, **think of someone whom you have neutral feelings toward,** such as a postal worker or a neighbor. Imagine sending that person warmth and light from your heart center. As you visualize this, repeat in your mind: *May you be free from suffering.* *May you be happy.* *May you be peaceful and at ease.* Continue repeating these phrases in your mind for 2 to 3 minutes as you imagine sending stronger and brighter light and warmth toward the person.
5.	Now, **think of someone whom you have negative feelings toward,** such as a boss or colleague or someone who makes you frustrated or upset. Imagine sending that person warmth and light from your heart center. As you visualize this, repeat in your mind: *May you be free from suffering.* *May you be happy.* *May you be peaceful and at ease.* Continue repeating these phrases in your mind for 2 to 3 minutes as you imagine sending stronger and brighter light and warmth toward the person.
6.	Finally, **extend that warm feeling toward all living beings.** Imagine spreading warmth and light from your heart center. As you visualize this, repeat in your mind: *May all be free from suffering.* *May all be happy.* *May all be peaceful and at ease.* Continue repeating these phrases in your mind for 2 to 3 minutes.
7.	If the full exercise feels too lengthy at first, start with sending compassion to yourself first and gradually add others over time.

Mantra Meditation (Week 6)

A mantra is a repeated sound, word, or phrase that can be used as a point of focus during meditation. You have probably heard of the most widely recognized yoga mantra *Om*, which is often chanted before or after a yoga session.

The Sa-Ta-Na-Ma Mantra Mudra Meditation combines both mantra and mudras in a simple meditation exercise. This important syllabic mantra meditation called *Kirtin Kriya*, or Sa-Ta-Na-Ma, is used in such yoga traditions as Kundalini yoga. Each syllable of the mantra is complemented by an active hand position on both hands. You can use any of the mudras that have the fingertips of your hands touching together. Figure out which mudra based on how you're feeling. Are you feeling cluttered or disconnected from your day? Try Connected Mind Mudra. Are you feeling tired and could use more energy? Try the Energy Mudra.

For other mantra meditations, try rhythmic breathing exercises (page 91) or mindful walking with mantras (page 243).

Table 9.8   Sa-Ta-Na-Ma Mantra Meditation

1.	Sit in a comfortable position.
2.	Close your eyes, and focus on strength and energy.
3.	Inhale and exhale deeply through your nose for 2 to 3 cycles.
4.	**Say these syllables out loud** in this sequence and coordinate movement with both hands: • **"Sa"** (rhymes with "Ma") Press your index finger and thumb together. • **"Ta"** Press your middle finger and thumb together. • **"Na"** Press your ring finger and thumb together. • **"Ma"** Press your little finger and thumb together.
5.	Visualize each sound coming out through the top of your head, releasing negative energy.
6.	On the next the Sa-Ta-Na-Ma cycle, **press your thumbs into your fingernails with each syllable,** instead of to your fingertips.
7.	Continue to **repeat Sa-Ta-Na-Ma, alternating every complete cycle between fingertips and fingernails.** Do 10 full cycles.
8.	For the next 10 cycles, whisper the syllables quietly. Continue to match your mudras to each syllable.
9.	For the final 10 cycles, silently repeat the syllables in your mind. Continue to coordinate the mudras with each syllable.
10.	Once you are done, let your breath return to normal.
11.	You can repeat for up to 3 sets of 10 to 15 exhalations as long as it feels comfortable.

Body Scan Meditation (Week 7)

Body scan meditation increases body awareness and relaxation and is particularly useful at the end of a long day or before bedtime to help with better sleep. A body scan meditation has immediate healing power for chronic pain.[30]

Table 9.9   Body Scan Meditation

1.	Lie in a comfortable position. You can also do this in a seated position if you prefer. Close your eyes if that is comfortable.
2.	Bring your attention into your body. Start to pay attention to your breath. Relax your face and jaw as you continue to breathe. Keep your face relaxed.
3.	**Observe whether there is any tension or pain in your body,** and start to let it relax. Notice if there are specific areas that you carry stress.
4.	**Let your body be heavy.** Notice where your body is touching the ground. Notice where your feet are touching the ground, your legs on the chair or ground. Soften and relax your body into those spaces.
5.	Bring your attention to the **bottom of your feet and ankles.** How do your arches or ankles feel? How do the tops of your feet feel? Continue to breathe as you notice the sensations. On your next inhalation, imagine your breath traveling like water streaming down your torso and legs to your feet. Exhale and let your feet relax into the ground.
6.	Shift your attention to the **knees and calves.** How do the front and back of your calves feel? How do your knees feel? Inhale and imagine your breath traveling down your torso to your knees and calves. Exhale and melt those areas into the ground.
7.	Move your attention to the **thighs, hips, and pelvis.** How do the front and back of your thighs feel? How do your pelvis and hips feel? How does your bottom and tailbone feel? On the next inhalation, imagine your breath traveling down your body into your thighs, hips, and pelvis. Exhale and release them into the ground.
8.	Bring your attention to your **lower back and abdomen.** How does your lower back feel? How does your abdomen feel? Inhale and imagine your breath traveling like cool water down your body into your lower back and abdomen. Exhale and soften and release those areas into the ground. Let them be heavy.
9.	Shift your attention to your **upper and middle back, shoulder blades, and chest.** Is there any tightness in those areas? Inhale and imagine your breath traveling like water to your upper torso. Exhale and release your shoulder blades into the ground and let your chest expand and relax.
10.	Bring your attention to your **fingers, wrist, forearms, and upper arms.** How do they feel? On the next inhalation, imagine your breath traveling like water through both arms. Exhale and let your arms be heavy.
11.	Bring your attention to your **neck, shoulders, and collarbone,** areas that commonly feel tension. Are they tense or tight? Inhale and imagine your breath traveling like cool water through your neck and shoulders. Exhale and let them soften and melt on the ground, widening your collarbone.
12.	Bring your attention to your **face, eyes, ears, mouth, jaw, and forehead.** Are they clenched or grimacing? Inhale and imagine your breath traveling like water through your face, eyes, ears, mouth, jaw, and forehead. Exhale and let them melt on the ground. Let your face relax.
13.	Finally, bring your attention to **top of your head.** Inhale and imagine your breath traveling like water to the top of your head. Exhale and let your head be heavy and relaxed.
14.	**Inhale to feel the wholeness and completeness of your entire body** as it expands. Exhale and relax your whole body.

Visualization Meditation (Week 8)

Visualization or guided imagery is a general technique that can be used to enhance specific feelings or prepare the mind. It has been used to help athletes perform better. In this exercise, you will be guided to a safe and comforting place where you can experience positive feelings, such as security and gratitude. If you're feeling that you're experiencing a lot of chaos or vulnerability, then this technique provides an anchor and safe harbor.

Table 9.10 Visualization Meditation

1.	Start in a comfortable seated, standing, or lying position.
2.	Begin to **notice your breath.** Breathe in smoothly and steadily 5 times.
3.	**Imagine that you are at the top of a short set of stairs.** At the bottom of the stairs, imagine a door.
4.	Inhale slowly. **Exhale and imagine stepping down slowly one step.** Inhale again and exhale as you imagine stepping another step down. With each step, your body is more relaxed and grounded. With each step, you exhale, and with each exhale, tension leaves your body. Repeat and continue pairing your breath with each step down for 10 steps.
5.	Once you are down these steps, imagine you **open the door.**
6.	The imagined space behind this door is any space of your choosing that you find to be the most comforting and relaxing. This can be an outdoor space under a tree or by the ocean. It can be your bedroom or living room or a combination of many different spaces that you would like. It is any space that you enjoy where you feel safest and most relaxed.
7.	Once you **"walk in" that space,** take a look around you. What is the light like? What are the textures of the items in the space, whether grass on the ground or the soft fabric of a couch or chair? Notice what is around you on the walls or in the sky. What are the colors? Do you hear any sounds? Is it quiet? Are there birds chirping or the gentle sound of a brook or ocean waves? What does it smell like? This space is yours to see and experience. Continue to breathe and look around you in this safe place.
8.	**Sit somewhere in that space.** Imagine feelings of security, peace, and gratitude. Can you notice a sense of security in this space? What else makes you feel this sense of security, such as people, activities, or experiences? Can you feel thankful for this space? What else do you feel thankful for in your life? Can you feel peaceful in this space? What else makes you feel peaceful?
9.	You can do this visualization in only a few minutes or for much longer, such as 30 minutes.
10.	When you're ready, bring your attention back to your body and breath. Move your fingers and toes to bring your mind back to your body. Open your eyes.

Additional Types of Meditation

We have included a few extra meditations so you can use them in case you find certain forms of meditations in our weekly program very challenging or just not enjoyable.

Om *Meditation*

Meditation doesn't have to be long. If you're looking for a supershort and simple meditation to clear your mind, try chanting a single *Om* out loud. It clears your mind of distractions with its simple vibration.

> If you're looking for a short and simple meditation to clear your mind, try chanting a single *Om* out loud.

Om is a common single-syllable mantra, or *bija* (seed) mantra. *Bija* mantras are thought to contain creative power and primordial energy, as a seed contains a tree. The *Om* syllable in Sanskrit is known as *aum* or *praṇava*, or "humming," a derivative of *pranu*, "to reverberate." The vibration seeks to cover the entire spectrum of human sound. You can do this before a yoga session. Try one or up to three *Oms* back-to-back, taking a breath in between. It is also a great way to bookend your practice so that you can transition both in and out of your yoga sequence.

Table 9.11   *Om* Meditation

1. Start in a comfortable seated or standing position.
2. Begin to notice your breath. Breathe in smoothly and steadily 5 times.
3. Inhale deeply through your nostrils.
4. On the exhale, chant the sound of the 4 parts of the **Om** mantra:
   - **a ("ah")** Open your mouth wide to start the sound at the back of the mouth and direct the stream of air toward the point between your eyebrows.
   - **u ("ooh")** The sound and breath should start to resonate through your mouth, throat, and chest and through your entire body.
   - **m ("mm")** Place the tip of your tongue on the roof of your mouth as you come to the end of your exhalation.
   - **ṁ ("mm" [nasal sound])** This is *Anusvara*, which means "aftersound."
5. Inhale and exhale.
6. Stop here, or repeat for 2 more times.
7. When you're ready, bring your attention back to your body and breath. Move your fingers and toes to bring your mind back to your body. Open your eyes.

Sending and Receiving (Tonglen) *Meditation*

Sending and receiving meditation, or *Tonglen*, is a form of Tibetan meditation. It is used to develop compassion and openness. It may be helpful if you're feeling stuck and want to feel more open, kind, and understanding toward yourself and others in your life.

Table 9.12   Sending and Receiving Meditation

1.	Sit in a comfortable position. You can keep your eyes gently open, looking forward or at a point on the ground in front of you.
2.	Start to notice your breath. Observe the natural rhythms of inhalation and exhalation.
3.	**Imagine with each inhalation, you inhale hot, heavy air.** You can imagine inhaling air that is the color of coffee.
4.	**Imagine as you exhale, you exhale cool, light air.** You can imagine exhaling air the color of ocean water.
5.	Find a situation in your life where you feel suffering—whether it is within yourself or another person you know is suffering. On the inhalation, imagine inhaling that suffering like a dark cloud. Let it dissolve and disappear in your heart. Then, exhale and send that person your cool, light breath.
6.	Continue for as little as 1 minute and up to 30 minutes or more. You can start with 2 to 3 minutes and gradually work up to 10 to 15 minutes.

Ego Eradicator

Ego Eradicator is a form of Kundalini meditation that boosts self-confidence and energy. Do it in the morning for 1 to 2 minutes. You can work toward longer periods of this meditation, but do not go beyond 9 minutes a day. Try this meditation before you have a big presentation, public speaking event, or important meeting. The meditation is very stimulating and energizing, so do it in the morning or midday. This exercise involves a rapid and intense breathing, called Breath of Fire (page 98), so don't do this meditation if you are pregnant or have such medical issues as asthma or other respiratory problems, high blood pressure, or anxiety or panic attacks.

Table 9.13   Ego Eradicator Meditation

1.	Start in a comfortable seated position.
2.	Sit with your spine tall, and make sure your neck and shoulders are relaxed.
3.	**Raise and straighten your arms** so they are positioned like the hands of a clock at 10 o'clock and 2 o'clock, both at 60 degrees from the ground. Your heart should be at the center of the clock.
4.	**Curl your fingers inward,** toward your palm, so your hands are in a thumbs-up position. Point your thumbs upward, as if plugging them into the sky.
5.	Close your eyes and take 4 or 5 slow, deep breaths to relax and tune into your breath and body.
6.	**Start Breath of Fire** using short, rapid exhalations from your nose (it will sound as if you're clearing your nose or panting), about 1 to 3 per second at a pace comfortable to you. Your abdomen should be drawn in with each exhalation. Inhalations should be passive and effortless in between each exhalation.
7.	If there is any pain or difficulty breathing with this exercise, stop immediately.
8.	As a beginner, start with 1 to 2 minutes of this exercise and, with experience, continue to extend the time to up to 9 minutes a day. Do not go beyond 9 minutes.
9.	At the end, open your hands and spread out your fingers actively. Inhale slowly as your bring your arms together overhead, thumbs touching. Exhale and relax your arms by your side.

Combining Meditation and Hand Mudras

Hand mudras (see Chapter 8) can be combined with mantra meditation in a simple and useful way. You can use mudras to enhance attention and focus during meditation. Here are two easy ways to combine mudra with meditation.

Pressure Mudra Meditation. The first way to combine mudra and meditation is simply to notice the pressure between your fingertips and hands in mudras. This method brings your attention to your hands as a focal point during meditation.

Table 9.14   Pressure Mudra Meditation

1.	Sit in a comfortable position.
2.	Figure out your intention: Is your intention to feel more relaxed? Grounded? Compassionate? Energetic?
3.	**Pick a mudra that fits your current intention.** For example, if you are feeling distracted and want to feel more settled, try Connected Mind Mudra. If you are feeling vulnerable and want to feel more reassured, try Heart Embrace Mudra. If you are feeling drained and would like more energy, try Life Mudra in both hands.
4.	Form the mudra with your hands.
5.	Close your eyes, and focus on your intention.
6.	Inhale and exhale deeply through your nose for 2 to 3 cycles using a breathing technique; for example, Victorious Breath or rhythmic breathing.
7.	**Notice where your fingers touch** and where your hands feel pressure.
8.	**Press firmly** and steadily in your mudra and focus on these points of pressure between your hands and fingers.
9.	Continue to **press hard enough that you feel heat building** between your fingertips, but nothing should be painful.
10.	Once you finish 10 full cycles of breath with this steady pressure of your mudra, release the mudra. Let your hands be separate and relaxed, and allow your breath to return to normal.

Pulsing Pressure Mudra Meditation. The second way is to pulse the pressure of your fingertips with the breath cycle. This simple exercise coordinates your breath with fingertip pressure.

Table 9.15   Pulsing Pressure Mudra Meditation

1.	Sit in a comfortable position.
2.	Figure out your intention: Is your intention to feel calmer? More open? Collected? Clear-minded?
3.	Pick a mudra that fits your current intention. For example, if you are feeling disconnected, try Wisdom Mudra with both hands. If you are facing challenges and would like to persevere, try Overcoming Mudra.
4.	**Form the mudra** with your hands.
5.	Close your eyes, and focus on your intention.
6.	Inhale and exhale deeply through your nose for 2 to 3 cycles using a breathing technique; for example, Victorious Breath or rhythmic breathing.
7.	Notice where your fingers touch and where your hands feel pressure.
8.	**Press firmly enough to build heat** between the fingertips.
9.	Now, **pulse your fingertips** by pressing your fingertips when you inhale, and releasing slightly as you exhale. Keep your fingertips touching when released.
10.	Continue to **press firmly during inhalation, and release gently during exhalation** for 10 breath cycles.
11.	Then, reverse the pattern for 10 breath cycles: Press your fingers firmly together during exhalation, and release during inhalation.
12.	When you are finished, relax and separate your hands, and let your breath return to normal.

✦

In our experience, some people are naturally drawn to certain types of meditation and it's easier for some than others. There isn't a right or wrong form of meditation. If you don't like a certain meditation, perhaps try it at another time to see whether it feels different. Or move on to a different form. Or even take a break from meditation altogether, and come back to it later when you're ready. Maybe you discover that your favorite and only form of meditation is simply paying attention to your breath, so stick with that.

I often troubleshoot over months with people to help them figure out the type of meditation that fits into their life and personality—and some people find that they just can't stick with meditation, no matter what kind. And that's all okay. As you read about in our own personal stories in Chapter 1, we each prefer different parts of yoga and choose to practice it differently. So, don't be discouraged if meditation doesn't seem to have the immediate effects you were hoping for or even if it doesn't have a place in your life now. It's all part of the process of figuring out what kind of practice you want to build for yourself.

CHAPTER 10

Putting It All Together: Our 8-Week Yoga Program

Yoga is 99% practice and 1% theory.

SRI K. PATTABHI JOIS

The following 8-week yoga program integrates yoga poses, breathing techniques, and meditation into a gradually progressive practice. As you'll see, we developed a particular *sequence* of poses for each week and organized them around themes, such as grounding, compassion, and strength.

Consistency is the key to the practice of yoga and its benefits. Self-compassion and awareness are its foundation. Stay aware of what the poses feel like, stop or adjust if you feel pain, and most of all, be kind to yourself as you learn. This isn't a contest, and we urge you not to judge yourself about what you can and can't do.

General Structure of Yoga Pose Sequence

There are many ways to do yoga poses, including a few poses at a time. You can also build your own sequences. Here is one approach to the basic structure of a yoga sequence.

1. **Integration.** Start with an *integration pose*. Observe your mind and body and pay attention to your breath in this pose. Integration is enhancing the connection and awareness of your mind, body, and breath. During this starting pose, form an intention, such as the goal to feel more grounded or to dedicate your practice to someone that you care about.

2. **Warm up.** Warming up the body is important to increase blood flow throughout the body and stretch the muscles and joints gradually, so as to prevent injury and ease your body into more intense poses. Sun Salutation A and B series are set ways to warm up the body.

3. **Standing poses.** The purpose of the standing poses section is to build heat and energy in your core muscles as well as strength and flexibility. Energy is at a peak during this section.

4. **Twisting poses.** Twists generate a lot of core heat in the body.

5. **Balance poses.** Balance poses improve concentration and confidence as well as proprioception. These poses are not aimed toward perfection, but embody the principle of letting go of perfection and self-judgment in yoga.

6. **Backbend poses.** Backbends are safer when your spine and body is already warmed up, since they require flexibility in your thoracic spine and shoulders.

7. **Hip opener poses.** Hip openers stretch your hip and pelvic muscles and release energy and tension in your body.

8. **Cool-down.** This section gradually winds down the energy in your body and mind. Cool-down poses include inversions or reclining poses.

9. **Final resting pose.** The last pose is typically Corpse Pose. Breath returns to normal in this pose as your body and mind experience deep relaxation.

Table 10.1 Order of Yoga Pose Sequence

General Order	Purpose	Examples
Integration Pose	Connect with breath, increase body awareness, form intention	Seated pose with mindful breathing Child's Pose Standing Forward Bend
Warm-up	Warm up the body (spine, joints, and muscles) to increase blood flow and decrease risk of injury or strain	Downward Facing Dog Pose High Plank Pose Sun Salutation A series Sun Salutation B series
Standing Poses	Build heat, strength, and flexibility in the body	Warrior I Pose Warrior II Pose Extended Triangle Pose Extended Side Angle Pose
Twisting Poses	Detoxify and energize core muscles	Revolved Lunge Pose Revolved Fierce Pose
Balance Poses	Create focus and improve balance and confidence	Tree Pose Half Moon Pose
Backbend Poses	Stretch chest, thoracic spine, and shoulders	Camel Pose Bridge Pose
Hip Opener Poses	Release hip and pelvic muscles	Half Pigeon Pose Bound Angle Pose
Cool-Down	Gradually wind down the pace and body temperature to relax the body	Reclining Spinal Twist Supported Bridge Pose Inversion: Legs up the Wall Pose
Resting	Full relaxation of body and mind	Corpse Pose

Table 10.2 Our 8-Week Yoga Program

Yoga Component	Week 1	Week 2	Week 3	Week 4	Week 5	Week 6	Week 7	Week 8
Theme	*Grounding*	*Compassion*	*Strength*	*Energy*	*Resilience*	*Balance*	*Stress Relief*	*Gratitude*
Starting Pose	Mountain Pose	Child's Pose	Easy or Hero Pose	Easy or Hero Pose	Child's Pose	Hero Pose	Child's Pose	Supported Fish Pose
Warm-up	Child's Pose	Mountain Pose	Mountain Pose	Downward Facing Dog Pose	Sun Salutation A modified x 2	Sun Salutation A modified x 2	Thread the Needle Pose	Sun Salutation A modified x 2
	Tabletop, Cat, and Cow Poses	Sidebending Mountain Pose	Sun Salutation A modified x 2	High Plank Pose	Sun Salutation A x 2	Sun Salutation A x 2	Standing Forward Bend	Sun Salutation A x 2
	Sun Salutation A modified x 3	Sun Salutation A modified x 3	Sun Salutation A x 2	Sun Salutation B x 2	Dolphin	Sun Salutation B x 1	Sun Salutation A modified x 3	Standing Forward Bend
Standing Sequence	Low Lunge Pose	Warrior I Pose	Warrior I Pose	Warrior II Pose, Reverse Warrior	Warrior II Pose, Reverse Warrior	High Lunge Pose	Low Lunge Pose	Low Lunge Pose
	Pyramid Pose	Warrior II Pose	Warrior II Pose	Extended Side Angle Pose	Revolved Lunge	Warrior II Pose	Wide-Legged Forward Bend	Extended Side Angle Pose
	Standing Forward Bend	Reverse Warrior Pose	Fierce (Chair) Pose	Extended Triangle Pose	Revolved Fierce (Chair) Pose	Extended Triangle Pose	Big Toe Pose	Pyramid Pose
Balance	Supported Warrior III Pose	Tree Pose	Side Plank Pose	Supported Warrior III Pose	Eagle Pose	Tree Pose	Goddess Pose with breath	Half Moon Pose

Table 10.2   Our 8-Week Yoga Program (*continued*)

Yoga Component	Week 1	Week 2	Week 3	Week 4	Week 5	Week 6	Week 7	Week 8
Backbend	Warrior III Pose	Supported Bridge Pose	Camel Pose	Warrior III Pose	Crocodile or Locust Pose	Locust, Bow Poses	Reverse Tabletop Pose with Lion's Breath	Camel Pose
Hip Opener	Yogi Squat	Reclining Bound Angle Pose	Goddess Pose with "ha" breath	Lizard Pose	Wide-Legged Forward Bend Pose	Reclining Pigeon Pose	Half Pigeon Pose	Half Pigeon Pose
Cool-Down	Reclining Hand to Big Toe Pose	Reclining Spinal Twist	Supported Shoulder Stand	Seated Spinal Twist	Bridge or Supported Bridge Pose	Seated Head to Knee Forward Bend	Crocodile Pose	Reclining Spinal Twist Pose
	Staff Pose	Happy Baby Pose	Fish Pose	Staff Pose, Seated Forward Bend	Reclining Spinal Twist	Seated Forward Bend	Bridge Pose	Knee to Chest Pose
Resting Pose	Corpse Pose	Corpse Pose	Corpse Pose	Legs up the Wall or Corpse Pose	Corpse Pose	Corpse Pose	Legs up the Wall or Corpse Pose	Supported Fish or Corpse Pose
Breathing Exercise	Breath Awareness, Victorious Breath	Victorious Breath, Even Rhythmic Breathing Beginner Level 1	Even Rhythmic Breathing Beginner Level 2 and 3	Lion's Breath, Even Rhythmic Breathing Beginner Level 4	Rhythmic Breathing Beginner Level 5	Alternate Nostril Breath, Rhythmic Breathing Intermediate Level 1	Lion's Breath, Victorious Breath, Left Nostril Breath	Humming Bee Breath, Rhythmic Breathing Intermediate Level 2
Meditation (*Beginner: 5 to 10 minutes Intermediate and up: 15 to 30 minutes*)	Breath Meditation	Mindfulness Body and Sound Meditation	Mindful Walking	Gazing Candle Meditation	Compassion Meditation, Sending and Receiving Meditation	Mantra Meditation	Body Scan Meditation	Visualization Meditation

Our 8-Week Yoga Program

Our program provides eight yoga pose sequences along with breathing and meditation exercises based on weekly themes. Although we recommend that you do our 45 minutes of poses and 15 minutes of breathing and meditation two to three times a week, explore what frequency feels right for you. On the other days of the week, we recommend doing 10 to 15 minutes of breathing or meditation.

Week 1: Grounding

Week 1 focuses on being grounded and aware.

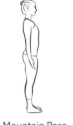

Mountain Pose

Yoga pose sequence:

1. Start in Mountain Pose for 5 breaths to integrate your body, mind, and breath. Feel grounded to the earth, rooting through all corners of your feet.
2. Start in Tabletop. Inhale to Cow Pose and exhale to Cat Pose, alternating for 5 rounds.
3. Next, learn Sun Salutation A and practice for 3 rounds.

Tabletop Pose

Sun Salutation A (Surya Namaskar A)

Sun Salutation sequence is a foundational warm-up sequence in yoga and has many variations. It is an ancient tradition. Start with the more supported version to warm up your body. To warm up your spine, it is generally safer to do the modified version for one to two rounds, since it has a gentler backbend of Baby Cobra or Cobra Pose, before progressing to the full Sun Salutation A version with Upward Facing Dog Pose (Week 3).

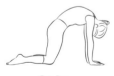

Cat Pose

Sun Salutation A Modified

1. Stand in Mountain Pose.
2. Inhale and lift your hands toward the sky in Upward Salute.
3. Exhale to bend forward to Standing Forward Bend.
4. Inhale to Standing Half Forward Bend.

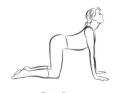

Cow Pose

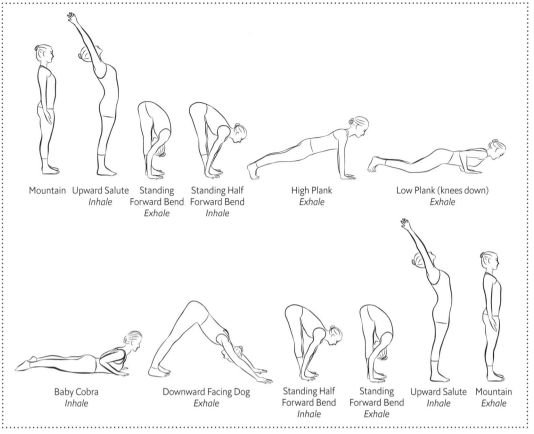

Mountain | Upward Salute *Inhale* | Standing Forward Bend *Exhale* | Standing Half Forward Bend *Inhale* | High Plank *Exhale* | Low Plank (knees down) *Exhale*

Baby Cobra *Inhale* | Downward Facing Dog *Exhale* | Standing Half Forward Bend *Inhale* | Standing Forward Bend *Exhale* | Upward Salute *Inhale* | Mountain *Exhale*

Figure 10.1   Sun Salutation A Modified

5. Exhale as you step back one foot at a time to High Plank Pose. Bring your knees down to the floor and lower to Low Plank Pose.
6. Inhale to Baby Cobra (or Cobra) Pose.
7. Exhale and press back to Downward Facing Dog Pose.
8. Inhale as you step both feet forward to Standing Half Forward Bend.
9. Exhale to fold forward to Standing Forward Bend.
10. Inhale as your hands rise to Upward Salute.
11. Exhale as you press your hands together in front of your chest and return to Mountain Pose.
12. Repeat for 3 cycles.

4. Continue to heat your body by doing Low Lunge and Pyramid Pose on both sides (5 breaths each side per pose).
5. Take a break in Standing Forward Bend (10 breaths).

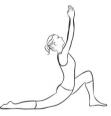

Low Lunge Pose

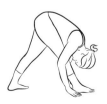

Pyramid Pose

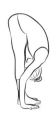

Standing Forward Bend

6. Balance with blocks in Supported Warrior III Pose for 5 breaths on both sides. If this feels comfortable, try balance in Warrior III without blocks on both sides.

7. Stretch your hips in Yogi Squat (10 breaths) with or without blocks.

8. Use a strap to get a better sense of your range of motion by doing Reclining Hand to Big Toe Pose on both sides. If able to lift your legs toward your chest to 90 degrees or closer, then you are able to sit safely in Staff Pose without straining your lower back. If not, stay in Reclining Hand to Big Toe with a strap (10 breaths).

9. Rest in Corpse Pose (3 to 5 minutes).

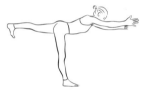

Supported Warrior III Pose

Breathing exercise: Breath Awareness (page 87), Victorious Breath (page 93)

Meditation: Breath Meditation (page 241)

Self-reflection journaling exercise: Write about why you want to do yoga. If you are new to yoga, what makes you interested in yoga? If you're someone who has done yoga for a while, think back to when you first started. Have your reasons for doing yoga evolved, and, if so, how?

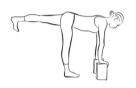

Warrior III Pose

Yogi Squat

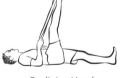

Reclining Hand to Big Toe Pose

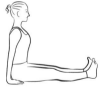

Staff Pose

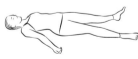

Corpse Pose

Week 2: Compassion

Week 2 focuses on self-compassion and kindness toward others.

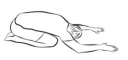

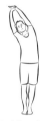
Child's Pose

Yoga pose sequence:

1. Start in Child's Pose (5 breaths).
2. Stand in Mountain Pose and stretch your sides in Sidebending Mountain Pose (5 breaths) on both sides.
3. Do Sun Salutation (modified version) for 3 rounds.
4. With your right foot forward, do Warrior I Pose (5 breaths). Exhale as you expand your arms to Warrior II Pose and adjust your feet. Inhale to stretch your side body in Reverse Warrior Pose. Exhale and return to Warrior II. Switch legs and repeat.
5. Focus on balance in Tree Pose (5 breaths each side).
6. Use a block to do Supported Bridge Pose (10 breaths) for a gentle backbend.
7. Relax your hips in Reclining Bound Angle Pose (10 breaths), using blocks under your knees.
8. Cool down with Reclining Spinal Twist and Happy Baby Pose (5 breaths).
9. Relax in Corpse Pose (5 breaths).

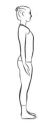
Mountain Pose

Breathing exercise: Victorious Breath (page 93), Even Rhythmic Breathing Beginner Level 1 (page 91)

Meditation: Mindfulness Body and Sound Meditation (page 242)

Self-reflection journaling exercise: What do you consider your weaknesses or imperfections? Write a letter to yourself from the point of view of a compassionate friend.

Sidebending Mountain Pose

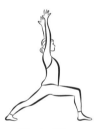
Warrior I Pose

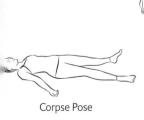
Corpse Pose

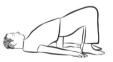
Reclining Spinal Twist

Supported Bridge Pose

Happy Baby Pose

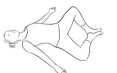
Reclining Bound Angle Pose

Tree Pose

Warrior II Pose

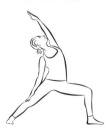
Reverse Warrior Pose

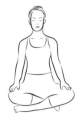

Easy Pose

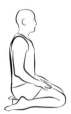

Hero Pose

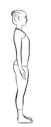

Mountain Pose

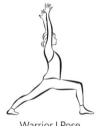

Warrior I Pose

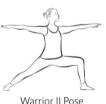

Warrior II Pose

Week 3: Strength

This week focuses on building strength and courage.

Yoga pose sequence:

1. Sit in Easy or Hero Pose (10 breaths) to connect to your breath.
2. Stand in Mountain Pose and warm up your body in Sun Salutation (modified version) for 2 rounds.
3. Next, do the full version of Sun Salutation A for 2 rounds.

Sun Salutation A

1. Stand in Mountain Pose.
2. Inhale and lift your hands toward the sky in Upward Salute.
3. Exhale to bend forward to Standing Forward Bend.
4. Inhale to Standing Half Forward Bend.
5. Exhale as you step back one foot at a time to High Plank Pose and lower to Low Plank Pose, bringing your knees down to the floor.
6. Inhale to Cobra or Upward Facing Dog Pose.
7. Exhale and press back to Downward Facing Dog Pose.
8. Inhale as you walk your feet (or step) forward between your hands to Standing Half Forward Bend.
9. Exhale to fold forward to Standing Forward Bend.
10. Inhale as your hands rise to Upward Salute.
11. Exhale as you press your hands together in front of your chest and return to Mountain Pose.
12. Repeat for 2 rounds.

A more vigorous version of Sun Salutation A for more advanced practitioners skips High Plank, and you jump back from Standing Half Forward Bend directly to Low Plank. It is important not to jump back to High Plank since this puts unsafe pressure onto your shoulder joints.

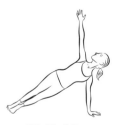

Fierce Pose

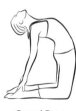

Side Plank Pose

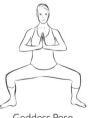

Camel Pose

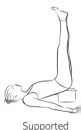

Goddess Pose

Supported
Shoulder Stand

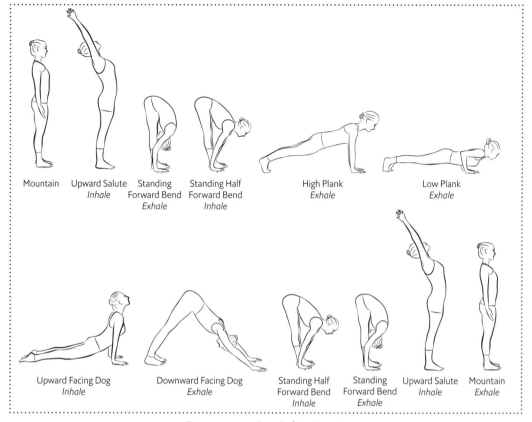

Figure 10.2   Sun Salutation A

4. With your right foot forward, do Warrior I Pose (5 breaths). Exhale to Warrior II Pose (5 breaths). Switch legs and repeat.

5. Build heat in Fierce (Chair) Pose (5 breaths).

6. Do Side Plank Pose (5 breaths each side).

7. Do Camel Pose against the wall or modified with blocks (5 breaths).

8. Stretch your hips in Goddess Pose with "ha" breath (5 breaths) to bring in positive strength.

9. Cool down with Supported Shoulder Stand with a block under your sacrum and Fish (or Supported Fish) Pose (10 breaths).

10. Relax in Corpse Pose (3 to 5 minutes).

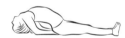

Fish Pose

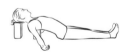

Supported Fish Pose

Breathing exercise: Even Rhythmic Breathing Beginner Levels 2 and 3 (page 91)

Meditation: Mindful Walking (page 243)

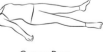

Corpse Pose

Self-reflection journaling exercise: What do you consider your three greatest strengths? When have you been courageous, and how did it feel?

Week 4: Energy

Week 4 energizes the body and mind.

Yoga pose sequence:

1. Sit in Easy or Hero Pose to become aware of your breath for 10 breaths.
2. Step back to Downward Facing Dog Pose. Build core heat and energy by alternating between Downward Facing Dog and High Plank Pose five times, staying in each pose for 5 Victorious Breaths.
3. Do Sun Salutation B for 2 rounds.

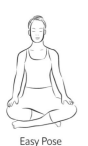

Easy Pose

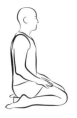

Hero Pose

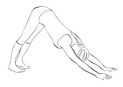

Downward Facing
Dog Pose

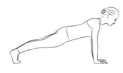

High Plank Pose

Sun Salutation B (Surya Namaskar B)

1. Stand in Mountain Pose.
2. Inhale and lift your hands toward the sky in Fierce (Chair) Pose.
3. Exhale to bend forward to Standing Forward Bend.
4. Inhale to Standing Half Forward Bend.
5. Exhale as you step back one foot at a time to High Plank Pose and lower to Low Plank Pose. Inhale to Cobra or Upward Facing Dog Pose.
6. Exhale and press back to Downward Facing Dog.
7. Step your right foot forward to Warrior I Pose and inhale.
8. Exhale as you place your hands on the ground to frame your front foot. Step back to High Plank and lower through Low Plank. Inhale to Cobra or Upward Facing Dog Pose.
9. Exhale and press back to Downward Facing Dog.
10. Step your left foot forward to Warrior I Pose and inhale.
11. Exhale as you place your hands on the ground to frame your front foot. Step back to High Plank and lower through Low Plank. Inhale to Cobra or Upward Facing Dog.
12. Exhale and press back to Downward Facing Dog.
13. Walk, step, or lightly jump your feet to the top of your mat for Standing Half Forward Bend.
14. Exhale to fold forward to Standing Forward Bend.
15. Inhale as your hands rise to Fierce (Chair) Pose.
16. Exhale as you press your hands together in front of your chest and return to Mountain Pose.
17. Repeat for 2 rounds.

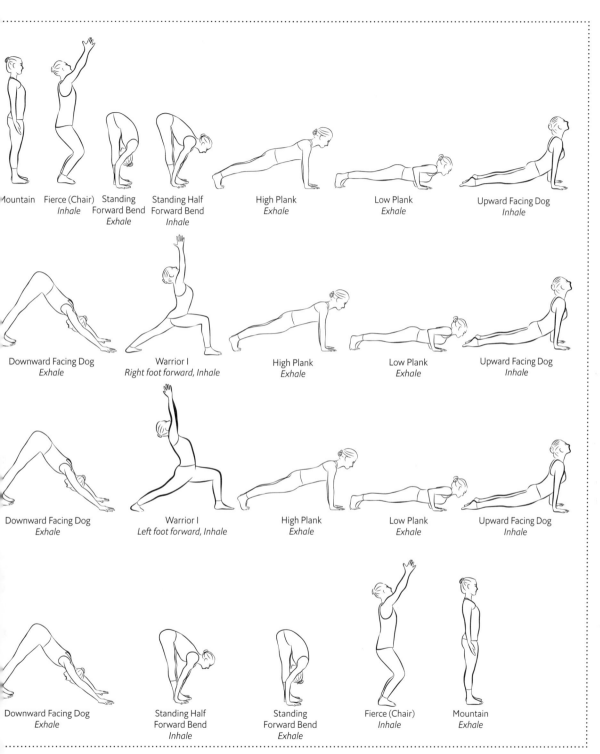

Mountain

Fierce (Chair)
Inhale

Standing
Forward Bend
Exhale

Standing Half
Forward Bend
Inhale

High Plank
Exhale

Low Plank
Exhale

Upward Facing Dog
Inhale

Downward Facing Dog
Exhale

Warrior I
Right foot forward, Inhale

High Plank
Exhale

Low Plank
Exhale

Upward Facing Dog
Inhale

Downward Facing Dog
Exhale

Warrior I
Left foot forward, Inhale

High Plank
Exhale

Low Plank
Exhale

Upward Facing Dog
Inhale

Downward Facing Dog
Exhale

Standing Half
Forward Bend
Inhale

Standing
Forward Bend
Exhale

Fierce (Chair)
Inhale

Mountain
Exhale

Figure 10.3   Sun Salutation B

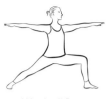

Warrior II Pose

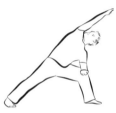

Reverse Warrior Pose

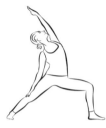

Extended Side Angle
Pose (Supported)

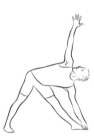

Extended Triangle Pose

4. Do Warrior II (5 breaths), inhale to Reverse Warrior, and move to Extended Side Angle (5 breaths) and then Extended Triangle Pose (5 breaths). Switch legs and repeat on the other side.

5. Practice balance with Supported Warrior III (5 breaths) and Warrior III Poses (5 breaths) on both sides.

6. Do Bridge Pose (5 breaths) and then stretch your hips with Lizard Pose (10 breaths) on both sides.

7. Cool down with Seated Spinal Twist on both sides, Staff Pose (5 breaths), and Seated Forward Bend (5 breaths).

8. Rest in Legs up the Wall or Corpse Pose (3 to 5 minutes).

Breathing exercise: Lion's Breath page 96), Even Rhythmic Breathing Beginner Level 4 (page 91)

Meditation: Gazing Candle Meditation (page 244)

Self-reflection journaling exercise: What activities give you more energy? Who are the people in your life who make you feel more energized after you spend time with them?

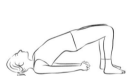

Warrior III Pose

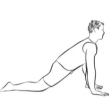

Bridge Pose

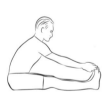

Lizard Pose

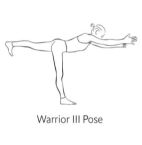

Seated Spinal Twist

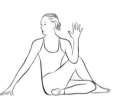

Staff Pose

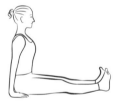

Seated Forward Bend

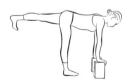

Supported Warrior III Pose

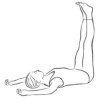

Legs up the Wall Pose

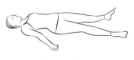

Corpse Pose

Week 5: Resilience

You're halfway through! Week 5 focuses on resilience and flexibility.

Child's Pose

Yoga pose sequence:

1. Start in Child's Pose to connect to your breath, body, and mind.
2. Do Sun Salutation A (modified version) for 2 rounds.
3. Do Dolphin Pose to build heat.
4. Exhale to Warrior II Pose and inhale to Reverse Warrior Pose, and alternate with breath between them for 3 rounds to create flexibility in the side body. Then do Revolved Lunge with the option to keep your knee up or down. Switch legs and repeat.
5. Do Revolved Fierce (Chair) Pose (5 breaths) on both sides.
6. Do Eagle Pose on both sides (5 breaths each side) for balance.
7. Lie prone to do Crocodile or Locust Pose (5 breaths).
8. Cool down with Wide-Legged Forward Bend (10 breaths), Bridge or Supported Bridge Pose (10 breaths), and Reclining Spinal Twist (5 breaths each side).
9. Rest in Corpse Pose (10 breaths).

Dolphin Pose

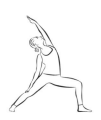

Warrior II Pose

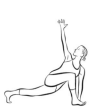

Reverse Warrior Pose

Breathing exercise: Rhythmic Breathing Beginner Level 5 (page 91)

Meditation: Loving Kindness Meditation (page 244)

Self-reflection journaling exercise: When was a time that you felt that you were frustrated or were up against a challenge but were able to overcome it? What things—perhaps people or your personal characteristics—allowed you to be resilient?

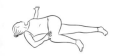
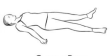

Reclining Spinal Twist

Corpse Pose

Wide-Legged Forward Bend

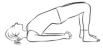

Bridge Pose

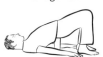

Supported Bridge Pose

Crocodile Pose

Locust Pose

Eagle Pose

Revolved Lunge modification

Revolved Fierce Pose

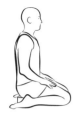

Hero Pose

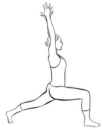

High Lunge Pose

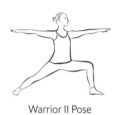

Warrior II Pose

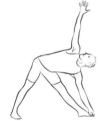

Extended Triangle Pose

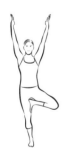

Tree Pose

Week 6: Balance

Week 6 explores how to achieve more physical and mental balance.

Yoga pose sequence:

1. Sit in Hero Pose (10 breaths) to connect with your breath, body, and mind.
2. Do Sun Salutation A modified twice, Sun Salutation A twice, and Sun Salutation B once.
3. With your right foot forward, balance in High Lunge Pose (5 breaths). Exhale to Warrior II Pose, bringing your back heel down and adjusting your feet. Inhale as you straighten your front knee and reach your right hand forward for Extended Triangle Pose. Switch legs, and repeat on the other side.
4. Balance in Tree Pose for 5 breaths each side.
5. Do Locust Pose (5 breaths) to warm up your spine, and then do Bow Pose.
6. Do Reclining Pigeon Pose (10 breaths on each side) to release your hips.
7. Cool down in Seated Head to Knee Pose (5 breaths each side) and then Seated Forward Bend (10 breaths).
8. Rest in Corpse Pose (3 to 5 minutes).

Breathing exercise: Alternate Nostril Breath (5 minutes), Rhythmic Breathing Intermediate Level 1 (5 minutes)

Meditation: Sa-Ta-Na-Ma Mantra Meditation (page 246)

Self-reflection journaling exercise: What areas of your life do you wish ha more balance? What are three things that nurture balance that you can do?

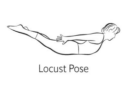

Locust Pose

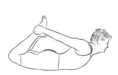

Bow Pose

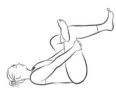

Reclining Pigeon on your back

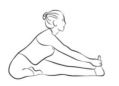

Seated Head to Knee Pose

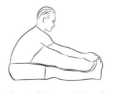

Seated Forward Bend

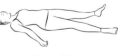

Corpse Pose

Week 7: Stress Relief

Week 7 focuses on stress relief and relaxation.

Yoga pose sequence:

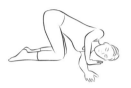

Child's Pose

1. Start in Child's Pose (10 breaths), rocking your forehead left and right to release tension in your forehead.
2. Release neck and shoulder tension in Thread the Needle Pose (5 breaths each side).
3. Relax your neck and shoulders in Ragdoll version of Standing Forward Bend (10 breaths).
4. Do Sun Salutation A (modified version) for 3 rounds.
5. Release your hips in Low Lunge Pose (5 breaths each side).
6. Relax your neck in Wide-Legged Forward Bend (10 breaths).
7. Stand in Big Toe Pose (10 breaths).
8. Do Goddess Pose with 5 rounds of releasing "ha" breath.
9. Exhale in Lion's Breath in Reverse Tabletop Pose 3 times.
10. Do Half Pigeon Pose (10 breaths each side), then Crocodile Pose (10 breaths).
11. Cool down in Bridge Pose (5 breaths).
12. Release all tension and rest in Legs up the Wall or Corpse Pose (3 to 5 minutes).

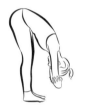

Thread the Needle Pose

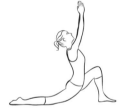

Standing Forward Bend
Ragdoll variation

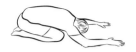

Low Lunge Pose

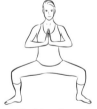

Goddess Pose

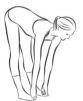

Big Toe Pose

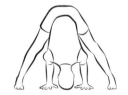

Wide-Legged Forward Bend

Breathing exercise: Lion's Breath (page 96), Victorious Breath (page 93), Left Nostril Breath (page 94)

Meditation: Body Scan (page 247)

Self-reflection journaling exercise: Can you think of or imagine a place where you feel most calm and relaxed? What does it look like; what are the details, textures, smells, or sounds of the place that feels calming?

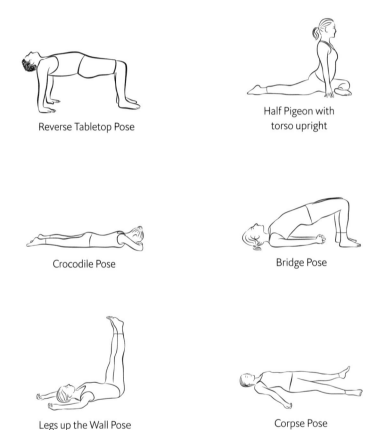

Reverse Tabletop Pose

Half Pigeon with torso upright

Crocodile Pose

Bridge Pose

Legs up the Wall Pose

Corpse Pose

Week 8: Gratitude

Week 8 promotes a sense of gratitude and acceptance.

Yoga pose sequence:

1. Start in Supported Fish Pose (10 breaths) to expand your chest.
2. Do Sun Salutation A (modified version) for 2 rounds.
3. Do Sun Salutation A for 2 rounds.
4. Rest and explore the feeling of gratitude in Standing Forward Bend (10 breaths).
5. Do Low Lunge Pose (5 breaths each side).
6. Reach actively in Extended Side Angle Pose (5 breaths each side).
7. Release your neck and stretch your hamstrings in Pyramid Pose (10 breaths each side).
8. Feel expansion and openness of your heart in Half Moon Pose (5 breaths each side).
9. Feel your chest broaden in Camel Pose (5 breaths).
10. Do Half Pigeon Pose (10 breaths each side).
11. Cool down in Reclining Spinal Twist (5 breaths each side), and Knee to Chest Pose (10 breaths).
12. Rest in Supported Fish or Corpse Pose (3 to 5 minutes).

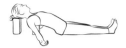

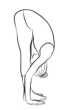

Supported Fish Pose

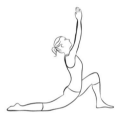

Standing Forward Bend

Low Lunge Pose

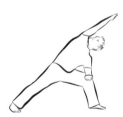

Extended Side Angle
Pose (Supported)

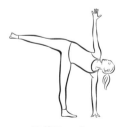

Half Moon Pose

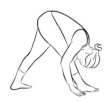

Pyramid Pose

Breathing exercise: Humming Bee Breath (page 94), Rhythmic Breathing Intermediate Level 2 (page 91)

Meditation: Guided Imagery Meditation (page 248)

Self-reflection journaling exercise: What are five things that you are grateful for? Who are five people that you are grateful for having in your life?

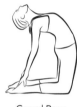

Camel Pose

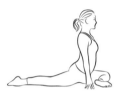

Half Pigeon with
torso upright

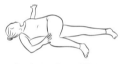

Reclining Spinal Twist

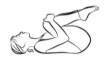

Knee to Chest Pose

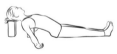

Supported Fish Pose

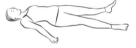

Corpse Pose

Beyond Our 8-Week Program

You may find that you start the program for a few weeks and get interrupted by normal everyday life. Or it might be too hectic to do meditation or breathing exercises every day. Our program is not intended to be rigid. It aims to give you a sample template to build your own yoga practice within your own time and to do so within the limitations of your schedule. Our program offers basic building blocks and tools to start your home practice. We encourage you to explore different yoga classes and styles as well, where you can experience personalized attention to your alignment and adjustments.

There will inevitably be times when you stop doing yoga for any number of reasons. The great thing about yoga is that it will be there when you're ready, and no one is checking to see when the last time you did yoga was and judging you for it. We understand how hard it is to go back to or do the things that you know are good for you—even the things you enjoy—once you've gotten out of the habit. We have also heard from the people who say, "I stopped doing yoga, and it's so hard to go back, because I'm just not as good as I was before," or "I'm not good at yoga." Don't let those thoughts stop you from coming back to yoga when you want to. In our opinion, there is no such thing as "being good at" yoga—it is what we learn and how we grow when we do yoga.

Yoga is a path of continual growth and change. We hope that our book has nourished your compassion, inspiration, and curiosity so that you may continue with yoga beyond our program. We are very grateful to have been able to share this part of your journey with you.

✦

Namaste.

Yoga for Specific Health Conditions

Yoga research for specific health conditions has proliferated in the last decade. Yoga can help the health conditions listed here, but we still recommend checking with your doctor first before trying yoga. We have suggested a few breathing exercises, poses, and meditations to consider, but these are not exclusive. Most studies do not specify the exact poses or exercises that they used but most are a gentle form of yoga that integrates poses, breathing, and meditations. If you have an active or moderate to severe health condition, you should consider working with a specialized yoga therapist (see page 17 on how to find a yoga therapist) in coordination with your doctor to create a plan that is tailored to you.

Physical Conditions

Arthritis

For people who have arthritis, exercise is especially important to help maintain range of motion, joint stability, and muscle mass. Three out of four people with arthritis are not active enough because the pain and stiffness of arthritis can make it difficult to exercise.[1] Yoga helps preserve and improve joint mobility while reducing stress, pain, and fatigue. Poses strengthen gluteus, quadriceps, and hamstring muscles to better support your knees. One study of 75 people with rheumatoid arthritis (RA) or knee osteoarthritis found that eight weeks of yoga (two 60-minute classes and one home practice per week) improved physical fitness, walking, flexibility, and quality of life.[2]

Consider: Standing Poses (pages 137–149), Bridge Pose (page 183)

Precautions: Rheumatoid arthritis can weaken the ligaments of the upper cervical spine and erode joints, leading to neck instability, leading to a higher risk of neck injury at the ligaments at the occipitoatlantal (occiput-C1) and atlantoaxial (C1–C2) joints, which are at the base of the neck. Poses that involve significant neck rotation or put pressure on the neck, such as full Shoulder Stand (we only teach in Chapter 7 the supported version), and Plow and Headstand (which we did not include in this book due to the increased risk of injury when done unsupervised) should be avoided. Standing poses, such as Extended Side Angle Pose, in which your neck is traditionally rotated so that you can gaze upward, should be modified so that your neck is not significantly rotated or strained.

Asthma and Respiratory Issues

Breathing exercises can improve quality of life for asthma patients. Preliminary small studies suggest that yoga can help improve lung function and general quality of life in adults with asthma. Lung expiratory volume for people with asthma improved after a 4-week Iyengar program of poses and breathing exercises, but more noticeable differences likely require longer practice. About half of the thirteen randomized controlled trials on breathing exercises and asthma have reported improved lung function in people with asthma, but all the studies that measured quality of life found that quality of life improved.[3] There are three categories of breath training for asthma: (1) exercises that retrain the pattern of breathing, (2) exercises that strengthen respiratory muscles, and (3) exercises that increase flexibility of the rib cage and improve posture. The retraining breathing techniques have the most current evidence of reducing asthma attacks. Given the diverse number of breathing exercises used in the different studies, it is uncertain what types of breath exercises are helpful. However, many of the types of breathing exercises used by physiotherapists for people with asthma overlap with yoga breathing techniques, including breathing that focuses on the use of the abdomen rather than upper-chest muscles as well as slow, controlled, paced breathing that emphasizes nasal breathing rather than mouth breathing.

Yoga training has also been studied in people with chronic obstructive pulmonary disease (COPD), a group of progressive lung diseases that block airflow and make it difficult to breathe. Five studies assessing people with COPD have found that yoga improves lung function, including the volume of forced expiration in one second and distance covered in six minutes of walking.[4]

Consider: Breath Awareness (page 89), Three-Part Breath (page 89), Rhythmic Breathing (page 91)

Precautions: Yoga, like any other type of exercise, can trigger or worsen asthma symptoms. Make sure that you have your bronchodilator inhaler with you and consider using it fifteen minutes before starting yoga. If you have respiratory diseases, such as asthma or COPD, you should avoid rapid or forceful breathing exercises, which may trigger difficulty breathing.

Cancer Survivors

Mindfulness-based therapies can be helpful to reduce anxiety, depression, sleep issues, fatigue, and overall quality of life in cancer survivors. There is growing evidence that yoga can help manage treatment-related side effects, such as nausea and fatigue, in cancer survivors. Several randomized controlled trials for cancer survivors have found that yoga can improve physical fitness and reduce cancer-related fatigue, stress, and depression.

Cancer-related fatigue can affect over a third of cancer survivors, with much higher rates for those undergoing chemotherapy or radiation. There is no standard medical treatment for cancer-related fatigue even though it is a very common and debilitating symptom. Reviews of randomized controlled trials—mostly in women with breast cancer—have found that yoga can improve cancer-related fatigue, as well as improve psychological health and quality of life.[5] A small study found that yoga breathing techniques could help people going through chemotherapy by improving sleep, anxiety, and overall quality of life.[6] A small study found that children and adolescents ages ten to seventeen who completed cancer treatment also benefit from yoga, experiencing lower anxiety after six weeks of yoga.[7] One major source of suffering for people undergoing chemotherapy is the anticipation of the fear and nausea of later treatments. Relaxation techniques and meditations can be used to reduce this fear.

Consider: Working with specialized yoga therapists and clinicians to develop individualized yoga sequences, hospital-based yoga programs

Chronic Pain

Acute pain and chronic pain are different. Acute pain is sudden and signals a need to fight or flee, to struggle or run. Chronic pain by contrast is not an adaptive survival response but a nuisance, a defense gone wrong. It's like car alarms in your neighborhood going off late in the night, signifying not theft but inept parking— solitary, unheeded, insistent, and typically useless. Chronic pain is defined as pain lasting longer than three months.

Several studies have shown that yoga can significantly improve chronic back and neck pain as well as pain from rheumatoid arthritis and osteoarthritis. For people suffering from chronic lower back pain, yoga has been shown to improve back function and spinal flexibility. Although a single yoga session is unlikely to reduce the pain, more regular sessions can be helpful and a weeklong intensive program of yoga with postures, breathing practices, and meditation has been shown to reduce pain. There is also encouraging evidence that guided imagery can help.

Over time chronic pain can lead to fear of movement, a sense of helplessness, and rumination, which can cause people to avoid any therapies that involves physical movement. If physical poses create too much anxiety, then try other limbs of yoga that might feel more accessible, such as nidra sleep, meditation, or breathing practices.

Consider: Mountain Pose (page 114), Upward Salute (page 120), Wide-Legged Forward Bend (page 134), Standing Forward Bend (page 129), Downward Facing Dog Pose (page 123), Bound Angle Pose (page 188), Body Scan Meditation (page 247), Mindfulness Body and Sound Meditation (page 242)

Precautions: If you are taking sedating or pain medications, stay alert, keep track of your breathing, and limit how long you hold poses (on average, less than 10 breaths per pose) so as to avoid falling asleep during a pose, which can cause nerve damage.

Connective Tissue Disorders and Other Disorders with Neck Instability

Marfan syndrome and Ehlers-Danlos syndrome are rare connective tissue disorders that lead to hypermobility of the atlantoaxial (C1–C2) joint in the neck and other joints. If you have a connective tissue disorder, you should talk to your doctor first before doing yoga. Other medical conditions are associated with neck instability, such as Down syndrome, neurofibromatosis, skeletal dysplasias, and less common syndromes. People with such medical conditions should avoid poses that put significant pressure on the neck (e.g., Plow, Shoulder Stand, Headstand) unless permitted by their physician.

Epilepsy

Yoga is also being explored as an option to reduce the frequency and duration of seizures in adults with epilepsy that cannot be controlled with medications alone. Approximately 30 percent of epilepsy cannot be fully treated despite antiepileptic medications. A few small studies have shown that yoga may help people be seizure free for longer and to have less frequent and shorter seizures.[8] There are many types of seizure disorders and these can originate in different parts of the brain. More focused research is needed to see whether yoga helps particular types of seizure disorders.

Consider: Working with specialized yoga therapists and clinicians to develop individualized yoga sequences, hospital-based yoga programs

Fertility Treatment

Yoga can also help couples facing the stress of fertility issues and treatments. In the United States, about 7 to 15 percent of couples are affected by infertility. Dealing with infertility can be very stressful for both people in the relationship. Up to 40 percent of women participating in in vitro fertilization (IVF) experience anxiety and depression. One study found that six weeks of yoga improved anxiety, depression, and quality of life for women awaiting in vitro fertilization. In addition, mindfulness skills can reduce self-judgment and feelings of shame in women coping with infertility. A 10-week mindfulness course at two hours weekly helped reduce feelings of being defeated, trapped, or ashamed. Both yoga and mindfulness can be powerful tools to help women who are considering IVF treatment.

Consider: Restorative yoga, Mindfulness Body and Sound Meditation (page 242), Mindful Walking (page 243), Breath Awareness (page 87)

Glaucoma

Glaucoma is a medical condition of increased pressure inside the eye. It can lead to optic nerve damage, resulting in vision loss. Headstand doubles the pressure inside the eye, so people with recent or chronic glaucoma should avoid performing Headstand, Shoulder Stand, and Handstand poses. More gentle inversion poses, such as Legs up the Wall Pose, can replace full inversions but should be discussed first with your medical doctor.

Headaches and Migraines

Yoga is also being studied as a complementary therapy for different neurological disorders, including headaches and migraines.[9] Many studies show that mind-body therapies, such as yoga and meditation, can reduce the severity and frequency of headaches and migraines.

Consider: Victorious Breath (page 93), Downward Facing Dog Pose (page 122), Standing Forward Bend (page 129), Wide-Legged Forward Bend (page 134),

Reclining Bound Angle Pose (page 189), Seated Forward Bend (page 199), Legs up the Wall Pose (page 207), Corpse Pose (page 209), Breath Meditation (page 241), Visualization Meditation (page 248)

Menopause

More than 88 percent of women during menopause will experience hot flashes or night sweats, which are called vasomotor symptoms. During menopause, women can also experience pain during sex, sleep and mood difficulties, low energy, and difficulty concentrating.

Yoga seems to help alleviate symptoms of menopause better than do other forms of exercise. A study of 355 healthy women aged forty to sixty-two years compared yoga and exercise for menopause symptoms.[10] The yoga group participated in ninety minutes weekly of cooling breathing, poses, and guided meditation and twenty minutes daily at home. Women who did twelve weeks of yoga had overall improved quality of life, fewer hot flashes or flushing symptoms, and better sexual functioning, while exercise did not lead to any improvement. Other studies have found that yoga can help ease fatigue, insomnia, and pain related to menopause.

Consider: Hero Pose (page 111), Downward Facing Dog Pose (page 122), Standing Forward Bend (page 129), Staff Pose (page 198), Bound Angle Pose (page 188), Reclining Bound Angle Pose (page 189), Seated Forward Bend (page 199), Yoga Nidra (page 44), Body Scan Meditation (page 247)

Metabolic Syndrome and Type 2 Diabetes

Metabolic syndrome is a combination of risk factors that together lead to grave long-term health consequences, such as heart disease, stroke, and diabetes. The risk factors include increased blood pressure, high blood sugar, high levels of triglycerides (a type of fat), and increased body fat around the waist. More than a third of American adults have metabolic syndrome. Lifestyle changes, such as a healthier diet and more exercise, are critical to prevent metabolic syndrome from becoming a more serious medical issue. Three months of weekly yoga practice has been shown to reduce waist circumference and lower blood pressure, cholesterol, and blood sugar levels in people with metabolic syndrome.

Yoga may also be a safe, low-cost way to prevent and manage type 2 diabetes. Several small studies with promising results show that yoga reduces body mass index, waist circumference, and weight, and improves blood sugar control and insulin sensitivity.

For people who want an accessible form of yoga, restorative yoga is a great option and has been rated highly by people with metabolic syndrome who are new to yoga. This style of yoga uses such props as bolsters, blankets, and blocks to help you support poses for longer than you can with other forms of yoga. The relaxing practice releases muscle tension, improves sense of well-being and energy, and decreases overall stress.

Consider: Sun Saluation A (page 264) and B (page 266) sequences, Bound Angle Pose (page 188), Reclining Bound Angle Pose (page 189), Camel Pose (page 178), Legs up the Wall Pose (page 207), Mindfulness Body and Sound Meditation (page 242), Mindful Walking (page 243), Breath Awareness (page 87)

Multiple Sclerosis

Multiple sclerosis (MS) is the most common autoimmune demyelinating disease affecting the central nervous system and a leading cause of disability in young adults. Symptoms can include fatigue, imbalance, chronic pain, impaired movement, and depression. Seven randomized controlled trials suggest yoga can help fatigue and mood in MS, similar to other forms of exercise.[11] More research is needed to find out if yoga can help with other MS symptoms.

Consider: Working with specialized yoga therapists and clinicians to develop individualized yoga sequences, hospital-based yoga programs

Osteoporosis

Osteopenia and osteoporosis, conditions of low bone mineral density, affects older adults, especially postmenopausal women. Gentle yoga can be safe for people with osteopenia and osteoporosis and improves bone density when done with caution or under supervision. With a little care, depending on the severity of osteoporosis, the benefits can outweigh the risks. When you strengthen the muscles that support your spinal column, you can improve balance, posture, and range of motion. Given the wide range of bone density among people with osteopenia and osteoporosis, there is no one-size-fits-all approach. You should speak with your doctor to find out whether yoga is safe for you.

Precautions: People with osteoporosis are at higher risk of fragility fractures in the spine.

Poses that involve extreme spinal flexion can cause compression fractures due to force on the vertebrae, so these poses should be avoided or modified for those with osteopenia or osteoporosis: Seated Forward Bend (page 199), Plow (page 68), Bridge (page 183), Camel (page 178), and Wheel (Figure Appendix A.1) Poses

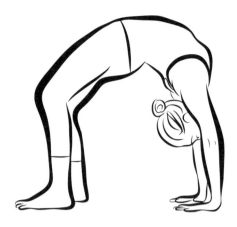

Figure Appendix A.1   Wheel

Parkinson's Disease

Yoga may also be able to help people with early stages of Parkinson's disease, a progressive neurodegenerative disease that leads to impaired movement, affecting muscle tone and flexibility, and can cause depression and a negative outlook. Small studies have found that yoga can help improve depression, blood pressure, body weight, and lung function. Some studies have also found that yoga was able to immediately reduce tremors associated with Parkinson's.[12] Improving balance is critical to help quality of life and health since Parkinson's disease doubles the risk of falls, and one third of falls can cause injuries and intensifies the fear of walking.[13] Yoga has also been incorporated in physical therapy to strengthen muscles and improve balance in Parkinson's disease.

Consider: Working with specialized yoga therapists and clinicians to develop individualized yoga sequences, hospital-based yoga programs

Premenstrual Syndrome

Premenstrual syndrome (PMS), also known as premenstrual tension (PMT), is a set of symptoms that occur one to two weeks prior to menstruation and can include mood swings, anxiety, fatigue, bloating, and headaches. During the premenstrual phase, the "fight-or-flight" system is overactive and leads to higher heart rate and blood pressure. Yoga has been shown to reduce this reactivity. A study of sixty women with premenstrual symptoms in India found that the breathing technique Alternate Nostril Breath (page 94), combined with yoga pose sequences, significantly decreases the rise in body weight, heart rate, and blood pressure. Yoga also reduced anger, depression, and anxiety in the premenstrual phase. Yoga nidra, a practice for deep relaxation sleep, has also been shown to help women with mild to moderate premenstrual symptoms, though it was not effective for more severe symptoms.

Consider: Victorious Breath (page 93), Hero Pose (page 111), Low Lunge (page 143), Standing Forward Bend (page 129), Half Moon Pose (page 161), Wide-Legged Forward Bend (page 134), Staff Pose (page 198), Seated Forward Bend (page 199), Bound Angle Pose (page 188), Reclining Bound Angle Pose (page 189), Body Scan Meditation (page 247), Gazing Candle Meditation (page 244)

Restless Leg Syndrome

Restless leg syndrome (RLS) is a burdensome nervous system and sleep disorder characterized by needing to move your legs, especially in the evening, and can interrupt sleep. This disorder causes a vague, unpleasant sensation—not quite pain, not quite itch, not quite pressure—that only goes away by getting up and walking around. It's subtle, but causes very real misery. Preliminary studies have found that eight weeks of gentle yoga can improve sleep, mood, and RLS symptoms.

Consider: Standing Forward Bend (page 129), Reclining Bound Angle Pose (page 189), Legs up the Wall Pose (page 207), Body Scan Meditation (page 247)

Stroke Rehabilitation

Yoga may be able to play an important role in rehabilitation after strokes. Strokes are the leading cause of disability in adults in the United States. Strokes occur when blood flow to an area of the brain is cut off, damaging brain cells. Depending on the area of the brain affected, strokes can result in muscle weakness, paralysis, difficulty speaking, and changes in mood. Recovery from stroke can be difficult, leading to anxiety and depression. Preliminary studies have found that yoga can help improve balance, mobility, depression, anxiety, and quality of life during rehabilitation for disabilities after strokes.

Consider: Working with specialized physical and yoga therapists to develop individualized yoga sequences, hospital-based yoga programs

Psychological Conditions

Addiction Recovery

In a 1974 study published in the *American Journal of Psychiatry*, researchers found that the longer people practiced meditation, the more likely they were able to cut back on or quit smoking marijuana. More than 50 percent were able to reduce or quit smoking marijuana within the first three months of meditation.

A more recent 2012 survey suggests the same trend. Over 12 percent of people who do yoga find that they cut back on or stop alcohol, and the effects are greater the longer yoga is practiced. Studies support the use of yoga in recovery from alcohol and opiate dependence. Yoga and mindfulness programs have been found to be equally—and in some cases more—effective in reducing relapse rates compared to cognitive-behavioral treatment and twelve-step programs. More important, yoga can also be combined with these programs as well.

Yoga and meditation provide several tools that can help addiction recovery. Yoga and its philosophy of self-awareness and self-compassion encourages awareness of triggers and cravings. Yoga also encourages tolerating experiences without needing to react immediately, which can help people in recovery, particularly in coping with stress and anxiety. By reducing stress, anxiety, and depression, yoga can help ease emotional states that can trigger relapses. Finally, yoga is built on a foundation of a nonjudgmental atittude, which vastly helps replace shame and stigma with hope and self-acceptance in addiction recovery.

Consider: Standing Forward Bend (page 129), Half Moon Pose (page 161), Reclining Bound Angle Pose (page 189), Bridge Pose (page 183), Legs up the Wall Pose (page 207), Mindfulness Body Sound Meditation (page 242), Gazing Candle Meditation (page 244)

Precautions: Alcohol can impair your awareness, balance, and reaction time as well as hasten dehydration—all aspects which can be harmful if combined with yoga. A new fad in San Francisco and Los Angeles, as well as in Colorado, combines marijuana with yoga in "cannabis-enhanced" classes. These "ganja yoga" or "pot yoga" classes are for people approved for medical marijuana and offer a smoking session before doing yoga postures.

There are no studies on whether marijuana use during yoga is safe. Cannabis can cause you to be less aware of pain, which could make you less able to know when you are exceeding your limit in poses. If you're not able to recognize pain early enough, you risk pushing yourself too far and potentially straining muscles and joints. Also, the only reported death linked to yoga in the medical literature is from a rare air embolism in a sixteen-year-old girl who was doing "voluntary mouth-to-mouth" yoga breathing with marijuana, antihistamines, and barbiturates in her system. She did a type of breathing that is not found in mainstream yoga practice, so it is unclear whether the forced breathing, or its combination with substances, caused her death. Other serious injuries have occurred when drugs are combined with yoga, including one case of nerve injury when someone passed out in a Seated Forward Bend while under the influence of opiates and sedating medication.

Anxiety

Anxiety is the most common mental health issue in the United States, affecting one in five people. Even though anxiety disorders are very treatable, less than a third of people suffering with anxiety actually receive treatment. Yoga is an effective way to reduce anxiety, including panic disorder, generalized anxiety, phobias, and obsessive-compulsive disorder.[14]

Think back to the last time that you felt anxious or nervous. Were you holding your breath? Did your breath then become shorter or irregular? Most likely, yes. When anxiety sets in, it is very easy to lose track of your breathing. When you're anxious, you may feel as if your breathing is out of control. You start to sweat, your heart races, and it becomes difficult to breathe, which is your fight-or-flight response. For people with panic disorder, this set of physical reactions can lead to a panic attack. Yoga is an effective tool to turn on the counteracting parasympathetic nervous system and to remind you to connect with your breath first before reacting. Being able to take a pause makes the difference to avoid an escalating path toward a panic attack. Instead, just being aware of your body's reactions can slow down your nervous system, reduce anxiety, remind yourself that you can get through the event, and prevent a panic attack from happening.

Yoga both reduces general anxiety and improves sleep and overall quality of life in people suffering from anxiety, in many cases independent of the underlying cause of the anxiety. It has been shown to be as equally effective as the standard talk therapy, such as cognitive behavioral therapy, for some anxiety disorders. Yoga reduces symptoms of panic disorder, improves bodily sensations that occur during panic attacks, and modifies the irrational beliefs that can occur during episodes of anxiety. Yoga by itself can be helpful, but it is even more powerful when combined with other forms of therapy like cognitive behavioral therapy.

Yoga is useful for anxiety because it gives you a tool that comes with far fewer negative side effects compared to commonly used medications, such as selective serotonin reuptake inhibitors or benzodiazepines. It can also be combined with medications safely and may reduce the need for or lower the dose of medications over time. Yoga reduces anxiety in all ages, including older adults as well as school-age children and teens.

Consider: Victorious Breath (page 93), Alternate Nostril Breathing (page 94), Mountain Pose (page 114), Standing Forward Bend (page 129), Extended Triangle Pose (page 148), Half Moon Pose (page 161), Seated Forward Bend (page 199), Bound Angle Pose (page 188), Bridge Pose (page 183), Legs up the Wall Pose (page 207), Corpse Pose (page 209)

Attention

Yoga improves attention in adults and children. Yoga has been studied in children with attention deficit/hyperactivity disorder (ADHD) with promising results. One small study found yoga and meditation was able to reduce ADHD symptoms in about 40 percent of children with ADHD and 90 percent of the children improved their academic performance.[15]

Consider: Victorious Breath (page 93); focused attention meditations, such as Breath Meditation (page 241), Mindfulness Body and Sound Meditation (page 242), and Mantra Meditation (page 246); Mountain Pose (page 114), Tree Pose (page 163), Eagle Pose (page 165), and other Standing and Balance Poses (pages 158–168)

Body Image and Eating Disorders

In an emerging area of research, there are a few small studies on eating disorders, including binge-eating disorder, with promising results that yoga can improve psychological well-being, self-image, and decrease preoccupations with food.[16] Spending more time "in" your body can shift treating your body like an object to feeling empowered. Mindful eating, or eating with full intention and attention, is becoming more popular to treat binge eating disorder and most studies show significant improvement of symptoms with this approach. Mindful eating and awareness can help you get in touch with feeling of being satisfied and satiated.

People who do yoga may be less at risk for developing eating disorders, but there are still considerations to make sure yoga doesn't trigger or worsen negative body image or self-esteem issues or contribute to exercising excessively. Eating disorders can fuel overexercising, an emphasis on thinness, perfection, or control. This tendency could make yoga turn into an exercise in perfection that is more harmful than beneficial, so it's important to pay attention to *how* you approach yoga.

Consider: We suggest working with a yoga therapist with a background in eating disorders. Try Breathing Meditation (page 241) and Compassion Meditation (page 245)

Depression

Depression affects one in ten Americans at some point during their lifetime. Depression is more common in women than men, with one in four women experiencing depression at some point. Symptoms of depression can include low energy, feeling unable to enjoy life, changes in appetite, difficulty sleeping, and poor concentration. Depression often comes with other conditions, such as alcohol or substance abuse, due to the urge to self-medicate when sad, angry, lonely, or upset. Many people do not seek treatment for depression because of the stigma associated with mental illness, or because they do not want to be on medication, especially women who may be thinking about becoming pregnant.

Yoga is an accessible practice that can be safely combined with all standard treatments for depression. A study of 124 men and women with depression or anxiety participated in an 8-week mind-body program at the Benson Henry Institute for Mind Body Medicine and found significantly less depression and anxiety. Several studies have shown that yoga can help reduce depressive symptoms in pregnant women and older adults. In a 2012 review of clinical trials, eight high-quality randomized control studies found that yoga reduced depression symptoms.

There is some early evidence that yoga could be helpful long-term with depression, even after you stop practicing. One small study showed that women with depression who participated in an 8-week yoga program continued to benefit from the program one year later.[17] Women said that they felt like yoga gave them "a tool in their toolbox" to combat depression and stress through breath, relaxation, and physical movement. Even though many of the women did not continue in classes because of financial or time constraints, they still reported that yoga had a long-term positive impact on their quality of life a year later.

Consider: Sun Salutation B (page 266), Child's Pose (page 112), Downward Facing Dog Pose (page 122), Cobra Pose (page 172), Standing Forward Bend (page 129), Wide-Legged Forward Bend (page 134), Half Pigeon Pose (page 193), Reclining Bound Angle (page 189), Happy Baby Pose (page 204), Corpse Pose (page 209), Mindfulness Body and Sound Meditation (page 242), Compassion Meditation (page 245)

Memory

Yoga helps with improving memory, processing speed, reaction times, and ability to make higher-level decisions.[18] A single session of yoga improves reaction times and performance accuracy compared to regular aerobic exercise.[19] Yoga improves memory and decision-making abilities of older adults as well.[20] Even yoga breathing techniques, such as Left Nostril Breathing and Alternate Nostril Breathing, for forty-five minutes daily for three days improves memory.[21]

Consider: Rhythmic Breathing (page 91), Left Nostril Breathing (page 94), Alternate Nostril Breathing (page 94); focused awareness meditation, such as Breath Meditation (page 241) and Gazing Candle Meditation (page 244)

Schizophrenia

In another emerging area of research, yoga and physical exercise may be helpful as an add-on therapy for people with schizophrenia to improve symptoms and overall quality of life.[22] Yoga could help improve cognitive symptoms and social skills. Often, medications that are commonly used to treat schizophrenia are associated with weight gain and risk of developing metabolic syndrome, so yoga could play an important role in preventing obesity and diabetes.

Consider: Hospital-based yoga programs

Precautions: There is one case of a young man with a history of psychosis who developed auditory hallucinations during an intensive Bikram yoga training program, possibly triggered by stress or dehydration. So, if you are experiencing symptoms that make it difficult to stay in touch with reality or might feel detached from your body or mind, then it's best to discuss yoga and meditation first with your doctor.

Smoking Cessation

Over a quarter of smokers who did yoga cut back on or even stopped smoking cigarettes altogether. Nicotine from cigarettes is one of the most addictive chemicals, as addictive as heroin and cocaine in research studies. Nicotine reaches the brain within ten seconds of inhalation of cigarette smoke, activating brain circuitry in pleasure areas reinforcing addiction. Yoga has the potential to reduce cravings in addictions. Cigarette smoking is the leading cause of preventable disease and death in the United States and accounts for the cause of death in one in five Americans. Even though current smoking rates are declining, 18 percent of Americans continue to smoke. Nearly seven out of ten smokers want to quit, but quitting on your own can be very challenging. Approximately 85 percent of people who try to quit on their own relapse within the first week.

Fourteen studies have found that yoga and meditation help people quit smoking and avoid relapse for longer periods of time compared to general wellness programs. How does yoga and meditation do this? One theory is that the mindfulness and attention developed through yoga and meditation help smokers become actively aware of triggers that cause them to smoke. One study used functional magnetic resonance imaging (fMRI) of the brain and found that meditation and mindful attention helped smokers reduce cravings in response to smoking images and reduced brain activity in areas associated with cravings.

Yoga also reduces anxiety and stress—conditions that often cause smokers to return to smoking. A study of women smokers found that participants in a yoga program reported less anxiety and improved overall well-being and health compared to those that participated in a general wellness program, and were more successful at quitting smoking six months later.[23]

Consider: Mindfulness Body and Sound Meditation (page 242), Gazing Candle Meditation (page 244), Balance poses (pages 158–168)

Trauma and Post-traumatic Stress Disorder

Post-traumatic stress disorder (PTSD) is a form of anxiety disorder following a life-threatening event, or at least something your brain registers as life-threatening. It consists of recurrent brief traumatic nightmares that reprise the death threat event, trancelike flashbacks triggered by other events evoking the original trauma, panic, depression, and of course the usual biological markers of psychiatric upheaval—difficulty falling asleep, difficulty staying asleep, despair in the morning, weight loss, fears of death while also wishing to be dead, and loss of one's usual ability to concentrate, have pleasure, or connect emotionally with other people. The evidence is that such life-threatening events can actually cause physical and chemical changes in the human brain that can sometimes go on to become permanent.

As many as 70 percent of adults in the United States experience a traumatic event in their lives; 20 percent of them go on to develop PTSD. One in nine women experience PTSD at some point during their lifetime. Approximately 8 percent of Americans (24.4 million people) are dealing with PTSD at any given time—this is equivalent to the number of people who live in the state of Texas.

Yoga and meditation can help reduce symptoms of post-traumatic stress disorder by connecting them with their body and breathing in a way that gives them a sense of control and empowerment and releases the physical and mental tension of helplessness and fear.

In a 2014 study published in the *Journal of Clinical Psychiatry*, researchers compared a 10-week yoga program with a health education class over three years in women with chronic PTSD who had not responded to standard medications or therapy. Yoga was better able to reduce PTSD symptoms both during the program and in the long term. At the end of the study, half of the women in the yoga group no longer showed any PTSD symptoms. The women in the yoga group stayed improved while PTSD symptoms in the health education class group returned.

Combat veterans are significantly affected by trauma, and up to 20 percent of war veterans returning from Afghanistan and Iraq suffer from PTSD. Even though promising treatments for PTSD are available, the stigma of mental illness makes access to mental health care very challenging. Also for some, going into treatment is experienced on some level as going back into battle. Dropout rates from PTSD treatment are over 60 percent for Afghanistan and Iraq war veterans.

The Veterans Health Administration and US Department of Defense recommend combining yoga and meditation along with standard treatment for PTSD. Meditation programs have helped reduce PTSD severity in veterans. Doing yoga for as little as one week to three weeks can help with PTSD symptoms. A small study published in the *Journal of Traumatic Stress* found that a group of veterans with PTSD that practiced meditation-based yoga had far fewer and less intense PTSD symptoms than did the group that did not practice yoga. The yoga group had less anxiety and slower breathing rates compared to the control group and also were better able to regulate their physical response on tests that measured startle reactions to noise. PTSD symptoms continued to be improved one year later, even though some of the participants had stopped practicing yoga. Another study that included nine sessions of Hatha yoga over three weeks showed that yoga helped veterans with combat stress and PTSD reduce anger and improve sleep and quality of life. Yoga nidra, a deep relaxation technique, has helped war veterans relax and is now integrated into the treatment program at the Walter Reed Army Medical Center.

Consider: Yoga Nidra (page 44), Breath Meditation (page 241), Mindfulness Body Sound Meditation (page 242); work with yoga teacher with training in trauma-sensitive yoga

Yoga and Pregnancy

Yoga can reduce depression, anxiety, stress, and pain during pregnancy and also help a mother bond with her baby. Women who practice yoga during pregnancy and after birth have lower cortisol levels, an indication of stress levels, and a more positive mood on the days that they practiced yoga. Studies have also found that yoga can reduce the pain, discomfort, sleep disturbances, and stress of pregnancy and improve the overall quality of life.

Over half of all pregnant women experience stress or anxiety at some point in their pregnancy, and these often spike in the third trimester. Anxiety during pregnancy can be associated with higher risk of preterm birth and long-term effects on the child's learning, behavior, and motor development, so reducing anxiety is important for the health of the mother and baby.

One study found that yoga during pregnancy could help women lower their stress hormones and improve anxiety after only a single session.[1] Anxiety continued to improve at the end of eight weeks of yoga. Yoga classes can also provide important social support during pregnancy. Both yoga and weekly support groups have been shown to equally lower cortisol, the stress hormone, and reduce depression, anxiety, and anger. Yoga can be combined with meditation or other mind-body activities, such as tai chi. Mothers who participate in yoga and mindfulness training, including body scan meditation, experience far less anxiety and negative feelings during their third trimester.

Yoga can also be a helpful option for women suffering from depression during and after pregnancy. About 13 percent of women experience clinical depression during pregnancy.[2] Many women may want to avoid or reduce doses of antidepressant medications during pregnancy, and yoga can be combined with standard treatment to help reduce depression during pregnancy. Yoga has also been shown to improve the sense of attachment between mother and child in pregnant women who are depressed.[3]

Up to one in every five pregnant women may experience depression after giving birth, or postpartum depression. Yoga can reduce depression and improve quality of life in women with postpartum depression. A randomized controlled trial of women with postpartum depression found that 78 percent of the women who did yoga two times a week for eight weeks were able to reduce depression and anxiety, and improve their overall quality of life.[4]

Yoga has also been shown to lower the pain intensity and time period of active labor and increase satisfaction after childbirth. Five clinical studies have found an association between yoga and lower rates of both preterm labor and low birth weight.

The studies in pregnant women have found that prenatal yoga is safe and have not reported any falls, injuries, or safety problems.

Here are some general tips on how to approach prenatal yoga based on the recent research findings:

1. Start early to reap the most benefits.

Talk to your doctor early about whether yoga could be a safe option during your pregnancy. Gentle prenatal yoga is generally safe for healthy women with uncomplicated pregnancies. If you have a pregnancy with medical issues, we recommend consulting your physician before pursuing prenatal yoga. Yoga has the potential to be more effective when started earlier in the pregnancy. Starting yoga in the first trimester has been shown to improve pregnancy-related pain, discomfort, and stress later on in the third trimester, a period when anxiety and pregnancy-related stress can spike. Women who did yoga earlier also had more personal confidence about their upcoming labor and delivery.

2. Do yoga poses, breathwork, deep relaxation, and meditation.

Breathing techniques, deep relaxation, and meditation have been found to be more effective in reducing stress, depression, and discomfort compared to physical poses alone or standard exercise, such as walking, during pregnancy. Avoid any rapid or intense breathing like Breath of Fire (page 98) and Bellows Breath (page 98) or holding your breath, which require significant contraction of the abdominal muscles.

3. Choose modifications for poses that emphasize stability and strength over flexibility and endurance.

During pregnancy, it's important to adjust to the changing center of gravity. Hormones during pregnancy, including high levels of estrogen and relaxin, loosen your muscles, ligaments, and connective tissues during pregnancy. This laxity starts as early as the first trimester, when relaxin is at its highest levels, so pregnant women have a higher risk of joint instability and overstretching ligaments. It's important not to push yourself too far. Use blocks, a chair, or the wall to add stability, if needed. Instead of trying to achieve flexibility or endurance, focus instead on *strength* and *stability* in each pose. Pregnancy can also lower your blood pressure, which can make you more vulnerable to dizziness and headaches, so take care during transitions between poses, from sitting to standing.

4. Practice in a thermally neutral environment.

Yoga in extreme heat is discouraged during pregnancy, given increased risks of overheating and dehydration. The combination of the heated environment and hormones that loosen the ligaments and tendons during pregnancy also means that your joints and muscles are at higher risk of overstretching, leading to injuries, so if you're considering this at all, it's important to speak to your doctor before doing hot yoga if you're pregnant.

It's not clear whether hot yoga is unsafe during pregnancy, since there are no studies on this topic. Hot yoga styles, such as Bikram yoga classes, have room temperatures reaching 104 to 105 degrees Fahrenheit (40 to 41 degrees Celsius) and a humidity of up to 40 percent. A small study has shown that internal body temperatures in hot yoga classes, such as Bikram yoga, can reach up to 103 to 104 degrees Fahrenheit (39.4 to 40 degrees Celsius). Early signs of heat intolerance, which precedes heat exhaustion, can start at around a core body temperature of 104 degrees Fahrenheit, so hot yoga comes with risks of overheating and dehydration. During the first trimester, overheating from other heated environments such as hot tubs and saunas or from extreme exercise have been shown to double the risk of defects or malformations in the baby. Also, heat can create additional laxity of muscles, ligaments, and connective tissue, which are already loosened by pregnancy hormones.

Given these potential risks to mothers-to-be and their babies and the lack of safety studies of hot yoga during pregnancy, we encourage those who haven't done hot yoga before to choose a thermally neutral environment during pregnancy. And if you've been doing hot yoga for a while and want to continue during pregnancy, speak to your doctor first.

5. Make space for the baby, and choose your positions based on your stage of pregnancy.

Prenatal yoga encourages you to modify poses to make space for the baby and avoid overstretching your abdominal muscles. In general, poses safe in prenatal yoga depend on your stage of pregnancy. Deep forward or backbends, deep twisting poses that put pressure on your abdomen, and intense core abdominal work should be avoided. Avoid inversions except for Downward Facing Dog. Intense backbends and inversions should be avoided as well. Standing Forward Bends can be modified with a wider stance of the legs to accommodate the growing belly. Bends should occur at the hip crease to avoid compressing the abdomen. Balance poses should be done close to the wall to ensure safety. In Sun Salutations, pregnant women should not jump back.

The third trimester is often when you experience more stress and anxiety, so prenatal yoga can be a useful and safe resource for uncomplicated pregnancies under the guidance of an experienced prenatal yoga teacher. A 2015 study in the journal *Obstetrics & Gynecology* provides encouraging results that many yoga poses may be safe during late stages of pregnancy, a time when pregnancy-related stress and anxiety can spike. The study closely monitored the vital signs of twenty-five women with healthy pregnancies between 35 and 38 weeks with varying levels of yoga experience. A certified yoga teacher led the moms-to-be through twenty-six different yoga poses, using modifications with props and the wall. There were no falls, injuries, or safety problems and vital signs for both moms-to-be and babies were normal. All the women reported feeling safe during the yoga poses and did not have any problems twenty-four hours later.

SIDE-LYING CORPSE POSE

During later weeks of pregnancy, when lying on your back can be uncomfortable, Corpse Pose can be modified with either a side-lying or inclined modification. Side-lying Corpse Pose modification should be done lying on the left side, to avoid putting pressure on the vena cava, a vein that circulates blood between the upper and lower parts of the body. You can place blankets under the right knee, arm, and head to feel more supported.

Sample Poses During Healthy Pregnancy

First Trimester: Warrior I Pose (page 140), Warrior II Pose (page 141), Extended Triangle Pose (page 148), Balance poses such as Warrior III Pose, Tree Pose, or Eagle Pose near a wall (pages 159–166), Bound Angle Pose (page 188), Wide-Legged Forward Bend (page 134), Reclining Bound Angle Pose (page 189)

Second Trimester: Warrior I Pose (page 140), Warrior II (can be modified with chair supporting body under front thigh) (page 141), Extended Triangle Pose (page 148), Extended Side Angle Pose (page 146), Fierce Pose (page 139), Balance poses such as Warrior III Pose, Tree Pose, Half Moon Pose (near a wall) (pages 159–164), Reclining Bound Angle (page 189)

Third Trimester: Cat Pose (page 117), Warrior I Pose (page 140), Warrior II Pose (page 141), Extended Triangle Pose (page 148), Extended Side Angle (page 146), Tree Pose (near wall) (page 163), Bound Angle Pose (page 188), Seated Wide-Legged Forward Bend (page 139), Side-Lying Corpse (page 296)

Breathwork: Relaxing breaths such as Victorious Breath (page 93), Alternate Nostril Breath (page 94), Humming Bee Breath (page 94)

Meditation: Body Scan Meditation (page 247), Mindfulness Meditation (page 242), Mantra Meditation (page 246)

Complicated Pregnancies

More research is needed on the risk and benefits of yoga during complicated pregnancies, so it is important to ask your physician to find out whether yoga is safe during pregnancy. There is some early evidence suggesting that yoga could help with improving birth weight in some types of complicated pregnancies. A study in India of 121 pregnant women with abnormal blood flow in the umbilical and uterine artery, a condition that can cause abnormally low birth weight, found that one hour of integrated yoga daily was better than walking for higher birth weight. Another study of women with high-risk pregnancies found that yoga three times a week was better than walking for fetal growth and mother-baby blood circulation. But this area of research is in its early stages, so it's best to consult with your doctor.

✦

It's important to practice yoga designed for different stages of pregnancy. Since the details of prenatal yoga go beyond the scope of this book, we encourage you to find prenatal yoga classes or resources.

Acknowledgments

We owe much gratitude to everyone who has helped make this book happen. Thank you to our Harvard Health Publications (HHP) team: editor in chief Dr. Gregory Curfman, Robert O'Connell, Nancy Ferrari, and Jill Mazzetta, as well as Patrick Skerrett, formerly at HHP. We thank our stellar literary agent, Linda Konner, and our phenomenal team at Perseus Books Group at Hachette, including Renée Sedliar, Caroline Pincus, Michael Giarratano, Miriam Riad, Michael Clark, Iris Bass, and Jeff Williams.

Dr. Wei

I am enormously grateful to Douglas Graham Purdy, my family (Ray, Ming, Lisa, David, Tiffany), Dr. Jennifer Mathur, Trang Dao, Dr. Julia Wood, Dr. Kathy Sanders, Dr. Rebecca Brendel, Dr. Felicia Smith, Dr. Judith Edersheim, Dr. Margaret Cramer, and Dr. Adele Pressman. Thank you to the yoga community, including Ossi Raveh, Be Shakti, Mikki Raveh, Dennis Teston, Greg Polvere, Allison Lamy, Natasha Giliberti, Brooke Farrell, Brittany Maschmeyer, Bonnie Varner, Allegra Romita, and Jessica Weiss. You all have been inspiring and supportive throughout the process of writing this book. And, last but certainly not least, I would like to thank Dr. Groves for his support and wisdom.

Dr. Groves

I would like to thank Frank Interrante, who handled questions of design, art, and aesthetics and rendered a thousand kindnesses; Annette Robinson, who organized both business and personal matters through the years, making life and writing possible; and John Daniel Groves, who was, of course, the reason for doing this book in the first place.

Together we thank Dr. Gregory Fricchione, Dr. Theodore Stern, Dr. John Denninger, and Dr. Jerrold Rosenbaum at Massachusetts General Hospital and Harvard Medical School for their support.

To us, an essential part of yoga is compassion and service, or *seva*. We are inspired by having the opportunity to be part of such nonprofit organizations as Exhale to Inhale, which provides yoga to survivors of domestic violence, and Kula for Karma, which offers yoga programs in hospitals and clinics.

We hope to continue to share yoga with many more and are grateful to all who have inspired us on this journey.

MARLYNN WEI, MD, JD
and JAMES E. GROVES, MD

Notes

Chapter 1: Why Do Yoga?

1. Holger Cramer, Romy Lauche, Jost Langhorst, and Gustav Dobos, "Is One Yoga Style Better Than Another? A Systematic Review of Associations of Yoga Style and Conclusions in Randomized Yoga Trials," *Complementary Therapies in Medicine* 25 (2016): 178–187.

2. M. Jay Polsgrove, Brandon M. Eggleston, and Roch J. Lockyer, "Impact of 10-Weeks of Yoga Practice on Flexibility and Balance of College Athletes," *International Journal of Yoga* 9 (2016): 27–34.

3. Barbara J. Stussman, Lindsey I. Black, Patricia M. Barnes, Tainya C. Clarke, and Richard L. Nahin, "Wellness-Related Use of Common Complementary Health Approaches Among Adults: United States, 2012," *National Health Statistics Reports* 85 (2015): 1–12, accessed July 23, 2016, http://www.cdc.gov/nchs/data/nhsr/nhsr085.pdf.

4. Ibid.

5. Ibid.

6. Neha P. Gothe, Arthur F. Kramer, and Edward McAuley, "The Effects of an 8-Week Hatha Yoga Intervention on Executive Function in Older Adults," *Journal of Gerontology* 69 (2014): 1109–1116.

7. Cramer et al., "Is One Yoga Style Better Than Another?" 178–187.

Chapter 2: Historical Frameworks of Yoga

1. Jayanta Bhattacharya, "The First Dissection Controversy: Introduction to Anatomical Education in Bengal and British India," *Current Science* 101 (2011): 1227–1232.

Chapter 3: The Modern Science of Yoga

1. Pamela E. Jeter, Jeremiah Slutsky, Nilkamal Singh, and Sat Bir S. Khalsa, "Yoga as a Therapeutic Intervention: A Bibliometric Analysis of Published Research Studies from 1967 to 2013," *Journal of Alternative and Complementary Medicine*. 21 (2015): 586–592.

2. Holger Cramer, Romy Lauche, and Gustav Dobos, "Characteristics of Randomized Controlled Trials of Yoga: A Bibliometric Analysis," *BMC Complementary Alternative Medicine* 14 (2014): 328.

3. Holger Cramer, Romy Lauche, Jost Langhorst, and Gustav Dobos, "Is One Yoga Style Better Than Another? A Systematic Review of Associations of Yoga Style and Conclusions in Randomized Yoga Trials," *Complementary Therapies in Medicine* 25 (2016): 178–187.

4. Michaela C. Pascoe and Isabelle E. Bauer, "A Systematic Review of Randomised Control Trials on the Effects of Yoga on Stress Measures and Mood," *Journal of Psychiatric Research*, 68 (2015): 270–282.

5. Manop Phoosuwan, Thanomwong Kritpet, and Pongsak Yuktanandana, "The Effects of Weight Bearing Yoga Training on the Bone Resorption Markers of the Postmenopausal Women." *Journal of the Medical Association of Thailand* 92 (suppl. 5) (2009): S102–S108.

6. Judith Balk, Melissa Gluck, Lisa Bernardo, and Janet Catov, "The Effect of Yoga on Markers of Bone Turnover in Osteopenic Women: A Pilot Study," *International Journal of Yoga Therapy*, 19 (2009): 63–68.

7. Paula Chu, Rinske A. Gotink, Gloria Y. Yeh, Sue J. Goldie, and M. G. Myriam Hunink, "The Effectiveness of Yoga in Modifying Risk Factors for Cardiovascular Disease and Metabolic Syndrome: A Systematic Review and Meta-analysis of Randomized Controlled Trials," *European Journal of Preventative Cardiology* (2014), accessed November 27, 2015, doi: 10.1177/2047487314562741.

8. Maria Rosario G. Araneta, Matthew Allison, Elizabeth L. Barrett-Connor, and Alka Kanaya, "Overall and Regional Fat Change: Results from the Practice of Restorative Yoga or Stretching for Metabolic Syndrome (PRYSMS) study," *Diabetes* 62 (2013): A1.

9. Rachel Neuendorf, Helané Wahbeh, Irina Chamine, Jun Yu, Kimberly Hutchison, and Barry S. Oken, "The Effects of Mind-Body Interventions on Sleep Quality: A Systematic Review," *Evidence-Based Complementary and Alternative Medicine* (2015), accessed December 4, 2015, doi: 10.1155/2015/902708.

10. R. Peters, "Ageing and the Brain," *Postgraduate Medical Journal* 82 (2006): 84–88.

11. Chantal Villemure, Marta Čeko, Valerie A. Cotton, and M. Catherine Bushnell, "Neuroprotective Effects of Yoga Practice: Age-, Experience-, and Frequency-Dependent Plasticity," *Frontiers in Human Neuroscience* 9 (2015): 281.

12. Sara W. Lazar, Catherine E. Kerr, Rachel H. Wasserman, Jeremy R. Gray, Douglas N. Greve, Michael T. Treadway, Metta McGarvey, Brian T. Quinn, Jeffery A. Dusek, Herbert Benson, Scott L. Rauch, Christopher I. Moore, and Bruce Fischl, "Meditation Experience Is Associated with Increased Cortical Thickness," *Neuroreport* 16 (2005): 1893–1897.

13. Britta K. Hölzel, James Carmody, Mark Vangel, Christina Congleton, Sita M. Yerramsetti, Tim Gard, and Sara W. Lazar, "Mindfulness Practice Leads to Increases in Regional Brain Gray Matter Density," *Psychiatry Research* 191 (2011): 36–43.

14. Chris C. Streeter, Theodore H. Whitfield, Liz Owen, Tasha Rein, Surya K. Karri, Aleksandra Yakhkind, Ruth Perlmutter, Andrew Prescot, Perry F. Renshaw, Domenic A. Ciraulo, and J. Eric Jensen, "Effects of Yoga Versus Walking on Mood, Anxiety, and Brain GABA Levels: A Randomized Controlled MRS Study," *Journal of Alternative and Complementary Medicine* 16 (2010): 1145–1152.

15. Sung-Ah Lim and Kwang-Jo Cheong, "Regular Yoga Practice Improves Antioxidant Status, Immune Function, and Stress Hormone Releases in Young Healthy People: A Randomized, Double-Blind, Controlled Pilot Study," *Journal of Alternative and Complementary Medicine* 21 (2015): 530–538.

16. Marian E. Papp, Petra Lindfors, Malin Nygren-Bonnier, Lennart Gullstrand, and Per E. Wändell, "Effects of High-Intensity Hatha Yoga on Cardiovascular Fitness, Adipocytokines, and Apolipoproteins in Healthy Students: A Randomized Controlled Study," *Journal of Alternative and Complementary Medicine* 22 (2015): 81–87.

17. Noriyuki Ouchi and Kenneth Walsh. "Adiponectin as an Anti-inflammatory Factor," *Clinica Chimica Acta* 380 (2007): 24–30.

18. Janice K. Kiecolt-Glaser, Jeanette M. Bennett, Rebecca Andridge, Juan Peng, Charles L. Shapiro, William B. Malarkey, Charles F. Emery, Rachel Layman, Ewa E. Mrozek, and Ronald Glaser, "Yoga's Impact on Inflammation, Mood, and Fatigue in Breast Cancer Survivors: A Randomized Controlled Trial," *Journal of Clinical Oncology* 32 (2014): 1040–1049.

19. Perla Kaliman, María Jesús Álvarez-Lópezb, Marta Cosín-Tomásb, Melissa A. Rosenkranzc, Antoine Lutzc, and Richard J. Davidsonc, "Rapid Changes in Histone Deacetylases and Inflammatory Gene Expression in Expert Meditators," *Psychoneuroendocrinology* 40 (2014): 96–107.

Chapter 4: Build Your Foundation

1. Jon Kabat-Zinn, *Wherever You Go, There You Are: Mindfulness Meditation in Everyday Life* (New York: Hyperion, 1994).

Chapter 5: How to Prevent Yoga Injuries

1. Holger Cramer, Lesley Ward, Robert Saper, Daniel Fishbein, Gustav Dobos, and Romy Lauche, "The Safety of Yoga: A Systematic Review and Meta-analysis of Randomized Controlled Trials," *American Journal of Epidemiology* (2015), doi: 10.1093/aje/kwv071.

2. Ibid.

3. Holger Cramer, Carol Krucoff, and Gustav Dobos, "Adverse Events Associated with Yoga: A Systematic Review of Published Case Reports and Case Series," *PLoS One* (2013), doi: 10.1371/journal.pone.0075515.

4. Holger Cramer, David Sibbritt, Jon Adams, and Romy Lauche, "The Association Between Regular Yoga and Meditation Practice and Falls and Injuries: Results of a National Cross-sectional Survey Among Australian Women," *Maturitas* (2015), doi: 10.1016/j.maturitas.2015.10.010.

5. Hemant Sharma, Narayan Singh Shekhawat, Sudhir Bhandari, Breda Memon, and Muhammed Ashraf Memon, "Rectus Sheath Haematoma: A Rare Presentation of Non-contact Strenuous Exercises," *British Journal of Sports Medicine* 41 (2007): 688–90, published online May 11, 2007, doi: 10.1136/bjsm.2007.036087.

6. Derek B. Johnson, Mathew J. Tierney, and Parvis J. Sadighi, "Kapalabhati Pranayama: Breath of Fire or Cause of Pneumothorax?: A Case Report" *Chest* 125 (2004): 1951–1952.

7. Wouter I. Schievink, "Spontaneous Dissection of the Carotid and Vertebral Arteries," *New England Journal of Medicine* 344 (2001): 898–906.

Chapter 6: Breathe More, Breathe Better: Yoga Breathing (*Pranayama*)

1. Richard Rosen, *The Yoga of Breath* (Boston: Shambhala, 2002), 20.

2. Allison N. Abel, Lisa K. Lloyd, and James S. Williams, "The Effects of Regular Yoga Practice on Pulmonary Function In Healthy Individuals: A Literature Review," *Journal of Alternative and Complementary Medicine* 19 (2013): 185–190.

3. B. K. S. Iyengar, *Light on the Yoga-Sutras of Patanjali* (San Francisco: Aquarian Press, 1993), 30.

4. Swami Niranjanananda Saraswati, *Prana Pranayama Pranavidya* (Munger, India: Bihar School of Yoga, 1994), chap. 2, verse 2.

5. William J. Broad, *The Science of Yoga* (New York: Simon and Schuster, 2012), 83–90.

6. Relu Cernes and Reuven Zimlichman, "RESPeRATE: The Role of Paced Breathing in Hypertension Treatment," *Journal of the American Society of Hypertension* 9 (2015): 38–47.

7. Michael R. Goldstein, Gregory F. Lewis, Ronnie Newman, Janice M. Brown, Georgiy Bobashev, Lisa Kilpatrick, Emma M Seppälä, Diana H Fishbein, and Sreelatha Meleth, "Improvements in Well-being and Vagal Tone Following a Yogic Breathing-Based Life Skills Workshop in Young Adults: Two Open-Trial Pilot Studies," *International Journal of Yoga* 9 (2016): 20–26.

8. Gopal Krushna Pal, Ankit Agarwal, Shanmugavel Karthik, Pravati Pal, and Nivedita Nanda, "Slow Yogic Breathing Through Right and Left Nostril Influences Sympathovagal Balance, Heart Rate Variability, and Cardiovascular Risks in Young Adults," *North American Journal of Medical Sciences* 6 (2014): 145–151.

9. Ananda Balayogi Bhavanani, Madanmohan, and Zeena Sanjay, "Immediate Effect of Chandra Nadi Pranayama (Left Unilateral Forced Nostril Breathing) on Cardiovascular Parameters in Hypertensive Patients," *International Journal of Yoga* 5 (2012): 108–111.

10. Shirley Telles, Meesha Joshi, and Prasoon Somvanshi, "Yoga Breathing Through a Particular Nostril Is Associated with Contralateral Event-Related Potential Changes," *International Journal of Yoga* 5 (2012): 102–107.

11. Peng Li, Wiktor A. Janczewski, Kevin Yackle, Kaiwen Kam, Silvia Pagliardini, Mark A. Krasnow, and Jack L. Feldman, "The Peptidergic Control Circuit for Sighing," *Nature* 530 (2016): 293–297.

12. Waleed O. Twal, Amy E. Wahlquist, and Sundaravadivel Balasubramanian, "Yogic Breathing When Compared to Attention Control Reduces the Levels of Pro-inflammatory Biomarkers in Saliva: A Pilot Randomized Controlled Trial," *BMC Complementary and Alternative Medicine* 16 (2016): 294.

13. Shirley Telles, Nilkamal Singh, and Raghuraj Puthige, "Changes in P300 Following Alternate Nostril Yoga Breathing and Breath Awareness," *Biopsychosocial Medicine* 7 (2013): 11.

Chapter 8: Deepen Your Practice: Muscle Locks (*Bandhas*) and Hand Expressions (*Mudras*)

1. Damien Keown, *A Dictionary of Buddhism* (New York: Oxford University Press, 2004), 182.

2. Dong Wook Han and Misook Ha, "Effect of Pelvic Floor Muscle Exercises on Pulmonary Function," *Journal of Physical Therapy Science* 27, no. 10 (2015): 3233–3235.

3. Ah Young Lee, Seung Ok Baek, Yun Woo Cho, Tae Hong Lim, Rodney Jones, and Sang Ho Ahn, "Pelvic Floor Muscle Contraction and Abdominal Hollowing During Walking Can Selectively Activate Local Trunk Stabilizing Muscles," *Journal of Muscle and Musculoskeletal Rehabilitation* (2016): 1–9.

4. Ah Young Lee, Eun Hyuk Kim, Yun Woo Cho, Sun Oh Kwon, Su Min Son, and Sang Ho Ahn, "Effects of Abdominal Hollowing During Stair Climbing on the Activations of Local Trunk Stabilizing Muscles: A Cross-Sectional Study," *Annals of Rehabilitation Medicine* 37, no. 6 (2013): 804–813.

5. Tista Bagchi, "The Signing System of *Mudra* in Traditional Indian Dance," *Paragrana* 19 (2010): 259–266.

6. Ahmer K. Ghori, Kevin C. Chung, "Interpretation of Hand Signs in Buddhist Art," *Journal of Hand Surgery* 32, no. 6 (2007): 918–922.

7. Gertrud Hirschi, *Mudras: Yoga in Your Hands* (Maine: Samuel Weiser, 2000), 121.

Chapter 9: Learn How to Meditate (*Dhyana*)

1. Pema Chödrön, *How to Meditate: A Practical Guide to Making Friends with Your Mind* (Boulder, CO: Sounds True, 2013).

2. Jon Kabat-Zinn, "An Outpatient Program in Behavioral Medicine for Chronic Pain Patients Based on the Practice of Mindfulness Meditation: Theoretical Considerations and Preliminary Results," *General Hospital Psychiatry* 4 (1982): 33–47.

3. Shian-Ling Keng, Moria J. Smoski, and Clive J. Robins, "Effects of Mindfulness on Psychological Health: A Review of Empirical Studies," *Clinical Psychology Review* 31 (2011): 1041–1056.

4. David R. Vago and David A. Silbersweig, "Self-Awareness, Self-Regulation, and Self-Transcendence (S-ART): A Framework for Understanding the Neurobiological Mechanism of Mindfulness," *Frontiers in Human Neuroscience* 6 (2012): 1–30.

5. Madhav Goyal, Sonal Singh, Erica M. S. Sibinga, Neda F. Gould, Anastasia Rowland-Seymour, Ritu Sharma, Zackary Berger, Dana Sleicher, David D. Maron, Hasan

M. Shihab, Padmini D. Ranasinghe, Shauna Linn, Shonali Saha, Eric B. Bass, and Jennifer A. Haythornthwaite, "Meditation Programs for Psychological Stress and Well-Being: A Systematic Review and Meta-analysis," *JAMA Internal Medicine* 174 (2014): 357–368.

6. Elizabeth A. Hoge, Eric Bui, Luana Marques, Christina A. Metcalf, Laura K. Morris, Donald J. Robinaugh, John J. Worthington, Mark H. Pollack, and Naomi M. Simon, "Randomized Controlled Trial of Mindfulness Meditation for Generalized Anxiety Disorder: Effects on Anxiety and Stress Reactivity" *Journal of Clinical Psychiatry* 74 (2013): 786–792.

7. Peter Lush, Peter Naish, and Zoltan Dienes, "Metacognition of Intentions in Mindfulness and Hypnosis," *Neuroscience of Consciousness* 1 (2016), accessed July 16, 2016, doi: 10.1093/nc/niw007.

8. Adam Moore and Peter Malinowski, "Meditation, Mindfulness and Cognitive Flexibility," *Consciousness and Cognition* 18 (2009): 176–186.

9. Alberto Chiesa, Raffaella Calati, and Alessandro Serretti, "Does Mindfulness Training Improve Cognitive Abilities? A Systematic Review of Neuropsychological Findings," *Clinical Psychology Review* 31 (2011): 449–464.

10. Cristiano Crescentini, Viviana Capurso, Samantha Furlan, and Franco Fabbro, "Mindfulness-Oriented Meditation for Primary School Children: Effects on Attention and Psychological Well-Being," *Frontiers in Psychology* 7 (2016), accessed July 15, 2016, doi: 10.3389/fpsyg.2016.00805.

11. Bethany E. Kok, Kimberly A. Coffey, Michael A. Cohn, Lahnna I. Catalino, Tanya Vacharkulksemsuk, Sara B. Algoe, Mary Brantley, and Barbara L. Fredrickson, "How Positive Emotions Build Physical Health: Perceived Positive Social Connections Account for the Upward Spiral Between Positive Emotions and Vagal Tone," *Psychological Science* 24 (2013): 1123–1132.

12. Julieta Galante, Ignacio Galante, Marie-Jet Bekkers, and John Gallacher, "Effect of Kindness-Based Meditation on Health and Well-Being: A Systematic Review and Meta-analysis," *Journal of Consulting and Clinical Psychology* 82 (2014): 1101–1114.

13. Jason C. Ong, Rachel Manber, Zindel Segal, Yinglin Xia, Shauna Shapiro, and James K. Wyatt, "A Randomized Controlled Trial of Mindfulness Meditation for Chronic Insomnia," *Sleep* 37 (2014): 1553–1563.

14. Gregory A. Tooley, Stuart M. Armstrong, Trevor R. Norman, and Avni Sali, "Acute Increases in Night-time Plasma Melatonin Levels Following a Period of Meditation," *Biological Psychology* 53 (2000): 69–78.

15. David S. Black and George M. Slavich, "Mindfulness Meditation and the Immune System: A Systematic Review," 1373 (2016): 13–24.

16. Richard J. Davidson, Jon Kabat-Zinn, Jessica Schumacher, Melissa Rosenkranz, Daniel Muller, Saki F. Santorelli, Ferris Urbanoski, Anne Harrington, Katherine Bonus, and John F. Sheridan, "Alterations in Brain and Immune Function Produced by Mindfulness Meditation," *Psychosomatics* 65 (2003): 564–570.

17. Atikarn Gainey, Thep Himathongkam, Hirofumi Tanaka, and Daroonwan Suksom, "Effects of Buddhist Walking Meditation on Glycemic Control and Vascular Function in Patients with Type 2 Diabetes," *Complementary Therapies in Medicine* 26 (2016): 92–97.

18. Katya Rubia, "The Neurobiology of Meditation and Its Clinical Effectiveness in Psychiatric Disorders," *Biological Psychology* 82 (2009): 1–11.

19. Kathi L. Heffner, Hugh F. Crean, and Jan E. Kemp, "Meditation Programs for Veterans with Posttraumatic Stress Disorder: Aggregate Findings from a Multi-Site Evaluation," *Psychological Trauma: Theory, Research, Practice, and Policy* 8 (2016): 365–374.

20. Mo Yee Lee, Amy Zaharlick, and Deborah Akers, "Impact of Meditation on Mental Health Outcomes of Female Trauma Survivors of Interpersonal Violence with Co-occurring Disorders: A Randomized Controlled Trial," *Journal of Interpersonal Violence* (2015), accessed July 15, 2016, doi: 10.1177/0886260515591277.

21. Cecilia Westbrook, John David Creswell, Golnaz Tabibnia, Erica Julson, Hedy Kober, and Hilary A. Tindle, "Mindful Attention Reduces Neural and Self-Reported Cue-Induced Craving in Smokers," *Social Cognitive and Affective Neuroscience* 8 (2013): 73–84.

22. Yi-Yuan Tang, Rongxiang Tang, and Michael I. Posner, "Mindfulness Meditation Improves Emotion Regulation and Reduces Drug Abuse," *Drug and Alcohol Dependence* 163 (2016): S13–S18.

23. Melissa A. Rosenkranz, Antoine Lutz, David M. Perlman, David R. W. Bachhuber, Brianna S. Schuyler, Donal G. MacCoon, and Richard J. Davidson, "Reduced Stress and Inflammatory Responsiveness in Experienced Meditators Compared to a Matched Healthy Control Group," *Psychoneuroendocrinology* 68 (2016): 117–125.

24. Sara W. Lazar, Catherine E. Kerr, Rachel H. Wasserman, Jeremy R. Gray, Douglas N. Greve, Michael T. Treadway, Metta McGarvey, Brian T. Quinn, Jeffery A. Dusek, Herbert Benson, Scott L. Rauch, Christopher I. Moore, and Bruce Fischl, "Meditation Experience Is Associated with Increased Cortical Thickness," *Neuroreport* 16 (2005): 1893–1897.

25. Britta K. Hölzel, James Carmody, Mark Vangel, Christina Congleton, Sita M. Yerramsetti, Tim Gard, and Sara W. Lazar, "Mindfulness Practice Leads to Increases in Regional Brain Gray Matter Density," *Psychiatry Research* 191 (2011): 36–43.

26. Jon Kabat-Zinn, *Wherever You Go, There You Are: Mindfulness Meditation in Everyday Life* (New York: Hyperion, 1994), 4.

27. Jennifer S. Mascaro, James K. Rilling, Lobsang Tenzin Negi, and Charles L. Raison, "Compassion Meditation Enhances Empathic Accuracy and Related Neural Activity," *Social Cognitive and Affective Neuroscience* 8 (2013): 48–55.

28. Tatia M. C. Lee, Mei-Kei Leung, Wai-Kai Hou, Joey C. Y. Tang, Jing Yin, Kwok-Fai So, Chack-Fan Lee, and Chetwyn C. H. Chan, "Distinct Neural Activity Associated with Focused-Attention Meditation and Loving-Kindness Meditation," *PLoS One* 7 (2012), accessed July 17, 2016, doi: 10.1371/journal.pone.0040054.

29. Helen Y. Weng, Andrew S. Fox, Alexander J. Shackman, Diane E. Stodola, Jessica Z. K. Caldwell, Matthew C. Olson, Gregory M. Rogers, and Richard J. Davidson, "Compassion Training Alters Altruism and Neural Responses to Suffering," *Psychological Science* 24 (2013): 1171–1180.

30. Michael Ussher, Amy Spatz, Claire Copland, Andrew Nicolaou, Abbey Cargill, Nina Amini-Tabrizi, and Lance M. McCracken, "Immediate Effects of a Brief Mindfulness-Based Body Scan on Patients with Chronic Pain," *Journal of Behavioral Medicine* 37 (2014): 127–134.

Appendix A: Yoga for Specific Health Conditions

1. Steffany H. Moonaz, Clifton O. Bingham, Lawrence Wissow, and Susan J. Barlett, "Yoga in Sedentary Adults with Arthritis: Effects of a Randomized Controlled Pragmatic Trial," *Journal of Rheumatology* 42 (2015): 1194–1202.

2. Ibid.

3. Diana A. Freitas, Elizabeth A. Holloway, Selma S. Bruno, Gabriela S. S. Chaves, Guilherme A. F. Fregonezi, and Karla M. P. P. Mendonça, "Breathing Exercises for Adults with Asthma," *Cochrane Database of Systematic Reviews* (2013), accessed December 6, 2015, doi: 10.1002/14651858.CD001277.pub3.

4. Xun-Chao Liu, Lei Pan, Qing Hu, Wei-Ping Dong, Jun-Hong Yan, and Liang Dong, "Effects of Yoga Training in Patients with Chronic Obstructive Pulmonary Disease: A Systematic Review and Meta-analysis," *Journal of Thoracic Disease* 6 (2014): 795–802.

5. Julie Sadja and Paul J. Mills, "Effects of Yoga Interventions on Fatigue in Cancer Patients and Survivors: A Systematic Review of Randomized Controlled Trials," *Explore (NY)* 9 (2013): 232–243.

6. Anand Dhruva, Christine Miaskowski, Donald Abrams, Michael Acree, Bruce Cooper, Steffanie Goodman, and Frederick M. Hecht, "Yoga Breathing for Cancer Chemotherapy–Associated Symptoms and Quality of Life: Results of a Pilot Randomized Controlled Trial," *Journal of Alternative and Complementary Medicine* 18 (2012): 473–479.

7. Mary C. Hooke, Laura Gilchrist, Laurie Foster, Mary Langevin, and Jill Lee, "Yoga for Children and Adolescents After Completing Cancer Treatment," *Journal of Pediatric Oncology Nursing* (2015), accessed December 5, 2015, doi: 10.1177/1043454214563936.

8. Mariangela Panebianco, Kalpana Sridharan, and Sridharan Ramaratnam, "Yoga for Epilepsy," *Cochrane Database of Systematic Reviews* (2015), last accessed December 5, 2015, doi: 10.1002/14651858.CD001524.pub2.

9. Helané Wahbeh, Siegward-M. Elsas, and Barry S. Okcn, "Mind-Body Interventions," *Neurology* 70 (2008): 2321–2328.

10. Katherine M. Newton, Susan D. Reed, Katherine A. Guthrie, Karen J. Sherman, Cathryn Booth-LaForce, Bette Caan, Barbara Sternfeld, Janet S. Carpenter, Lee A. Learman, Ellen W. Freeman, Lee S. Cohen, Hadine Joffe, Garnet L. Anderson, Joseph C. Larson, Julie R. Hunt, Kristine E. Ensrud, and Andrea Z. LaCroix, "Efficacy of Yoga for Vasomotor Symptoms: A Randomized Controlled Trial," *Menopause* 21 (2014): 339–346.

11. Holger Cramer, Romy Lauche, Hoda Azizi, Gustav Dobos, and Jost Langhorst, "Yoga for Multiple Sclerosis: A Systematic Review and Meta-Analysis," *PLoS One* 9 (2014): e112414.

12. Neena K. Sharma, Kristin Robbins, Kathleen Wagner, and Yvonne M. Colgrove, "A Randomized Controlled Pilot Study of the Therapeutic Effects of Yoga in People with Parkinson's Disease," *International Journal of Yoga* 8 (2015): 74–79.

13. Monika Rudzińska, Sylwia Bukowczan, Joanna Stożek, Katarzyna Zajdel, Elżbieta Mirek, Wiesław Chwata, Magdalena Wójcik-Pędziwiatr, Krzysztof Banaszkiewicz, and Andrzej Szczudlik, "Causes and Consequences of Falls in Parkinson Disease Patients in a Prospective Study," *Neurologia i Neurochirurgia Polska* 47 (2013): 423–430.

14. G. Kirkwood, H. Rampes, V. Tuffrey, J. Richardson, and K. Pilkington, "Yoga for Anxiety: A Systematic Review of the Research Evidence," *British Journal of Sports Medicine* 39 (2005): 884–891.

15. Sanjiv Mehta, Vijay Mehta, Sagar Mehta, Devesh Shah, Ashok Motiwala, Jay Vardhan, Naina Mehta, and Devendra Mehta, "Multimodal Behavior Program for ADHD Incorporating Yoga and Implemented by High School Volunteers: A Pilot Study," *ISRN Pediatrics* (2011), accessed December 6, 2015, doi: 10.5402/2011/780745.

16. Dianne Neumark-Sztainer, "Yoga and Eating Disorders: Is There a Place for Yoga in the Prevention and Treatment of Eating Disorders and Disordered Eating Behaviours?" *Advances in Eating Disorders* 2 (2014): 136–145.

17. Patricia Anne Kinser, R. K. Elswick, and Susan Kornstein, "Potential Long-Term Effects of a Mind–Body Intervention for Women with Major Depressive Disorder: Sustained Mental Health Improvements with a Pilot Yoga Intervention," *Archives of Psychiatric Nursing* 28 (2014): 377–383.

18. Neha Gothe and Edward McAuley, "Yoga and Cognition: A Meta-Analysis of Chronic and Acute Effects," *Psychosomatic Medicine* 77 (2015): 784–797.

19. Neha Gothe, Matthew B. Pontifex, Charles Hillman, and Edward McAuley, "The Acute Effects of Yoga on Executive Function," *Journal of Physical Activity and Health* 10 (2013): 488–495.

20. Neha P. Gothe, Arthur F. Kramer, and Edward McAuley, "The Effects of an 8-Week Hatha Yoga Intervention on Executive Function in Older Adults," *Journal of Gerontology* 69 (2014): 1109–1116.

21. Rinku Garg, Varun Malhotra, Yogesh Tripathi, and Ritu Agarawal, "Effect of Left, Right and Alternate Nostril Breathing on Verbal and Spatial Memory," *Journal of Clinical and Diagnostic Research* 10 (2016): CC01–CC03.

22. N Gangadhar Bangalore and Shivarama Varambally, "Yoga Therapy for Schizophrenia," *International Journal of Yoga* 5 (2012): 85–91.

23. Beth C. Bock, Kathleen M. Morrow, Bruce M. Becker, David M. Williams, Geoffrey Tremont, Ronnesia B. Gaskins, and Ernestine Jennings, "Yoga as a Complementary Treatment for Smoking Cessation in Women," *BMC Complementary and Alternative Medicine* 21 (2010): 240–248.

Appendix B: Yoga and Pregnancy

1. James J. Newham, Anja Wittkowski, Janine Hurley, John D. Aplin, and Melissa Westwood, "Effects of Antenatal Yoga on Maternal Anxiety and Depression: A Randomized Controlled Trial," *Depression and Anxiety* 31 (2014): 631–640.

2. US Department of Health and Human Services, Office of Women's Health, "Depression During and After Pregnancy Fact Sheet." (2009), accessed December 1, 2015, https://www.womenshealth.gov/publications/our-publications/fact-sheet/depression-pregnancy.html.

3. Maria Muzik, Susan E. Hamilton, Katherine Lisa Rosenblum, Ellen Waxler, and Zahra Hadi, "Mindfulness Yoga during Pregnancy for Psychiatrically At-Risk Women: Preliminary

Results from a Pilot Feasibility Study," *Complementary Therapies in Clinical Practice* 18 (2015): 235–240.

4. Melissa M. Buttner, Rebecca L. Brock, Michael W. O'Hara, and Scott Stuart, "Efficacy of Yoga for Depressed Postpartum Women: A Randomized Controlled Trial," *Complementary Theories in Clinical Practice* 21 (2015): 94–100.

Index